The Art of JAMA

One Hundred Covers and Essays From

The Journal of the

American Medical Association

THE GREAT FIGURE

Among the rain

and lights

I saw the figure 5

in gold

on a red

firetruck

moving

tense

unheeded

to gong clangs

siren howls

and wheels rumbling

through the dark city.

—William Carlos Williams

(See page 104)

William Carlos Williams: Collected Poems, 1909-1939. Vol. I.
©1938 by New Directions Publishing Corp, New York, NY;
reprinted by permission of New Directions.

The Art of JAMA

One Hundred Covers and Essays From

The Journal of the

American Medical Association

M. Therese Southgate, MD

Senior Contributing Editor
The Journal of the American Medical Association
Chicago, Illinois

with 104 full-color illustrations

American Medical Association
Physicians dedicated to the health of America

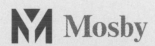 Mosby

St. Louis Baltimore Boston Carlsbad Chicago Naples New York Philadelphia Portland
London Madrid Mexico City Singapore Sydney Tokyo Toronto Wiesbaden

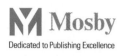
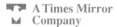

American Medical Association

Physicians dedicated to the health of America

Vice President and Publisher Anne S. Patterson
Editor Susie Baxter
Developmental Editor Anne Gunter
Project Manager Linda McKinley
Production Editor Catherine Bricker
Composition Specialist Peggy Hill
Designer Elizabeth Fett
Manufacturing Manager Theresa Fuchs

American Medical Association Editor Jane Piro
JAMA Editors Kate Whetzle, Roxanne K. Young

Composition by Mosby Electronic Production
Lithography by Color Associates, Inc.
Printing/binding by Grafos S. A., Barcelona, Spain

Mosby–Year Book, Inc.
11830 Westline Industrial Drive
St. Louis, Missouri 63146

International Standard Book Number 0-8151-0994-6
29462

96 97 98 99 00 / 9 8 7 6 5 4 3 2 1

To Josie and Tom

FOREWORD

George D. Lundberg, MD

Editor, *JAMA*

Art and science, science and medicine, medicine and humanities, humanities and art. Where does one end and the other begin? Are they seamless or joined at the corners? Do they form a circle or a square? Or are they perhaps more like a tapestry whose threads are inextricably intertwined?

For the first 80 years or so of publication and through nine editors, the cover of *The Journal of the American Medical Association* displayed only its table of contents. In the early 1960s, its tenth editor, John H. Talbott, MD, liked the fine arts and experimented with placing a small picture on the cover. Gradually he increased both the size of the image and the frequency of its appearance, until in 1964 the four-color, fine arts covers of *JAMA* were established.

Some years later, Robert Moser, MD, then at the *JAMA* helm, invited a young senior editor on the staff to assume responsibility for selecting the fine arts covers. Art was a field that was new to her, so she approached it cautiously. She decided to study art as systematically as she had studied medicine—in place of the textbooks of medicine, she began studying the art history textbooks whenever there was a free moment. To stay current with new developments, she subscribed to the art journals. Where once she had rounded on the wards, she now rounded in the galleries at the Art Institute of Chicago, accompanied at times by one of their curators. She also used the superb resources of the Art Institute's Ryerson Library for additional research. From time to time she would share with *JAMA* readers what she was learning, at first in the form of small, anonymous notes on that week's painting, placed in the issue wherever blank space could be found. Slightly longer pieces identified with her initials were then developed, which finally became the essays with the now familiar byline, *M. Therese Southgate, MD*. The approach worked, readers responded, and the idea flowered and flowered and flowered. Since 1974, Terry Southgate has

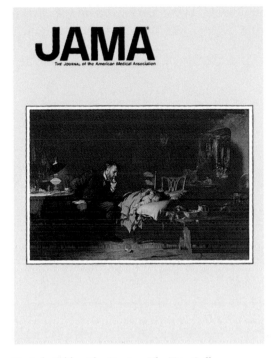

Sir Luke Fildes, The Doctor. *The Tate Gallery, London, England.*

chosen the art for more than one thousand *JAMA* covers and has herself written more than 500 essays and supervised another 350.

When I assumed the editorship of *JAMA* in 1982, one of my early decisions was whether to retain the art on the cover. I had enjoyed the covers for years as a *JAMA* recipient and later as an Editorial Board member, but there had always been pressure to remove the art. Scientific purists have frequently asked for a full table of contents on the cover. Advertising sales staff have expressed longing to put ads on the cover. I decided to keep the art. I'm glad I did.

As I travel around the world, I am frequently approached by *JAMA* readers who wish to discuss portions of the journal. More often than not, they will start off with praise for the *JAMA* art covers and ask about Dr. Southgate, especially how she as a physician learned so much about art. I tell them Terry trained as a journalist first and then as a physician but that in art history and art crit-

icism she is self-taught. Readers marvel at the insights in her essays and the eloquence with which she points out critical elements of a painting and its background that they had never thought of or recognized before, even in more familiar works of art.

JAMA's current critical objective number seven reads, "to inform readers about non-clinical aspects of medicine and public health, including the political, philosophic, ethical, legal, environmental, economic, historical, and cultural" (*JAMA* 270:1248-1249, 1993). Our *JAMA* art covers and cover stories help us meet that objective every week. In fact, they formed the beginning of our whole *JAMA* initiative to emphasize the humanities in medicine, and we now include essays, poems, and historical accounts nearly every week.

For many years, the art on the *JAMA* covers has been chosen simply because it is great art; it has no relation to the content of the issue, although often the image does have a seasonal relationship. I never see the selections until they are ready for print because I trust Terry completely. But about five times a year on special theme issues, the covers do relate to the journal's content, and I am sometimes consulted. Theme covers have drawn the reader inside issues on such subjects as alcoholism, adolescence, boxing, sports medicine, women's health, medical education, genetics, black American health, Hispanic health, violence, and of course, caring for the uninsured (repeated four times), prevention of nuclear war (repeated eleven times), Contempo (repeated annually but with varied art), and tobacco (repeated eight times but with a different painting each time).

Of course, the meaning of any painting is determined by the individual observer. Thus many times readers perceive cover themes when none are intended. Two covers of this ilk stand out in memory. The January 8, 1988, *JAMA* cover was *Comtesse d'Haussonville* by Ingres. Contained in that issue was the one-page essay "It's Over, Debbie" that began a raging debate about death, dying, and pain relief. Many thought the female figure on the cover represented Debbie. It did not. The October 28, 1988, *JAMA* was a theme issue dedicated to the Harvard Resource Based-Relative Value Scale, a creative method for paying physicians. The cover was *Harlequin* by Cézanne—and not intended to be related to the journal's content—but many physicians have come to refer to that issue as *The Clown Issue*, a relationship easy to discern, albeit spurious.

Not many busy physicians can make it to the Chicago Art Institute, the Tate Gallery, the Louvre, the Hermitage, or even the art museum in their own city very often. But they can look at the *JAMA* cover art and read the graceful and stimulating Southgate essay every week, thereby adding cultural enrichment and introspective repose to their busy professional lives.

Just as my favorite *JAMA* issue is always this week's *JAMA*, my favorite *JAMA* cover is this week's cover. Terry's selections and interpretations never cease to impress and, I believe, enlighten and often uplift. Terry Southgate seems to get more fan mail than all the rest of the *JAMA* editors put together. For more than a decade her readers have asked that she publish a collection of her favorite covers and cover stories, so here it is. Physicians and patients, be educated; be rounded; be inspired; enjoy.

Science and art, art and humanities, humanities and medicine, medicine and science—a full circle, a tapestry of life itself.

FOREWORD

Professor William H. Gerdts

PhD Program in Art History, City University of New York

T he covers and their associated essays that have appeared in *The Journal of the American Medical Association* since 1974 and the involvement of M. Therese Southgate, MD with the journal have provided an amazing resource for the journal's readers and initially probably a very surprising one. This resource consists of high-quality reproductions of works of art, which are usually oil paintings but also include some graphic work as well, produced by artists of many European and American countries from medieval times to the present, encompassing a full variety of classes of subject matter and rendered in strategies from the traditional to the then avant-garde. The great French academic William Bouguereau is represented here, as well as his antithesis, the Post-Impressionist Vincent van Gogh.

But, the philistine might argue, art belongs in art publications—in art magazines—along with books and catalogues; what role can these pictures possibly play in the function of a medical journal? Well, the answer is not difficult to discern, for the lives of the readers of the journal, those of medical professionals and laypersons alike, are involved with more than medical practice, and their interests go beyond the office and the hospital. Furthermore, members of the medical profession have often been in the lead among patrons of the fine arts. The history of our own country has witnessed not only the close friendships of physicians and surgeons with painters and sculptors but also the leadership of American art organizations by medical professionals—individuals who often became the spokespersons in both word and print concerning interrelationships of the arts with the political, cultural, economic, and moral fabric of American society.

Dr. Southgate has drawn upon public, private, and commercial sources that are almost all within the United States to round out a comprehensive survey of Western two-dimensional art. Certain individual collections stand out—the Kimbell Art Museum in Fort Worth, Texas, and the Art Institute of Chicago—so the reader comes away not only with a succinct art history but a sense of deep familiarity with these collections. But the richest source for these paintings is the National Gallery in Washington, DC, a repository of great works of art which are indeed not only the legacy of Western achievement but also the patrimony of the nation. In a sense, these works belong to all Americans, and this volume can only increase our awareness of our own heritage.

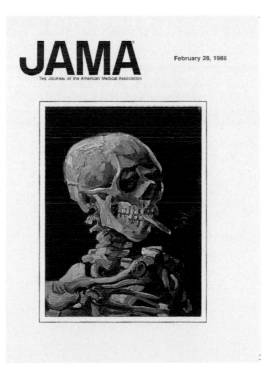

Vincent van Gogh, Skull with Cigarette. *The National Museum of Vincent van Gogh, Amsterdam, The Netherlands.*

Although this volume achieves artistic inclusiveness, it is also geared to some extent to its primarily American medical audience, in both aesthetic sympathies and thematic concerns. From the point of view of the art historian, I am amazed by numerous illustrations that might be considered by the uncritical to be offbeat. The California artist

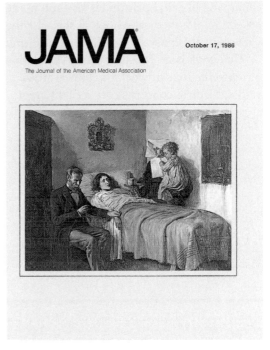

Pablo Picasso, Science and Charity. *Museo Picasso, Barcelona, Spain.*

Wores, who has been the subject of several *JAMA* covers reproducing works from the extensive collection of Drs. A. Jess and the late Ben Shenson, is represented by his *Chinese Fishmonger*, certainly one of his most distinguished works and one that bespeaks both his Munich training and his San Francisco background.

Then there are the pictures with obvious medical relevance, such as *Sister Juliet* of 1918 by the great turn of the century Irish artist Sir John Lavery. A particularly offbeat yet brilliant choice for inclusion here is Pablo Picasso's very early *Science and Charity* of 1897. This offers especially incisive comparison with a work that was painted only a few years earlier and is perhaps the most famous and certainly the most popular "doctor picture" ever created—*The Doctor*—by the late 19th-century English specialist in pictures of social relevance, Sir Luke Fildes. In a balance with this is the most famous American medical picture, Thomas Eakins'

1875 portrait of Professor Gross in *The Gross Clinic*, which many believe to be the greatest picture ever painted by an American artist. In addition, it is owned by a medical institution, The Jefferson Medical College in Philadelphia. Eakins devoted a great part of his career to detailing the appearance and lives of physicians and surgeons, so his later *The Agnew Clinic* of 1889 also takes its place here. It is only slightly less famous than *The Gross Clinic*, and like that painting is also still in the collection of a medical school, in this case the University of Pennsylvania School of Medicine.

This book is no "postage stamp" collection of reproductions of works by only famous artists. Medical concerns of a very different nature are also addressed in the delightful *First Aid* by the American Francis William Edmonds, a genre specialist little known today. But pictures of medical relevancy are only a small part of the *JAMA* covers and their selection here. I have a suspicion that Dr. Southgate shares with me an especial fondness for still-life pictures of fruits and flowers, judging by both the numbers and the quality of those presented, but these too are also very much in the minority. And the landscapes—particularly "pure" landscapes without significant figures—are quite rare. What appears to be the overwhelming and unifying theme here is the human figure, whether integrated with a landscape or urban setting or more commonly seen up close. There are figures of all ages, from children to the elderly, and all walks of life, from the very wealthy to the comfortably middle class to the urban and rural poor. Some are extremely passive, some are very active; some are heroic, some are timid; some have specific individuals, some have generic types. Both men and women contemplate, interrelate, and alienate, though men (and skeletons!) smoke while women mother. Figures work, play outdoor games, read, play cards, stroll, fish, drink, fight, make music, make love, and even make telephone calls. People, after all, are the concern of the medical profession, and they enjoy primacy here.

PREFACE

Since I took over the task, more than two decades ago, of selecting the fine arts reproduction that appears on the cover of *The Journal of the American Medical Association* each week, the question I have been asked most frequently is: "Why art on the cover of a medical journal and what has art to do with medicine?" It is a question I had also been asking myself repeatedly, and so I began to study each painting I selected and write a little essay about what I found—a process not too different, it turns out, from the way a physician approaches a new patient. When readers responded, I was encouraged to continue. Twenty years later I am convinced of what I sensed only vaguely at the time—that deep affinities exist between medicine and the visual arts. However, sometimes these relationships are easier visualized than verbalized. What follows then, is word and image: one hundred of the *JAMA* covers that appeared between December 1974 and December 1987 along with the essay that accompanied each. I do not pretend to have answered the question—I am not sure that the question ever can be fully answered— only to suggest that medicine and the visual arts are as intimately and inextricably related as psyche and soma, body and spirit.

But first, my disclaimers. I am not a trained art professional. I am an amateur but an amateur in the truest sense of the word: an amator, a lover; for that, I hope, many sins will be forgiven. Second, although I carefully researched each painting at the time I wrote the essay, scholarship is not static; not only does it constantly move forward, but in art history as in medicine it has moved at an accelerating pace. Thus these essays should not by any means be considered definitive or even scholarly. Rather, they are simply attempts to share with readers what I learned while I looked at a work of art. I hope that what comes through is not only facts and information but the sense of joy that comes from the discovery of a new dimension of one's life.

As distant as the two notions—medicine and art—may at first seem, they do share a common goal: the goal of completing what nature has not. Each is an attempt to reach the ideal, to complete what is incomplete, to restore what is lost. The search is for harmony as well as for form. In a painting the visible elements—color, form, and line—exist in a complete harmony of parts as determined by the artist. So too is a human person a complex harmony of body, spirit, and environment. When each is properly ordered to the other we have a work of art, a whole and healthy person. In a word, each concerns relationships and their ability to be communicated to another.

Again, as each strives toward their common goal, both medicine and art work with a common substrate: the physical world. This world is mostly visible to the human eye, but in some cases it is known only by special instruments or by its effects, being more felt than seen. Medicine, for example, deals with the human body and the quality of its functioning. Art, on the other hand, may choose a tree, a stream, a mountain, a human face— even pure line and color as its object. The one strives to bring the human body to that ideal state where its spirit may use and enjoy all of its various qualities: understanding, love, tenderness, compassion, mercy, forgiveness. The other tries to transform the world into one that can be comprehended and enjoyed by the spirit.

Besides these similarities between the visual arts and medicine, there are perhaps not surprisingly even deeper affinities between the practitioners of each, between artists and physicians. The first and perhaps the most obvious is observation, keen observation. Observation is a skill that can be learned like any other. Keenness, on the other hand, comes from practice—from the constant stepping back to look at and listen to the things of our experience. It ranges from the way a physician listens to the patient's initial statement and notes demeanor, facial expression, posture, and the like to the way the artist's eye sees the light on the leaf or notes the angle of a branch where it meets a tree trunk, the shades of mauve in a sunset, the thickness of paint on a canvas. However, less obvious than observation is a second skill, also learned, that artists and physicians hold in common. Even more important than the first because it determines the quality of the first, it is the necessity of attention. Simone Weil describes this attention exactly: it is the ability to suspend our thought before the object of our observation, to leave our thought "detached, empty, waiting, ready to be penetrated by the object." Attention does not seek anything, nor does it impose itself on what is before it. It simply waits in a state of readiness to receive; what it receives is the truth of the object before it. In the case of the artist the faculty of attention can perhaps be more readily understood, for it is with the artist that we most commonly associate such qualities of being as stillness or contemplation. But physicians have the power too, by birthright. Does not our very language acknowledge it every time we use the phrase "attending physician" or say, "The physician attends the patient"? "Attention" and "attend" have the same Latin root.

These are some of the more obvious affinities between medicine and art: a common goal, an involvement with the physical world, and similar practitioners. But there is more. If each is to be effective at all in its goal of reaching the ideal for which the world is intended, each has need of all that science and technology can offer. In medicine the need is obvious and in art perhaps less so, but consider Piero della Francesca's 15th-century treatise on perspective and Michel Eugène Chevreul's 19th-century work on color theory. Consider how many artists, from Leonardo to Eakins, knew human anatomy at least as well as students of medicine, perhaps even better. And not to discount the role of technology in the visual arts, consider the collapsible paint tube.

Without it would we have had the great flowering of plein air painting of the late 19th century? Would we now be enjoying the sparkling, sunshine-filled canvases of Monet, Renoir's dappled nudes, Sisley's sun-drenched villages, Pissarro's rural workers?

In the end, both art and medicine are about seeing: one looks first with the eyes of the body, next considers with the eye of the mind, and finally, if one has been attentive enough, one begins to see with the eye of the soul. If we remain in this vision—are patient enough, and still enough—we begin to hear as well, somewhere in the depths beyond where words are formed. Perhaps this is why art is counted as one of the humanities: it is a wedding of all humans, across all barriers—time, distance, culture, race, even across the language of words. Perhaps this suggests why medicine and art have such a keen affinity for each other. It is in this same wordless language of the human spirit that the physician sees not just a disease nor even a patient but the person. It is a person who, as so eloquently put by Simone Weil, has been afflicted, just like the physician. It is in that moment that healing begins. Paradoxically, the healer is healed as well. That perhaps is the art of medicine.

As the years have passed since these essays were begun, so too has the number of persons to whom I am indebted increased. Virtually everyone on the staff of the journal and many in other areas of the American Medical Association as well has made a contribution at one time or another. I am especially grateful for the stimulating and at the same time congenial working environment provided by the successive leadership of the three *JAMA* editors under whose aegis these essays were developed: Robert H. Moser, MD, (1973-1975); William R. Barclay, MD, (1975-1982); and George D. Lundberg, MD who took over in early 1982 and a decade and a half later continues his enthusiastic support. There are numerous other heroes, unsung and mostly anonymous, who had a hand in these covers, from copy editors and proofreaders who so often caught and mended my infelicitous phrases and errors before they got to print, to those who never failed to offer a comment on the most recent cover. One of the nicest expressions of this are the many offices and workspaces decorated with favorite *JAMA* covers.

Some of those who have assisted me in specific ways, principally in bibliographic research but in other editorial tasks as well, are Marsha Meyer, Lori Burnette, and Charlene Breedlove, who also edited the section for a time. Throughout much of the time Mary Cannon was my very capable editorial assistant. All are, happily, still colleagues at the AMA, though long since gone on to other responsibilities. I also had the research abilities for a time of Virginia Hinze and then medical student Susie Reitz. The staff of the former AMA archive library under the directorship of Susan Crawford were not only always unfailingly gracious but supersleuths as well when it came to finding that obscure bit of information I needed (and often did not even realize I did until one of them suggested it) and masters at getting it all by yesterday. For this I wish to mention in particular Mary Jo Dwyer, Mary Devlin, Jean Fox, Marie Bates, Barbara Hopper, Ann Weller, Phyllis McClaren, and Martha Bier. For translations from the many languages I cannot read, including French, German, Italian, Portuguese, and Dutch, among others, I am grateful to Victoria Bigelow, Jane Larkin, Arthur Hafner, Elizabeth Missimer, Mary Ann Eiler, Robert Rinaldi, Kathleen London, and Alfons Van Cleven.

Several persons whose field is the fine arts rather than medicine and journalism must also be named. J. Patrice Marandel, then curator of European Painting at the Art Institute of Chicago, guided me on my first real tour of an art museum and taught me what to look for on its walls. In many ways that tour set the tone for future museum visits. Patrice also provided me access to information not readily available in reference texts and a quiet place to peruse it. John Keefe, then curator of Decorative Arts at the Art Institute, performed a similar service for his own department. It was from him that I first learned Roentgen is a familiar name in art as well as medicine: the Art Institute possesses a beautiful wood cabinet made by Roentgen, whose surname is the same as the discoverer of x rays, although the degree of kinship (if any) is as yet unknown. The entire staff of the Ryerson Library at the Art Institute, and in particular Cecelia Chin, now at the National Portrait Gallery, have been and continue to be very helpful. Arthur Wheelock, curator of Northern Baroque Painting at the National Gallery of Art, was always available to answer my many often naive questions about the gallery's collections and likewise alerted me to the many little nuances the Dutch like to hide in their paintings. Ira Bartfield, also at the National Gallery, made accessible and provided suggestions on hundreds of transparencies for possible *JAMA* covers and always made sure they arrived on time.

Back in Chicago, when we were unable to obtain a transparency for a cover, the AMA's own photographer, Joe Fletcher, did the photography. One of the high points in the early days was watching Joe set up and shoot after hours in an otherwise dark and eerily silent Art Institute. To Bonnie Van Cleven, still a member of the *JAMA* staff, special thanks must be given. She oversaw much of the administration, editing, and scheduling in those early days and on not a few occasions things turned out well because she made them turn out well.

Finally, there is one person more than any other perhaps, who has shared both the work and the joy of these covers with me for more than two decades, from 1974 until he retired last year: Thomas J. Handrigan, who, among his numerous other production duties for *JAMA*, served as color manager. It is Tom who has been responsible for the excellent reputation we have enjoyed with museums and readers alike in the design and layout of the covers and in the oft-noted quality of our color reproduction. By training and avocation an artist as well, Tom was most generous in sharing his own expertise and knowledge in painting, answering my many questions, alerting me to details in a work I might otherwise have missed, and even providing me with a minieducation in the graphic arts. Another high point of those early days was visiting the Art Institute with Tom, who, armed with a lightbox and a sharp eye, compared the transparency to the original work on the wall. Over the years, I learned that when Tom's eye and the rulebook were at odds, it was Tom's eye that was invariably correct. As Tom's successor, Charl Richey-Davis had not only a tough act to follow but came in near the end of a lengthy process when everything had to be done at once. Even under these difficult circumstances, Charl was able to reconstruct for this volume some 20 of the plates that could not be retrieved from the archives.

However, the gestation process is one thing, and delivery is another. Even when it is normal, gestation seems to be interminable. But one day labor begins and it is then that, regardless of time or distance, one summons the midwife. I was fortunate to have two on call: Roxanne K. Young, associate editor of *JAMA*, herself gravida 2, para 1 with the popular "A Piece of My Mind" collection, and Kate Whetzle, *JAMA* assistant editor, who was in constant attendance throughout the entire labor and delivery process. For one "pregnant with book," Kate has all the qualities of the perfect midwife, not the least being, besides her editorial knowledge and expertise, a general cheerfulness, an unflagging optimism, and an indomitable will to keep things moving. Moreover, it was Kate who took on the monumental task of tracking down and contacting the current owners of each painting, obtaining permissions (and new transparencies when necessary), verifying credit lines, and rechecking vital data on each artist, not to mention shepherding contracts and invoices through their labyrinthine ways and overseeing all the other editorial and administrative tasks that remain unnoticed except when they are not done perfectly. The labor was long and frequently seemed stalled; credit for the safe and happy delivery must go to the midwives. On the other hand, any shortcomings in the offspring belong to the author.

However, in the end it is the support, encouragement, and enthusiasm of the *JAMA* readers that have brought the pregnancy to term. The continuing existence of the *JAMA* covers themselves are due in fact to all those readers who have written over the years. Some wrote to share a thought, thank me, take me to task for a cover they did not like, give me information I had not had, or most important, correct the information I did have. The idea to collect the covers and their essays into a book and to publish them in this coffee-table format came from the readers in a steady and continuing flow of letters over the years. Therefore it is to them that the book ultimately owes its origins. Sadly, I could not answer all of the letters. Another cover story always seemed due at the printer's. So here instead, with thanks to all the *JAMA* readers, are the cover essays that importuned.

M. Therese Southgate, MD
Chicago, April 27, 1996

THE ART OF JAMA

The Art of **JAMA**

One Hundred Covers and Essays From
The Journal of the
American Medical Association

WILLIAM MULREADY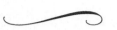

The Fight Interrupted

Though often classified with the Victorian painters, William Mulready (1786-1863) completed the bulk of his work before 1837, when Victoria's reign began, and though he did paint in London, he is, in fact, Irish. Mulready was a genre painter, a type found commonly in Dutch works of the 17th century and typified by scenes from everyday life presented in a realistic manner. Though portraying charm and sentimentality in good hands, in less skilled hands and with less sensitive imitators, genre can descend into banality and bathos, into what is sometimes, with not very complimentary intention, called "calendar art." But Mulready is saved by his composition and color.

Mulready has been called a typically "English artist," meaning that he relied heavily on narrative for his paintings, being tied especially to the literature of the time. Mulready did indeed, like so many of the artists of the time, do the illustrations for a book, the 1840 edition of Oliver Goldsmith's *The Vicar of Wakefield*.

...we see a homely, homefront anecdote, a frozen frame of some bloody action...

In *The Fight Interrupted*, which was painted in the same year that Napoleon and Wellington were at Waterloo, and which won Mulready the greatly coveted and financially advantageous election to the Royal Academy, we see a homely, homefront anecdote, a frozen frame of some bloody action, which, though hardly as important to us as Wellington and Napoleon, was not less important to the boys—nor, evidently, to the schoolmaster. Mulready is at home here: he was himself a well-known boxer and the father of four sons between the ages of 5 and 11, some or all of whom are undoubtedly shown in the painting.

Not to gainsay the charm of his subject, it is probably his color technique, however, that puts us in the greatest debt to Mulready. Forsaking the somber, all-over-brown tone that was heavily influencing contemporary English painting, Mulready applied his brilliant oils over a white ground; the technique culminated eventually in *The Fight Interrupted*, where his glazes of color are so thin that the white ground shows through—a technique that gives oils the transparency of watercolor and a brilliance heretofore unknown in English painting, one that the Pre-Raphaelites would later co-opt and develop.

William Mulready (1786-1863), *The Fight Interrupted*, 1816, Irish. Oil on panel, on a gesso ground. 71.8 × 93.2 cm. Painted for Viscount Whitworth, Lord Lieutenant of Ireland. Courtesy of the Board of Trustees of the Victoria and Albert Museum, London, England.

JAMA

THE JOURNAL of the American Medical Association

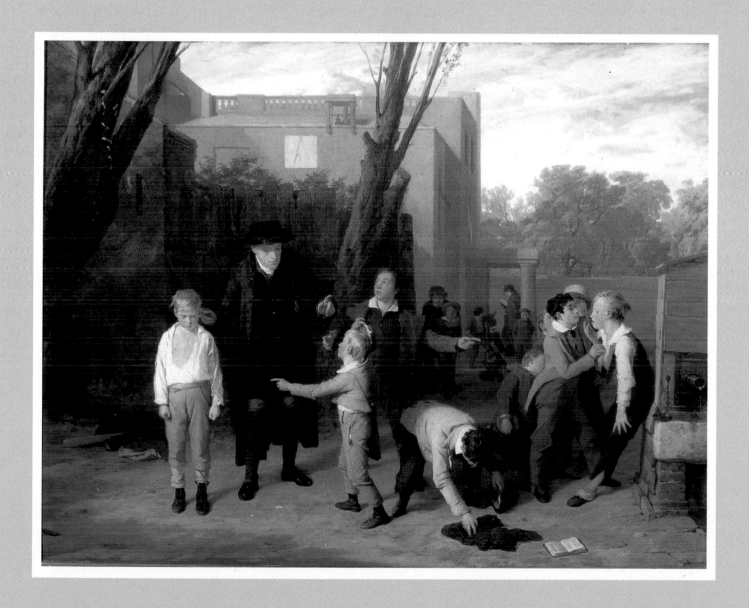

December 16, 1974

NICOLAS POUSSIN

Landscape With Saint John on Patmos

Nicolas Poussin (1594-1665), French painter of the classical school, was a consummate landscape artist without whom, art historians generally agree, Seurat and Cézanne could not have painted their distinctive landscapes. But early as he was in the genre of landscape painting, Poussin was still no pioneer. He was heavily influenced by the Venetian Bellini, teacher of Titian.

As Sir Kenneth Clark notes in *Landscape Into Art*, the chief difficulty of landscape painting was to bring logical form out of the disorder of natural scenery. This Poussin conceived could be done by a harmonious balancing of horizontal and vertical lines, meeting, he insisted, at right angles, a device that has caused his art to be called Cartesian or Pythagorean. Yet landscape is essentially horizontal, and if nature does happen to place any verticals they are not always at right angles to the horizon. This Poussin solved by introducing architecture to

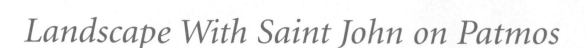

...to bring logical form out of the disorder of natural scenery.

provide the verticals, as in the temple columns and obelisk seen in *Landscape With Saint John on Patmos*. Moreover, if lines inclined away from the vertical, as does the slope of the mountain in the left background, Poussin introduced other verticals inclining just enough from the horizontal to intersect the landscape at right angles, as in the line of St John's back or the extended line from his hip to his knee. And, since penetration of space is the essence of landscape, Poussin conducts the eye to the background by his skillful use of subordinated diagonals, each stage in the slope to the sea marked

by a cadence of diminishing verticals—a promontory, a tree, a column. He unifies the entire scene with one of his favorite devices—a diagonal path that turns back on itself at two-thirds the height of the canvas.

Yet, though Poussin has imposed his own logic on the happenstance of nature, he still conveys, as John Maxon observes in his catalogue notes, a "grace and passion that are breathtakingly intense." Poussin's landscapes are rather like a classical symphony, in which the carefully constructed harmonies become fused into a single, grand work, so that it is always a surprise when one stops to identify the separate voices.

Nicolas Poussin (1594-1665), *Landscape With Saint John on Patmos*, 1640, French. Oil on canvas. 101.7 × 136 cm. Courtesy o f The Art Institute of Chicago, Chicago, Illinois; A. A. Munger Collection, 1930. Photograph © 1995 The Art Institute of Chicago, all rights reserved.

JAMA

THE JOURNAL Of the American Medical Association

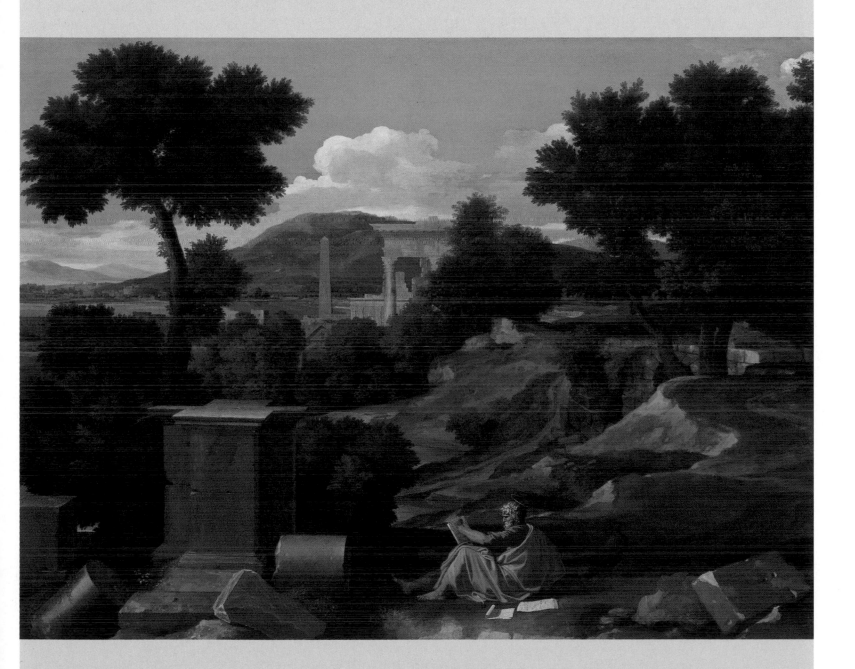

March 31,1975

GUSTAVE CAILLEBOTTE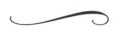

Paris Street; Rainy Day

Perhaps the most neglected of the early Impressionist painters has been Gustave Caillebotte (1848-1894). Indeed, until only a few years ago, he was appreciated more for his collection of Impressionist paintings than for his own work. He was independently wealthy and supported his friends, Monet and Pissarro among them, by buying their paintings.

Paris Street; Rainy Day was painted when Caillebotte was only 29 and is today considered his masterpiece—although Émile Zola said of it in 1877, the year it was completed, "When his talent has matured a little M Caillebotte will certainly be among the bolder members of the [Impressionist] group."

Caillebotte's training as a civil engineer is apparent in the draftsman-like quality of many of his paintings. In *Paris Street; Rainy Day*, for example, the focal lamppost exactly bisects the canvas, but the figures are so balanced that the eye does not immediately per-

> *"Grimy April only Maketh bloom the fire-escapes…"*

ceive this. Yet in spite of this mathematical precision, the painting still manages to catch the feel of a city spring: cold and wet, where the rain will water not a single blade of grass, open a bud, or nourish a tree. Steven Vincent Benét had it right: "Grimy April only Maketh bloom the fire-escapes, … Maketh winter coats and capes suddenly worn and shabby …"

The painting's title has an interesting history. For many years the work hung in the Art Institute of Chicago as *Place de l'Europe on a Rainy Day* until a visitor to the gallery, recently returned from a trip to Paris, called attention to the fact that the Place de l'Europe is actually a railroad bridge near the Gare Saint-Lazare (a scene also painted by Caillebotte, a year earlier, and now in Geneva at the Petit Palace.) The scene of the Art Institute's painting is actually some 200 meters to the northeast, at the intersection of rue de Moscou, rue de Turin, rue Clapeyron, rue Bucarest, and rue Leningrad. The essentials of the scene are little changed, wrote the visitor, except that the lamppost is gone, there are two traffic islands, the paving blocks have been covered over with asphalt, and "the crossing is choked by cars, moving and parked, like all of Paris."

JAMA

THE JOURNAL of the American Medical Association

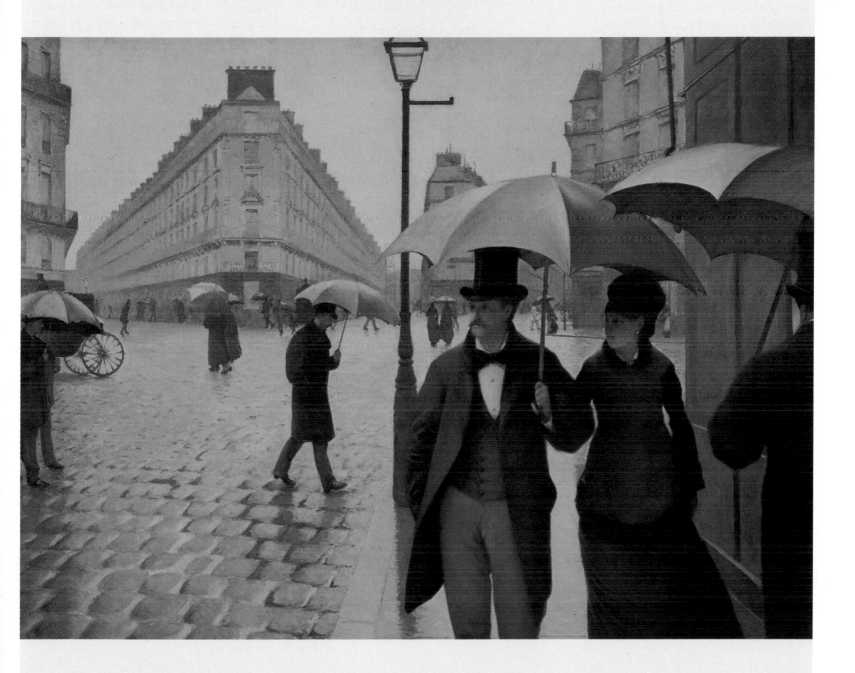

April 14, 1975

JAN HAVICKSZ STEEN

The Family Concert

The contemporaries Jan Havicksz Steen (c 1626-1679) and Jean-Baptiste Poquelin (Molière) are often compared for their comic genius, the one expressing it through his genre paintings of Dutch life, the other through his stage dialogues of common French speech. Hypochondria and the pomposity of the physician were favorite targets: Steen has several paintings entitled *The Doctor's Visit*, while Molière's last play was *Le Malade Imaginaire*. (He died during a performance while playing the title role.) Both men were *farceurs* of the highest order, choosing to satirize the universal human vices, especially hypocrisy and pretentiousness, but always with a deep sense of humanity so that even as we laugh, we feel sympathy for the characters.

Steen's *The Family Concert*, for example, is anything but a musical event, despite the

> *...even as we laugh, we feel sympathy for the characters.*

evidence of the various musical instruments—the lute, the recorder, the viola, the hunting horn, the double-bass viol. From the evidence of the empty jugs and glasses, the painting might better be called *In Their Cups*. The young couple in the background are completely innocent of any music making, while for the other young woman the songbook is merely a prop that permits her to demur from the attentions of cavalier and callow youth alike, shrewdly, meanwhile, holding the desires of both.

Incongruously, the largest instrument of all is played by a dwarf, whose beatific expression belies—or perhaps explains—the fact that he bows it with his meerschaum pipe. On the table is an open songbook, but the right-hand page is covered not with musical clefs, but with the notation "JSteen, 1666." And finally, the almost obscured gentleman in the rear with the benign facial expression is probably the artist himself, not quite part of the scene, yet overseeing all the foibles and idiosyncrasies of the family of mankind with kindness, gentleness, and forbearance.

JAMA

THE JOURNAL OF the American Medical Association

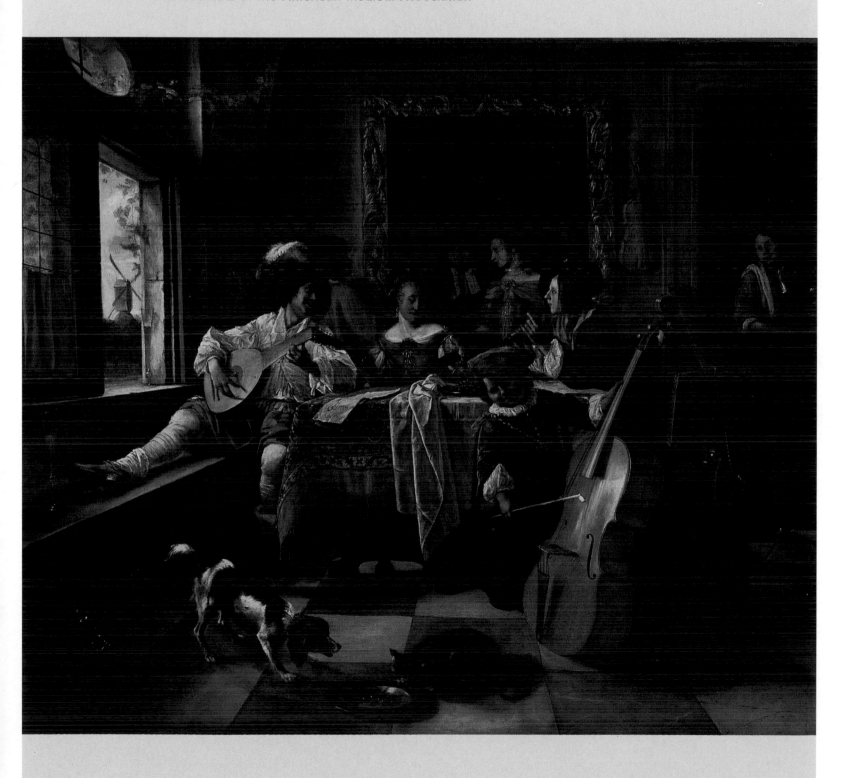

June 23, 1975

CLAUDE MONET

Arrival of the Normandy Train, Gare Saint-Lazare

When Claude Monet (1840-1926) painted *Arrival of the Normandy Train, Gare Saint-Lazare* (formerly *Old Saint-Lazare Station, Paris*) he was 37 years old and firmly identified as an "Impressionist." His more conventional paintings, such as *The Beach at Sainte-Adresse* (inset), belonged to the decade past; his "series"

*"Only an eye...
but my God,
what an eye!"*

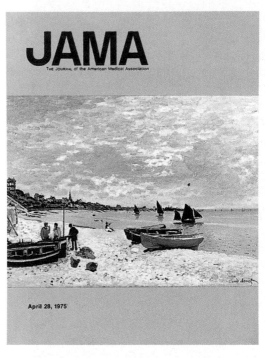

*The Beach at Sainte-Adresse
(la plage de Sainte-Adresse)*

paintings—the haystacks, the poplars, the Rouen cathedrals, the London and Venice views—were not to be seen for almost another decade and a half, when Monet would be already in his 50s. And the famed water lilies, which were to do for our concept of space what his early paintings had done for our concept of light, were yet more than 40 years away—many a person's entire life span at that time.

The steam locomotive (which had come to France only eight years before Monet's birth) and railway shed were "naturals" for a painter such as Monet. He painted the Gare Saint-Lazare many times; each instant of billowing smoke, bustling crowd, glass-broken light, panting engine, and limpid sky that accompanied the arrival of the train from Normandy was to him a new now. It was also from this station that Monet often went to his home in Le Havre, or later to Argenteuil.

Curiously, the several paintings of the Gare Saint-Lazare, which today typify the Impressionist movement, also presaged its end. From trying to capture a fleeting impression of a scene by painting it at different times of day and different seasons of the year, Monet went to the concept of capturing a single aspect of a scene on a single canvas. He was no longer interested, for example, in painting *a* haystack, but rather *an aspect* of a haystack. Toward that end, he set up canvases in a row—a "series"—and moved from one to the other as the scene changed. In Rewald's words, He "pursued a race with light." In Monet's words, he sought *instantaneity*. But his colleagues were unimpressed. Degas called him "a skillful, but not profound, decorator." Cézanne said: "Only an eye," but added, "but my God, what an eye!"

JAMA

THE JOURNAL of the American Medical Association

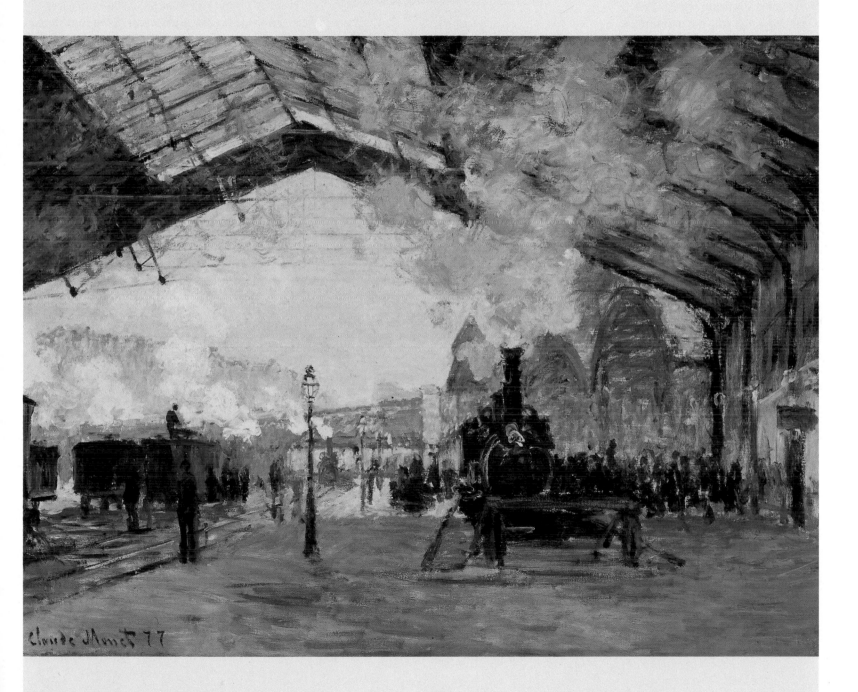

Claude Monet 77

July 21, 1975

WILLIAM MICHAEL HARNETT

Just Dessert

William Michael Harnett (1848-1892) is generally acknowledged as America's foremost still-life painter. Eat often enough in public dining rooms and you will most certainly see a Harnett reproduction: artful compositions of violins, musical scores, meerschaum pipes, half-read letters, books in worn leather bindings, pewter tankards, overturned inkwells, ashes glowing on a forgotten newspaper—in short, all the accoutrements of the gentleman's world of business and leisure in late 19th-century America.

Harnett's forte was *trompe l'oeil* (deceiving the eye); the illusion of a third dimension is so strong that the viewer, against all reason, feels constrained to touch the objects—to brush the glowing ashes off the tablecloth, to close the door, to feel the coldness of a copper mug. *Just Dessert* is atypical in that it is a fruit painting and also the only known painting of the copper

> *...the viewer, against all reason, feels constrained to touch the objects...*

pitcher. For the rest, Harnett used the same objects over and over in new compositions. Indeed, the pewter tankard is known, from other paintings, to have a dent on the opposite side, and the coconut was found among Harnett's effects after his death (although presumably the grapes were not).

Harnett was enormously popular at the turn of the century, but then went into eclipse until the mid-1930s. Since then his popularity (and price) have grown steadily. *Just Dessert*, valued at $1500 in 1942, was credited at $12,000 in 1958; another painting, missing for 70 years, was found in the basement of a Haight-Asbury house in 1971 and priced at $350,000. Moreover, two thirds of Harnett's work is thought to be still missing. It is difficult to explain this new popularity for *trompe l'oeil*, except if it be, as Frankenstein, a Harnett authority quips: "Our pleasure arises … from the realization that our *oeil* has been *trompe'd*." As always, though, caveat emptor: forgeries have been few, but misattributions many. And what of Harnett? With his delight in deceit and penchant for punning, he would have enjoyed the astronomical rise in prices: One of his favorite *trompe's* was painting stock market quotations and $5 bills so realistically that once he was arrested.

William Michael Harnett (1848-1892), *Just Dessert*, 1891, American. Oil on canvas. 56.5 × 68.0 cm. Courtesy of The Art Institute of Chicago, Chicago, Illinois; Friends of American Art Collection, 1942. Photograph © 1995 The Art Institute of Chicago, all rights reserved.

JAMA

December 1, 1975

THE JOURNAL of the American Medical Association

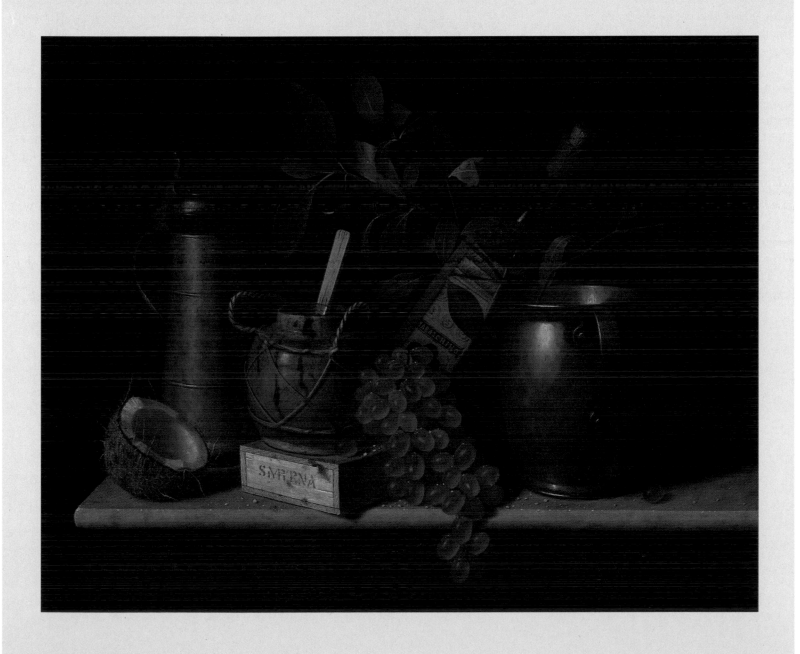

FRANÇOIS BOUCHER

Pensent-ils au raisin?
(Are They Thinking of the Grape?)

Louis XV reacted to the formality and grandeur of his predecessor's court by building a set of separate apartments at Versailles to permit privacy and discreet withdrawal from public duties. Likewise, the art of the period, much of it commissioned by a favorite of the King, Antoinette Poisson (also known as Marquise de Pompadour), followed the same intimate style, and because of its graceful ovals, resembling seashells, came to be known as "rococo."

Preeminent among Madame de Pompadour's protégés was François Boucher (1703-1770), whose *Pensent-ils au raisin?* (freely translated, "Are they thinking about the grape?") illustrates the qualities of this period. The theme is pastoral, the setting idyllic and intimate. The composition is

> *...the struggles of the young shepherd's heart and mind: bashful, timid, silly— and lecherous.*

oval and is developed by curving lines until the eye is led to the single, round grape in the young woman's hand. With his ruddy complexion and the bold, assertive primary colors of his costume, the shepherd is very much of this earth; the young woman, on the other hand, with her delicate pale skin

tones and the subtle mauve of her dress, is a spiritual, idealized creature. And tucked off to the side is Pan, the god with the goat-like visage, ruler of forests and shepherds.

Pensent-ils au raisin? Perhaps. But it should be remembered that into this sylvan setting Boucher has placed both sheep and goats, symbols perhaps of the struggles of the young shepherd's heart and mind: bashful, timid, silly—and lecherous. It is no wonder that Boucher, often called frivolous and amoral, was a favorite of the urbane court of 18th-century France.

François Boucher (1703-1770), *Pensent-ils au raisin? (Are They Thinking of the Grape?)*, 1747, French. Oil on canvas. 80.8 × 68.5 cm. Courtesy of The Art Institute of Chicago, Chicago, Illinois; Martha E. Leverone Endowment, 1973. Photograph © 1995 The Art Institute of Chicago, all rights reserved.

JAMA

THE JOURNAL of the American Medical Association

February 9, 1976

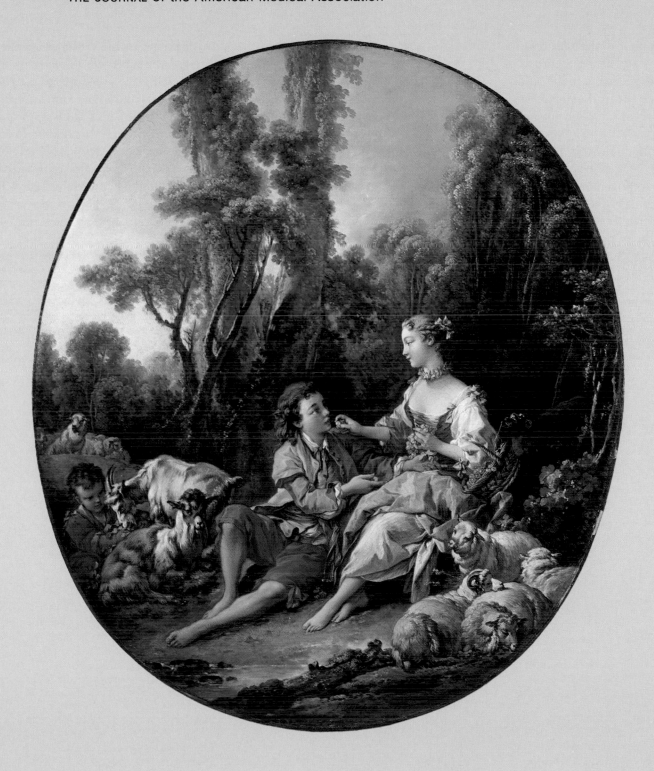

REMBRANDT HARMENSZ VAN RIJN (OR FOLLOWER)

Young Woman at an Open Half-Door

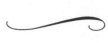

T he Dutch Republic of the 17th century was the Athens of Northern Europe. Not only did it prosper economically and politically, but it left the world an intellectual and cultural legacy not often equaled: in philosophy, Descartes and Spinoza; in mathematics, Stevin; in physics, Huygens; in microscopy, van Leewenhoek and Swammerdam; and in painting, more well-known artists than perhaps any other country. Yet the young republic would have been well remembered had the work of only one come down to us: the paintings of Rembrandt van Rijn (1606-1669), son of five generations of millers.

Rembrandt was approaching 40 when he painted *Young Woman at an Open Half-Door*. It is not known who the subject is,

> *…that very simplicity belies a complexity that engages the viewer in a dialogue…*

although the girl is dressed in the state costume of the orphans of North Holland. Some say she is Hendrickje Stoeffels, who became Rembrandt's third wife.

Artistically, Rembrandt's style has reached its maturity. His paintings have become calmer, simpler, more dignified. Yet that very simplicity belies a complexity that engages the viewer in a dialogue—with the subject, with the artist, with oneself—and even gives him a glimpse into the truth of the human spirit. Thus, while the still lifes, landscapes, and genre paintings of the Dutch masters of the 17th century will always be admired for such qualities as their sense of order, of balance, of tranquility and certitude, it is Rembrandt who reaches beyond the viewer's eye and intellect and brushes the soul.

JAMA

THE JOURNAL OF the American Medical Association

February 16, 1976

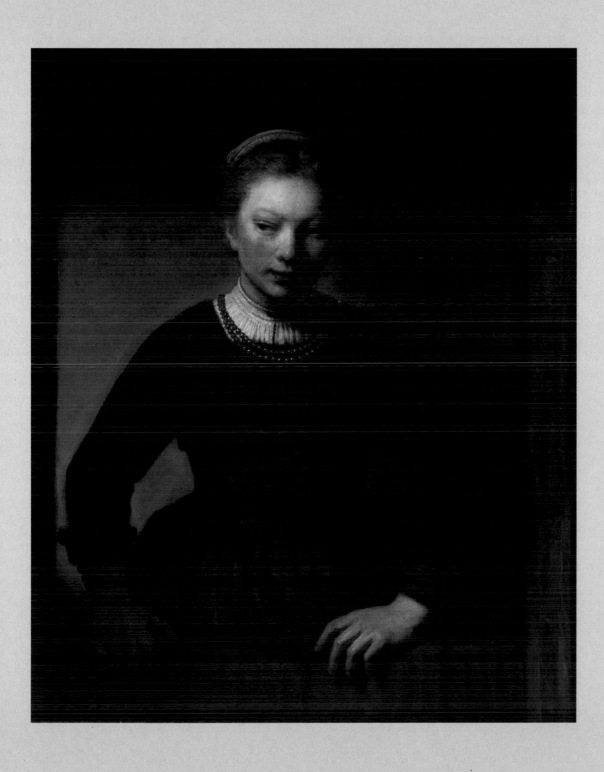

ADRIAEN VAN DER SPELT 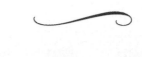 FRANS VAN MIERIS

Trompe-l'Oeil Still Life With a Flower Garland and a Curtain

E xcept that he was born in Gouda, worked for a time at the German court, and was a flower painter of 17th-century Holland, little else is known of Adriaen van der Spelt (1630-1673). Few of his paintings remain, but *Trompe-l'Oeil Still Life With a Flower Garland and a Curtain* (formerly "The Blue Curtain") clearly places him among the best of the "little Dutch masters."

Although flower painting dates well back into ancient history, it was only in the latter part of the 16th century that it became recognized as an independent category, and then largely because of the social, political, religious, and economic structure of the time. The Dutch, after breaking from Spain, had become a world maritime power. The people were frankly wealthy, but having little opportunity to buy land, they turned to speculation in such things as tulip bulbs, newly imported from Turkey (the word *tulipomania* dates from the 1630s, when

> *"…that deceptive truth which Dutch painters frequently delight in."*

the fever for speculating in these exotic bulbs reached its peak and the market crashed), or to buying status symbols: portraits of their new country—of the countryside, of the interiors of their homes, of themselves, or simply of artful arrangements of various objects such as food, glassware, and flowers. (Indeed, the term *still life* also dates back to this time, being derived from the Dutch *stilleven*, coined to describe these groupings of "still standing objects.") Until this time, artists had depended on a patron for subsidy, but with the rise of the wealthy Dutch middle class, the market became the patron, and

painters painted what they thought they could sell. Among all the painters, flower painters were the highest paid.

For all their hard realism, however, and their demand for faithful detail, it is to the credit of the Dutch burghers that they allowed their painters artistic license. Where in nature, for example, can one find a garland of simultaneously blooming tulips and roses, daffodils and carnations, marigolds, poppies, peonies, periwinkle, and columbine? Yet exactly by departing from the literal, van der Spelt has, as Waagen notes, "attained that deceptive truth which Dutch painters frequently delight in."

Adriaen van der Spelt (1630-1673) and Frans van Mieris (1635-1681), *Trompe-l'Oeil Still Life With a Flower Garland and a Curtain*, 1658, Dutch. Oil on panel. 46.5 × 63.9 cm. Courtesy of The Art Institute of Chicago, Chicago, Illinois; Wirt D. Walker Fund, 1949. Photograph © 1995 The Art Institute of Chicago, all rights reserved. Original photograph by Joe Fletcher.

JAMA

March 8, 1976

The Journal of the American Medical Association

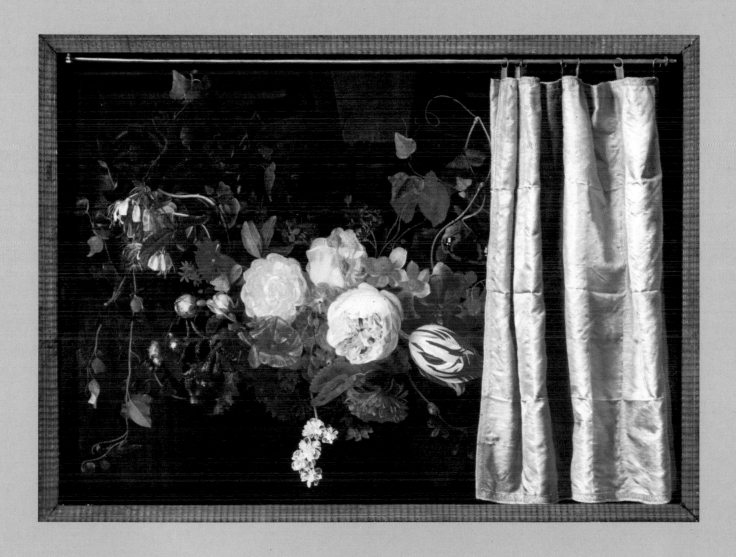

JOSEPH MALLORD WILLIAM TURNER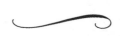

Valley of Aosta—Snowstorm, Avalanche, and Thunderstorm

If, as Sir Kenneth Clark has noted, landscape to the Englishman is religion, then certainly John Constable and his contemporary J. M. W. Turner (1775-1851) are its high priests. Born but a year apart, both were part of the Romantic school, and both turned to Nature in search of ultimate truth. But there the similarity ends. Constable was a Wordsworthian contemplative, approaching nature quietly, humbly, and passively and leaving us gentle, though somber, cow-eyed scenes of the English countryside. Turner, on the other hand, was the Byron, Keats, and Shelley of the palette. His Nature was a majestic, awesome, terrible god who overwhelmed men with floods and avalanches or sucked them into the vortex of a violent wind. The great Victorian, John Ruskin, describes the two men thus:

"The bad painter gives the cheap deceptive resemblance [to truth]. The good painter gives the precious non-deceptive resemblance. Constable perceives in a landscape that the grass is wet, the meadows flat,

> *...landscape to the Englishman is religion...*

and the boughs shady; that is to say, about as much as, I suppose, might in general be apprehended between men, by an intelligent faun and a skylark. Turner perceives at a glance the whole sum of visible truth open to human intelligence."

Though an influential writer, Ruskin has never been accused of impartiality.

Valley of Aosta—Snowstorm, Avalanche, and Thunderstorm was painted when Turner was in his 60s and had returned from his second trip to the Italian Alps. A sudden, violent whirlwind sweeps down the valley, pushing before it thunderous torrents of floodwater and rushing snow. The tiny figures in the right foreground are plucked from their pursuit of the ordinary affairs of life and forced to flee before the omnipotent

tempest. And though the mountains and the valley will remain after the storm has passed, it is obvious that for the puny figures, there is no contest.

Such whirling storms were Turner's typical way of expressing his profound pessimism, hopelessness, and essential powerlessness before man's fate. Yet if Turner is truly to be called the Shelley of the canvas, and although he may say in his ode to the wind, "Thou...Yellow and black, and pale, and hectic red...Thou dirge Of the dying year, ...dome of a vast sepulchre," is he not also compelled in truth to add, "O Wind, If Winter comes, can Spring be far behind?"

JAMA

THE JOURNAL OF the American Medical Association

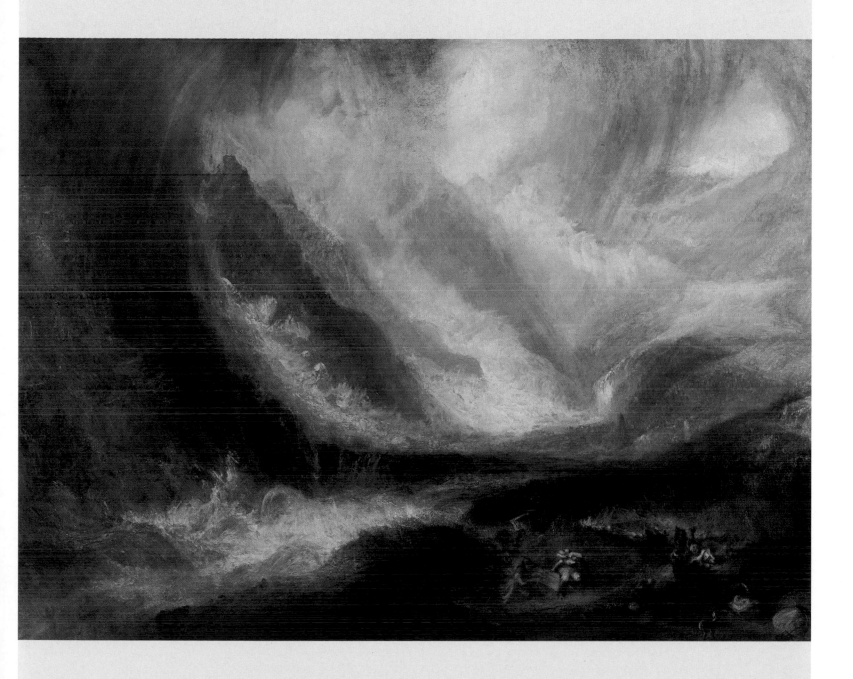

January 10,1977

MASTER OF THE FEMALE HALF-FIGURES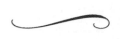

Mary Magdalene

Had Dickens been alive at the beginning of the 16th century, he would have called it, too, the best of times and the worst of times. On the throne of England sat Henry VIII, and Charles V was Emperor of Europe. Muskets were introduced into modern warfare, and Rome was sacked. The mystic and reformer, Teresa of Avila, was born, as were the two Reformer Johns, Calvin and Knox. Luther posted his 95 theses and Sir Thomas More wrote his *Utopia*. Columbus had long since returned from America and died, and Magellan was dead in the Philippines. Copernicus was a doctor of canon law and Ambroise Paré was performing surgery. Europe was having its first taste of pineapples, chocolate, and coffee, and the pocket handkerchief came into use. In Spain the slave trade was beginning, and plague was sweeping England. Michelangelo was painting the ceiling of the Sistine Chapel and da Vinci the portrait of the wife of a Florentine banker. Correggio, Raphael, and Titian were doing Madonnas. And someone we know today only as "Master of the Female Half-Figures" was doing Magdalenes. The High Renaissance was well under way.

Mary Magdalene is only one of more than a score of similar paintings left by

Simply a beautiful lady— no one in particular, everyone in general.

this anonymous Flemish master, who flourished between 1500 and 1530, probably in Antwerp. Truly secularized painting had not yet reached the Low Countries, but a clever painter could satisfy the popular taste by painting Madonnas and saints without halos—and especially saints who had once been "real sinners," such as a woman caught in adultery. Thus the artist could present a Magdalene engaged in any number of worldly occupations (other than motherhood), such as reading, writing, and playing musical instruments. He could also dress her in the most sumptuous and elegant gowns, gowns of rich velvet with voluminous sleeves that draped in precisely painted folds, and a décolletage that could barely contain the creased bosom above it. He would cover the head as befitted a modest young lady, but still somehow a tiny fringe of perfectly curled hair would escape to

frame an equally modest face with its downcast eyes, delicately molded alae, protruding upper lip and color reflecting the blush of the bosom. But always, the Master keeps our mind on penance, which is symbolized by the ornate ointment jar in the foreground. Further, the tiny landscape seen through the window signifies our pilgrimage from the earthly city below to the heavenly Jerusalem on high.

No Mona Lisa is our Mary Magdalene (and no Leonardo was the Master of the Female Half-Figure). Yet for nearly 500 years she has remained what she was intended to be: Simply a beautiful lady—no one in particular, everyone in general. She has all the warmth and passion of a porcelain figurine, but she is pleasant to look at, and she does not offend. *Mary Magdalene* is the kind of painting that could be hung above the fireplace of a 16th-century French inn, and it probably was.

JAMA

THE JOURNAL of the American Medical Association

February 28, 1977

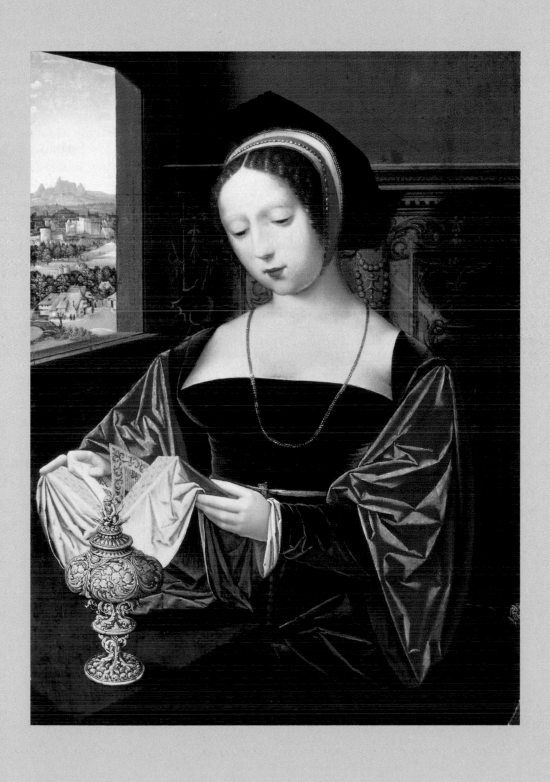

PAUL CÉZANNE

The Basket of Apples

Early in his career Paul Cézanne (1839-1906) worked closely with the Impressionists, especially Camille Pissarro, with whom he often painted out of doors. From the late 1870s on, however, their paths diverged and the Post-Impressionist Cézanne entered an uncharted wilderness; his efforts were eventually to map the way directly to Cubism and to much of modern, 20th-century painting.

Unlike the Impressionists, Cézanne no longer wished to paint the impressions of a moment, but to paint solid, lasting structures. This he did by disregarding light as the principal character in a painting and concentrating instead on the properties of color. Moreover, he heretically threw out both linear perspective and chiaroscuro (literally, light, dark), the two classic devices for putting a three-dimensional scene onto a two-dimensional surface, and instead chose color alone to accomplish these functions. To this he added an architectural design so simple, yet so intricate, that, like a Bach invention or a sonnet of Shakespeare, not a line can be subtracted or even moved without destroying the whole.

...like a Bach invention or a sonnet of Shakespeare, not a line can be subtracted...

The Basket of Apples is a masterpiece of this maturity. The shapes are simple: spherical apples, cylindrical bread and bottle, rectangular table, elliptical openings of plate and basket. Three-dimensional space is defined solely by color, with the warm colors (red, yellow) advancing toward the viewer and the cool colors (green, blue) receding. Even the apples are given volume simply by their multiple variations in color, each color a separate and carefully considered brushstroke. So painstaking and so deliberate was each stroke Cézanne put on a canvas that a contemporary critic called his work "a meditation, brush in hand." The elements of the design are less obvious, but a few minutes with straight-edge and pencil will demonstrate the interlocking cones and planes on which the painting is constructed.

Yet when we view this still life our impression is not of the anatomy, or ribs, of the design, but of color, brightness, cheerfulness, warmth. If one looks a little longer there is the sensation of actually having just come into someone's kitchen, with its smell of warm, freshly baked bread and apples and newly opened wine. There is an ephemeral quality to the painting—the bread will cool—and yet there is permanence and hope—there will always be moments like this.

Cézanne's genius was to take the color of the Impressionists and the design principles of the Classicists and to forge them into a unique creation. Not only has he profoundly affected all painting since that time, but he has given the 20th century a new way of seeing.

JAMA

March 7,1977

THE JOURNAL of the American Medical Association

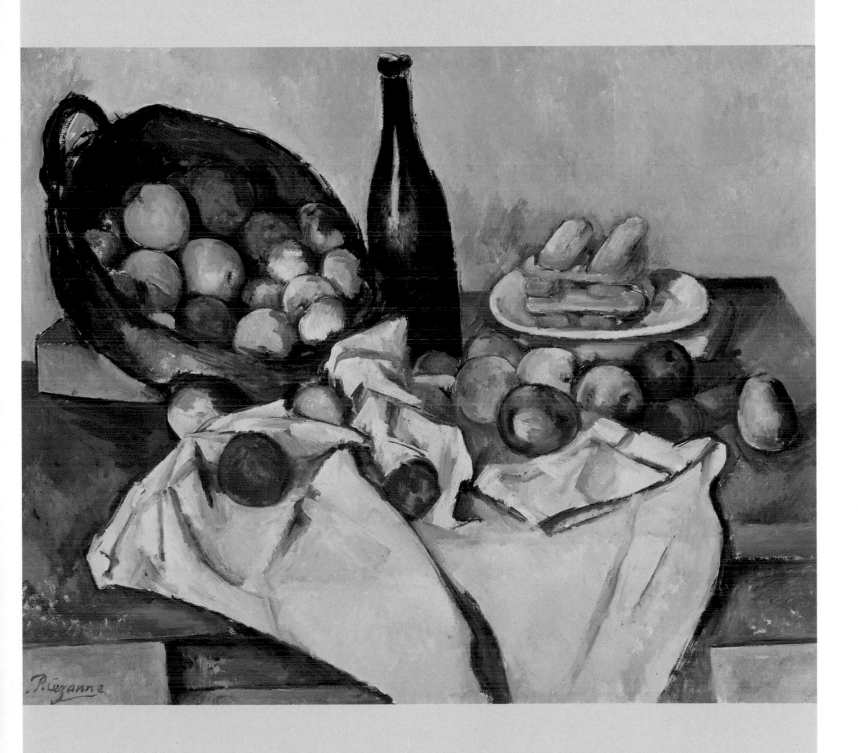

P.Cezanne

NICOLAI FECHIN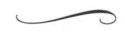

Manuelita With Kachina

If the term "cosmopolitan" can be applied to painting, then it is certainly Nicolai Fechin (1881-1955) who provides the definition. As a boy in his birthplace of Kazan, the capital city of the Tatar Republic, he helped his father carve icons and altar pieces. Later he studied with the Russian Realist Ilya Repin and also traveled throughout Europe, where he was most influenced by the Impressionists. As a result of the Bolshevik revolution, he came, in 1923, to New York City, where he was immediately in demand as a portrait painter. (Lillian Gish, in her costume as "Ramola," and Willa Cather were among his subjects.) Unhappy with city life, however, Fechin traveled west and finally, at the age of 46, settled in Taos, New Mexico, in the shadow of the Sangre de Cristo Mountains. Later, he was to move yet once more, to California, where he opened an art school in Hollywood. He died in Santa Monica in 1955, but it is Taos that he loved and with Taos that he is identified; indeed, his widow still maintains his studio in Taos.

> *...a meticulous draftsmanship, belied by the graceful pose of the subject...*

Manuelita With Kachina (formerly *Indian Maid Seated*) was painted probably around 1927, shortly after Fechin settled in Taos. The model is a young girl of the Taos tribe who sat for many of the well-known painters there. In her arms she cradles kachina dolls, carved from wood by the men of the Pueblo tribe and meant to represent one of their many supernatural beings. Perhaps because of the carved icons of his boyhood, Fechin was fascinated with the kachina dolls, and the ones pictured are from his own collection.

Though many consider his other works to far surpass *Manuelita With Kachina*, this painting is certainly among Fechin's most loved and popular works. In it are many of the attributes for which he is known: a meticulous draftsmanship, belied by the graceful pose of the subject; anatomical faithfulness, a subject he knew better than most doctors, said one critic; "biting colors" but always saved by a "cello-tone of gray," said another; and careful, though seemingly casual, brushwork. (He used many brushes, of all shapes and sizes, as well as a knife, and he never allowed anyone to clean his brushes but himself.) Most of all, however, Fechin has left us what he found and loved in the southwestern United States, in its confluence of the Indian, Spanish, and Anglo-American cultures: the exotic faces and vivid costumes of a people who reminded him of those he had known and painted in his Volga birthplace so many years before.

Nicolai Fechin (1881-1955), *Manuelita With Kachina*, c 1926-1930, American (born Russian). Oil on canvas. 51.4 × 40.9 cm. Courtesy of the San Diego Museum of Art, San Diego, California; gift of Mrs Henry A. Everett.

JAMA

April 11, 1977

THE JOURNAL of the American Medical Association

FELICE FICHERELLI (IL RIPOSO)

Judith

Apocryphal though it may be, few narratives can equal the Old Testament book of Judith for sheer drama. All of the elements are there: on the one hand, a contest between vastly unequal forces, a seemingly hopeless situation, the juxtaposition of sharply defined opposites; yet, on the other hand, risk, suspense, and a tension that finally, just at its breaking point, resolves in the wholly unexpected triumph of the weak over the strong. It is perhaps precisely because of the richness of these dramatic elements that so many sculptors and painters have chosen the biblical Judith as their subject. She has been portrayed, for example, by Donatello, Botticelli, Titian, and Cranach, among others. Michaelangelo used one of the four corners of the Sistine Chapel ceiling for the story of Judith. Even Chaucer had a go at it in verse.

Judith, once attributed to the 17th-century Florentine Giovanni Martinelli, is now thought to be the work of his contemporary, Felice Ficherelli (1605-1669), called Il Riposo, presumably for his quiet nature. Except for the qualities evident in his paintings, little else is known about him. Ficherelli chooses to portray his Judith in the moments just

> *...its very presence is a reminder of the discord of violence.*

after she has beheaded Holofernes with his own sword. Though she still remains in the Assyrian camp, her face betrays no fear. Rather, it is radiant, becoming the source of the light that creates the aura of the heroine about her head; she is thus apart from her maidservant, who represents all other women. By contrast, the severed head of Holofernes has lost its light completely and would not be visible at all did it not catch a little of the light from Judith's face.

Judith's enigmatic facial expression is reminiscent of that of the *Mona Lisa*, with which Ficherelli could have been familiar. Reminiscent also of da Vinci is the triangular format of the figure of Judith, its solid base tapering upward in blue and white billows until the eye rests at its apex—Judith's calm brow. The drama of the moment is emphasized by the brief, but sharp, accents of red. The tension

is illustrated by the placement of the maidservant just outside the triangle, so that not only is the perfect balance of the triangle disturbed, but the viewer's eye is pulled back and forth between the faces of the two women, unable to come to rest. Finally, in the lower right corner, the head of Holofernes, nearly lost in shadow though it is, creates a discord. Not only does it further disrupt the harmony of the triangle, but its very presence is a reminder of the discord of violence.

It matters little to the viewer that the events of the book of Judith could not have happened—at least not from a geographical or historical standpoint. What matters is that Ficherelli has taken the narrative of the heroic woman and transformed it into a visible drama of color, light, and shadow—and the abiding quality of a masterpiece, mystery.

JAMA

THE JOURNAL of the American Medical Association

July 18, 1977

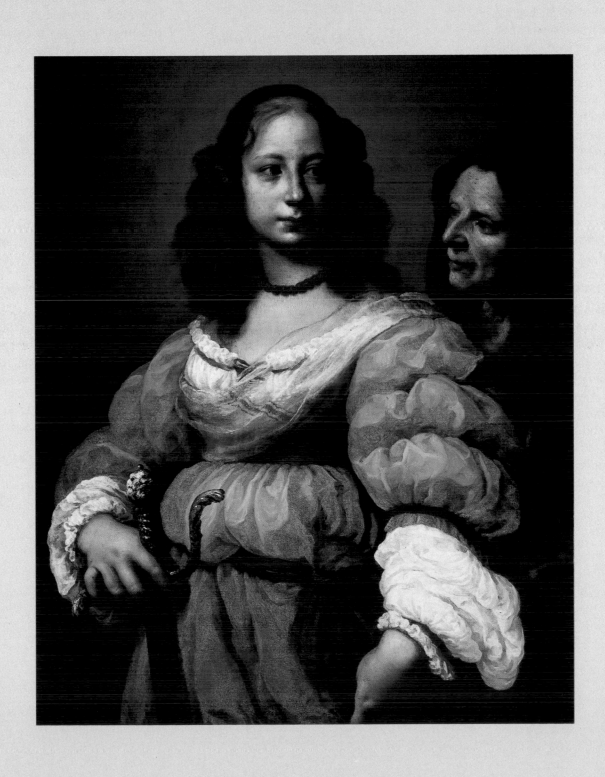

MARY CASSATT

Mother and Child

Only when she was nearing 40 did Mary Cassatt (1844-1926) begin to paint the subject with which she has become most closely identified, women and children. Prior to that time she had served a characteristically disciplined apprenticeship, studying first at the Pennsylvania Academy of the Fine Arts and then, at her own insistence, in Paris. She also thoroughly studied the works of Correggio in Italy, the paintings of Rubens in the Prado and in Antwerp, and also those of Franz Hals in Holland. Finally, back in Paris, she became the only American to exhibit with the Impressionists. She also became a lifelong and close friend of Edgar Degas, a relationship that has been much discussed, since neither ever married. Of Miss Cassatt, Degas said, "I would have married her, but I could never have made love to her [as a mistress]." Of Degas, Cassatt said that his criticism could "demolish me completely." Yet, in spite of this vulnerability to Degas' criticism, Mary Cassatt was seen as a "self-assured woman, stubborn and determined, indomitable and forceful, vibrant and optimistic in disposition." A family friend who saw her in 1901 described her as a "tall, slender, erect, scrupulously well-tailored

...the child's first dim realization that the world lies elsewhere than in her mother's eyes...

American spinster in her mid-fifties," impatient and annoyed at delays. And in 1905, just about the time she was painting *Mother and Child*, an art student who visited her in her Paris studio found her to be a "fiery and peppery lady, a very vivid, determined personality, positive in her opinions. I was scared to death of her."

Perhaps it was these very elements of her character and personality, plus the fact that she would never have children of her own, that enabled Miss Cassatt to keep the certain cool detachment necessary to portray the maternal theme without the sentimentality that can so easily destroy it. For example, the moments she captures are so intimate and the subjects so un-self-conscious that the viewer is perforce obliged to remain outside. To enter the scene would be to

destroy what is happening at that moment between the mother and her child. In her paintings of infants, the mother and child are characteristically absorbed in each other, gazing into each other's eyes, to the exclusion of the entire world. In the paintings of slightly older children, such as *Mother and Child*, the two are still completely absorbed in each other, but this time, the child, who is looking into a mirror held by her mother, begins to see her image reflected back at herself in something other than her mother's eyes. It is a painting of the child's first dim realization that the world lies elsewhere than in her mother's eyes, and, in the tenderness of this scene, that it is a good world as well.

Nowhere, perhaps, can the mother-child relationship be studied more profitably than in a catalogue raisonné of the hundreds of paintings Mary Cassatt did on this theme. Certainly, she surpasses all those who have attempted to put it into words.

Mary Cassatt (1844-1926), *Mother and Child*, c 1905, American. Oil on canvas. 91.3 × 63.8 cm. Courtesy of the National Gallery of Art, Washington, DC; Chester Dale Collection, 1963. © 1995 The Board of Trustees of the National Gallery of Art.

JAMA

August 1, 1977

THE JOURNAL of the American Medical Association

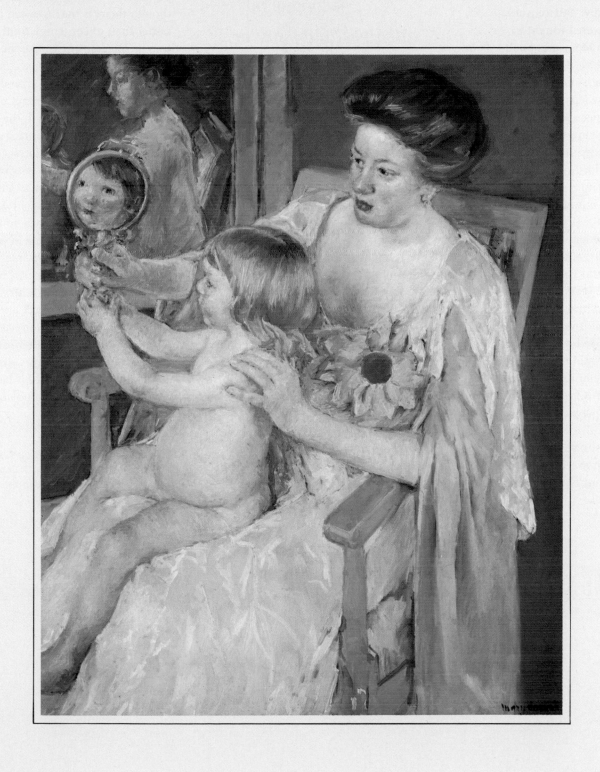

THEODORE WORES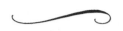

A Lesson in Flower Arrangement

Many artists of the late 19th century were influenced by 18th-century Japanese prints, which were brought to Europe along the new trade routes established with Japan. In the work of Degas, Cassatt, and other Impressionists, for example, one can see the Japanese influence in the organization of space, the unusual perspective, the odd viewing angles, and the flat planes, without depth.

The American Theodore Wores (1859-1939), who saw these prints in England, was likewise fascinated, but not so much with the prints as with the people who had made them. Thus it was that, with a little prodding from his friend James McNeill Whistler, Wores sailed into Yokohama Harbor in 1885, only 32 years after Commodore Perry had sailed into Uraga Harbor. Wores arrived at the beginning of his favorite season, spring. He had intended to stay three months; he stayed nearly three years. Not only is he one of the first Western painters to visit Japan, but he is probably the first to live "among the people," as he says, learning the language and adopting the customs, even to the costume. But Wores did not go to Japan so much to learn Japanese painting as to learn Japan. Thus, he retained

"Man has made no attempt to supplant or to improve nature, and has been but a loving assistant."

the bold, broad brushwork of his Munich training, except that in a happy marriage of his own temperament and the Japanese landscape, his colors become considerably brighter, even brilliant: "sunlit," "the tint of life and beauty," "noon-day," the critics later wrote. While many Western artists were influenced by the Japanese style, it can be fairly said that Wores brought the Western style to Japan, especially the use of light and shadow to give dimension.

A Lesson in Flower Arrangement is characteristic of Wores' Japanese paintings. It is a moment of life in a Japanese home in which a young girl, about to assume the responsibilities of womanhood, is being initiated into the highly symbolic and formal art of flower arranging. Two younger children,

perhaps her siblings, are equally absorbed, though theirs is the attention of curiosity rather than of contemplation. The composition of the painting is, like the flowers, at first glance unstudied. A second glance shows, in fact, a careful arrangement: the nine main chrysanthemums and two accessory ones direct the eye to the corresponding three main subjects (woman, vase of flowers, and girl) and two accessories (children).

For a painter who so passionately loved nature in its "natural state," a carefully arranged bouquet of cut chrysanthemums would seem to be contrary to his temperament. Yet, during his time in Japan, Wores had an important insight into beauty and its relationship to the artist: "Japan," he said, "more than any other country, perhaps, owes much of its general beauty and attractiveness to the hand of man…Man has made no attempt to supplant or to improve nature, and has been but a loving assistant." Especially in the light of his later California paintings, Wores, too, can be called "nature's loving assistant."

Theodore Wores (1859-1939), *A Lesson in Flower Arrangement*, 1885, American. Oil on canvas. 63.8 × 91.3 cm. Collection of Drs Ben and A. Jess Shenson.

JAMA

THE JOURNAL of the American Medical Association

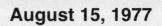August 15, 1977

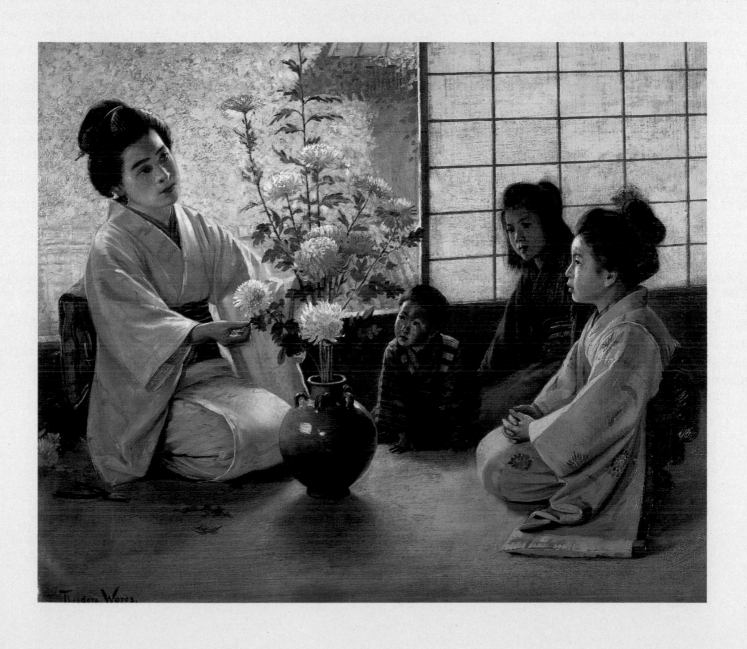

MAURICE DE VLAMINCK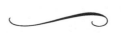

The River

Maurice de Vlaminck (1876-1958), born in Paris into a family of musicians, had but a single passion: to find a way of expressing the deep and powerful emotions he felt. In the beginning, the method was unimportant. Thus, he was at various times a gypsy violinist, a racing cyclist, a novelist, and finally, as he at last found his mode, a painter. He had had no training. "I composed by instinct, clumsily," he said. "I put colors there…to say what I felt. I painted stutteringly…I heightened every tone. I transposed all the emotion which I perceived inside of me into an orchestration of pure colors. I was a barbarian both tender and full of violence…I crushed and bungled ultramarines and vermilions, although they were very expensive…"

Vlaminck's father was unimpressed with his son's painting: "You'll never earn enough," he predicted, "to buy the salt to put in your soup." He was wrong. In 1905, Vlaminck, along with his friends Derain and Matisse, became known as the founders of the first new art movement of the 20th century, named "Fauvism." Like "Impressionism,"

…behind the mauve-tinted clouds a thousand tons of anger waits to explode…

the term was coined by a Paris journalist and was intended to be derogatory. The critic, startled by the intensity of their colors and the discords of the reds and greens, blues and oranges, referred to the artists in his review as "fauves," "wild beasts." Fauvism was short-lived but far-reaching; its principal offshoot was Cubism.

The River is but one of many scenes Vlaminck painted along the Seine, from Châtou to Havre. The colors of his Fauve days have become slightly muted, and there is just the barest flirtation with "Braque's little cubes." Most important, Vlaminck has been able to bridle the raw emotion of a van Gogh with the disciplined composition of a Cézanne, himself becoming a bridge between the two painters he most admired.

But the expression remains Vlaminck. The river is deceptively calm. It is in reality one of T. S. Eliot's "strong brown gods," "patient [only] to some degree," "almost forgotten," but "implacable," "intractable," and full of fury in its deepest currents. Likewise, behind the mauve-tinted clouds a thousand tons of anger waits to explode, here controlled only because it is Vlaminck who holds the brush. The trees speed past in blurred, slapdash strokes of green, while the houses simply wait, dumb and silent. The entire scene is one of foreboding. Within a short time World War I was to break over this northern French landscape.

Unlike the Impressionists, Vlaminck did not seek to record the emotion a landscape aroused in him; rather, he used nature to express the feelings he already had. His expression is simple, vivid, direct, and intense.

JAMA

August 22, 1977

THE JOURNAL of the American Medical Association

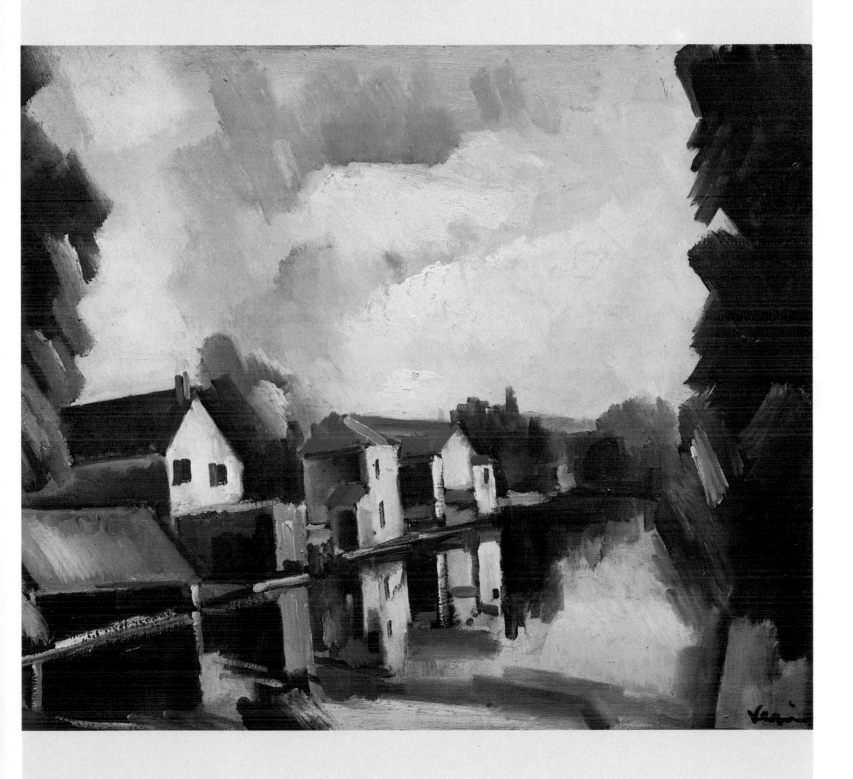

HENRI MATISSE

Apples

Until the 20th century, the last great revolution in painting belonged to the Renaissance. Brought to birth by Masaccio and given its identity by da Vinci, it taught humans to see in terms of light and dark and linear perspective. From then on, painting was largely a variation on, and a development of, these themes until, with the Impressionists, light became itself no longer the means, but the subject of the painting. From there it was only a short step to the 20th century, where reality is no longer the product of chiaroscuro and vanishing points, but a differential calculus of time and space with an infinitude of variations. What was a moment ago, is not now, and what is now, will not, in a moment, be. In a sense, each painter's truth is his own, and what he sees at this moment no longer exists, even as he touches the brush to the canvas. At the same time, all that is past and present and to come in what he paints is already contained in the object. Thus it is that Paul Klee can say, "An apple tree in bloom is in effect a complex of stages of growth, its roots, the rising sap, its trunk, the cross-section with the annual rings, the blossom, its structure, its sexual function,

What was a moment ago, is not now, and what is now, will not, in a moment, be.

the fruit, the core with its seeds," while at the same time, Gertrude Stein can insist that "A rose is a rose is a rose," and each can be expressing an equal truth.

The first of the revolutions in this new art, whose language is mathematical and whose expression is geometric, was Fauvism; its best known practitioner was Henri Matisse (1869-1954). While Fauvism itself was finished within five years and most of the so-called Fauves moved on into other, more radical expressions such as Cubism and Dadaism, Matisse continued to manipulate color and shape. He fit each to the other and each to itself until he got the "feel" he wanted. This, rather than the visually accurate representation of a particular object, marked the completion of the painting.

Apples, with its echoes of Cézanne's "cylinders, spheres, and cones," is such an essay in color. Its visual reality is a dish of apples sitting on a Louis XVI table, but Matisse has adjusted colors and shapes until what we actually see is his expression of the essence of apples. But if what we see is the residue left on the canvas after the scene has passed through the artist's experience, *how* we see presupposes an even more dynamic relationship. For, if we accept that what we are now is not what we were a moment ago, then the painting, too, is changing constantly in its meaning as our perspective shifts.

With the 20th century, the Renaissance is complete; its gift was to enable us to see in a new way. The newest gift, from the 20th-century artists, is to hand on yet another way to look at things, and eventually, to see.

JAMA

October 31, 1977

THE JOURNAL of the American Medical Association

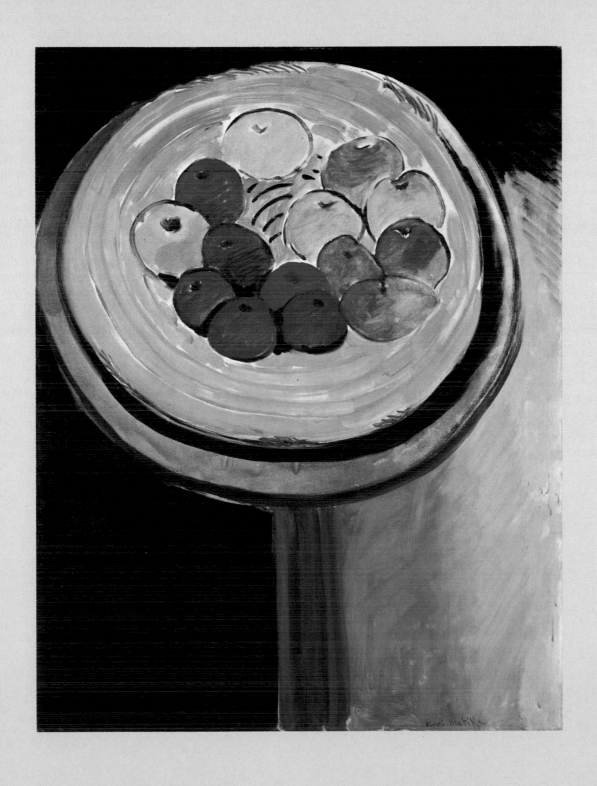

FILIPPINO LIPPI

Portrait of a Youth

Had Filippino Lippi (c 1457-1504) left not a single painting, he would still have had his place in history. He was the son of the lusty Carmelite Fra Filippo Lippi, himself a painter of note, who eloped with his model for the Virgin, the beautiful nun Lucretia, on the feast of the Girdle of Our Lady in 1456. It is a delicious scandal told with obvious relish, and probably not a little embellishment, by the 16th-century painter and biographer Vasari in his *Lives of the Artists* and retold for the 19th-century Romantics by Robert Browning in his poem "Men and Women." But Filippino has greater claim to fame in his own right. Like his father, he was a painter; unlike his father, he was apparently possessed of greater self-discipline.

Filippino lived at the very apogee of the Renaissance in the city that had invented the Renaissance. It was Florence whose painters discovered the new laws of perspective, whose architects built the perfect dome, and whose sculptors chiseled the perfect David. Its bankers made the florin the monetary standard for the world, and its poets made its dialect the language of Italy. Its Medici invented the income tax.

> *Florence is his stage;*
> *the world is his backdrop.*

Portrait of a Youth was painted when Filippino was 28 years old. The name of the youth is unknown, but from the cut of the cloth, he is a nobleman, perhaps a Medici— perhaps even the beautiful Piero, son of Lorenzo. In spite of his youth, his look is the look of confidence, the calm self-possession of a man who knows himself to be the standard against which others are measured. It is the look of an heir. Florence is his stage; the world is his backdrop. True, he is flawed by the merest touch of arrogance in the gaze, by a tinge of conceit, by the barest edge of a sneer about to break over his face. But he is, after all, only human. He is perhaps also too young to have learned to veil these defects of Everyman's soul from the artist's brush.

Filippino's work combines the flowing lines learned from Botticelli with the delicate modeling adopted from Masaccio. Produced by the interplay of light and shadow, this modeling is most evident in the protruding upper lip, the pronounced line of the jaw, and especially in the flaring nostrils—for some reason a preoccupation of Renaissance portraitists. Typically, the youth is framed by a window, although unlike others, this one does not open onto a distant landscape. Most characteristic of the new Renaissance manner, however, is our involvement with the painting. We no longer gaze in a detached awe, as at those remote, wooden Mothers of God of the Byzantine style, nor even in a "mustn't touch" wonder, as at the lovely, limpid Madonnas of Botticelli, but with a direct flesh-and-blood involvement. This 500-year-old youth will not take his eyes off us, nor can we take ours off him. If we were to meet him on the street tomorrow, we would speak to him—or pass him by if we still owed him the rent money. We like him, or we do not. Either way, he has become part of our lives.

Filippino Lippi (c 1457-1504), *Portrait of a Youth*, c 1485, Florentine. Oil on panel. 51 × 35.5 cm. Courtesy of the National Gallery of Art, Washington, DC; Andrew W. Mellon Collection, 1937. © 1995 The Board of Trustees of the National Gallery of Art.

JAMA

THE JOURNAL of the American Medical Association

November 14, 1977

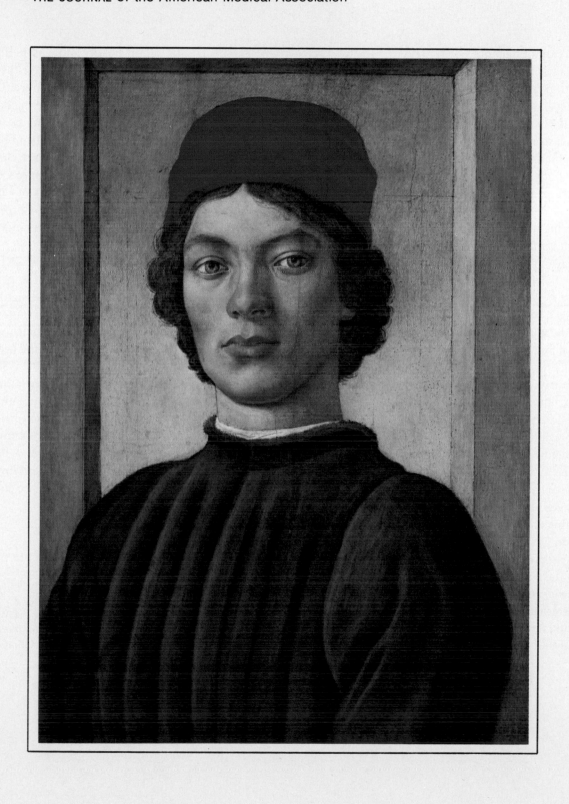

ORAZIO GENTILESCHI
GIOVANNI LANFRANCO

Saint Cecilia and an Angel

Novelists, it is claimed, cannot help but write autobiographically. One wonders if the same does not apply to painters as well. *Saint Cecilia and an Angel* was painted not long after Orazio Gentileschi (c 1563-1639) had been involved in a scandalous lawsuit concerning his daughter, and just a few years after St Cecilia's body had been unearthed in Rome, where Gentileschi was working at the time.

According to legend, Cecilia was a wealthy maiden of the third century who was married to a Roman pagan, Valerian, against her wishes. She told Valerian that she had vowed her virginity to God and that she was protected by an angel, whereupon Valerian demanded to see the angel. When the angel appeared, Valerian and, later, his brother were converted to Christianity. Ultimately, all three were martyred.

Gentileschi's daughter, Artemisia, had a somewhat different experience. According to court records of 1608, Orazio brought suit against his friend and fellow painter Tassi because Artemisia, then 15 years old, had been "deflowered by force and known in the flesh many a time by Agostino Tassi, painter…Also involved in this obscene affair was Tassi's hangeron Cosimo Quorli." One has the impression, however, that the major point of litigation was over Tassi's refusal to subsequently marry Artemisia, and was at least equalled by the concern that "the said Cosimo has also, with his lies, wrung from the hands of said maiden several paintings

> *…as delicate and as fragile as the girl's youth and beauty.*

by her father, and especially a Judith of considerable size." Eventually, after Artemisia was tortured to test the truth of her story and Tassi was temporarily imprisoned, the case was dismissed and Orazio and Tassi were reconciled. Two years later Orazio painted *Saint Cecilia and an Angel*; Artemisia was the model for the martyred virgin.

Living just at the end of the Renaissance era and the beginning of the Baroque period, Gentileschi preferred to identify himself as a Florentine. He is best known as a follower of the Lombard Caravaggio, who shocked his contemporaries with his introduction of *tenebrism*, the violent contrast of lights and darks. While retaining Caravaggio's brilliance of lighting, Gentileschi has muted his tones just enough to turn what could have been an assault on the senses into a simple and striking scene. The modeling of the figures is as delicate and as fragile as the girl's youth and beauty. Realism is introduced by the contemporary setting—the third-century Roman maiden has the hairstyle and gown of a 17th-century Florentine girl. Even the music notation is contemporary, perhaps a Palestrina motet. Still, for

all the beauty and near perfection, we have not a drama that engages us but merely a theatrical scene to admire. This is not a vulnerable and nubile maiden guarded by an angel with a flaming sword but a beautiful, breakable porcelain figurine watched by a rather simple-faced, china-like angel. Rather than being rapt in Cecilia's celestial music, he has the look of a dull-witted urchin impatient to get back to the streets. Still, it is a lovely scene, much as the legend of Cecilia is lovely.

In his later years Orazio became court painter to Charles I of England; he died in London in 1639. His daughter, Artemisia, went on to become a painter in the Caravaggesque style, specializing in scenes of violence; Judith with the head of Holofernes was a favorite. Her fame is said to have surpassed even that of her father. St Cecilia, meanwhile, whose authenticity is in serious doubt, has managed to retain her place in the Roman calendar of saints, despite its revision, and continues to be revered as the patron of musicians and inventor of the organ. Her feast day is celebrated on November 22.

Orazio Gentileschi (c 1563-1639) and Giovanni Lanfranco (1582-1647), *Saint Cecilia and an Angel*, c 1617-1618 and c 1621-1627, Roman and Parmesan. Oil on canvas. 87.8 × 108 cm. Courtesy of the National Gallery of Art, Washington, DC; Samuel H. Kress Collection, 1961. © 1995 The Board of Trustees of the National Gallery of Art.

JAMA

November 21, 1977

THE JOURNAL of the American Medical Association

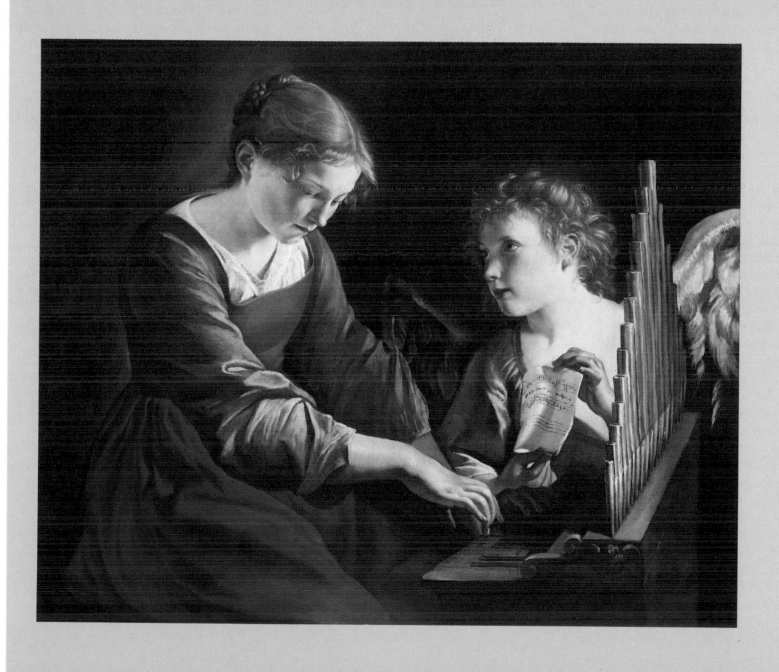

ÉDOUARD VUILLARD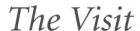

The Visit

To "take the thing just as it is and put it before us [is to be] deficient in mystery," says Mallarmé: "[the mind is deprived] of the delicious joy of believing that it is creating. To name an object is to do away with the three quarters of the enjoyment of the poem which is derived from the satisfaction of guessing little by little: to suggest it, to evoke it—that is what charms the imagination."

(Jean-) Édouard Vuillard (1868-1940) was one of the group of young French painters (self-named "Nabis," from the Hebrew word for prophet) who were heavily influenced by both Gauguin and the Symbolist poet Mallarmé. Vuillard's early paintings were such simple and unpretentious scenes of domestic interiors—which he painted in exquisite detail on panels often no larger than the lid of a cigar box—that his style came to be known as Intimisme. André Gide, in 1905, called Vuillard the most personal and the most intimate of storytellers. "M Vuillard speaks almost in a whisper—we have to bend over towards him to hear what he says." A year earlier Marcel Proust had spoken of Vuillard's "admirable talent, which has so often kindled my memory." But later critics have lamented that from about 1920 on Vuillard's work became retrogressive, sacrificing much of the intimacy of his turn-of-the-century paintings to the mere recording of detail.

The Visit belongs to these later years. It is a portrait of Mme Marchand, done for her husband, the playwright M Léopold Marchand. The setting is the Hessel drawing room, long familiar to Vuillard, with its velvet walls hung with paintings by Bonnard, Degas, and Renoir. Mme Hessel, whose husband was the art dealer M Josse Hessel, sits at the far right. Their adopted daughter Lulu stands before Mme Marchand. The time is 1931. Beyond that, however, for all the almost Proustian detail, Vuillard is silent. We are left with the delicious joy of creating the rest of the story. Our enjoyment comes from having to guess little by little what is going on.

The Visit is a quiet, serene, almost timid scene we might have glimpsed—or thought we had glimpsed—a hundred times before from the street on a winter's afternoon through half-open blinds and only barely noticed. Or, perhaps we are in the cinema and the film has become stuck: the action has been stopped, the sound has been temporarily lost. The last-spoken words still hang in the air. But in a moment the reel will continue unwinding, the lips will move again, the conversation will be resumed; perhaps Lulu will curtsy, the teacups will be cleared, and Mme Marchand will pull on her gloves and take her leave. Or is there another story, another meaning? Vuillard does not say. He allows his sitters to keep their secrets and our imagination to be charmed.

> *We are left with the delicious joy of creating the rest of the story.*

Vuillard was a shy and retiring man who never married. He lived with his mother until she died when he was 60. "Maman was my muse," he told his nephew Saloman in 1920. Beyond what we can read from his paintings, we know little else that is personal about this quiet man. Even his private journal was sealed until 1980. "I was never more than a spectator," he said. Again, in response to criticism about his later works, "I don't paint portraits. I paint people in their homes." Had he known Teilhard de Chardin, he might have replied, "What I paint is the milieu, which is as inseparable from the person as is the body and the spirit. I paint the whole person in its mysterious trinity of body-soul-environment."

A tragic footnote unfortunately attends the provenance of *The Visit*. Within ten years after the painting had been completed, Mme Marchand, who was Jewish, committed suicide, just before the German occupation of Paris in June 1940. Her husband could no longer bear to have the painting and disposed of it to an art dealer, whence it eventually found its way to the collector Chester Dale and to the National Gallery. Vuillard, elderly and in failing health, was persuaded to leave Paris ahead of the advancing German army but died, shortly after, on June 21, 1940, at La Baule as he was seeking refuge.

JAMA

THE JOURNAL of the American Medical Association

December 12, 1977

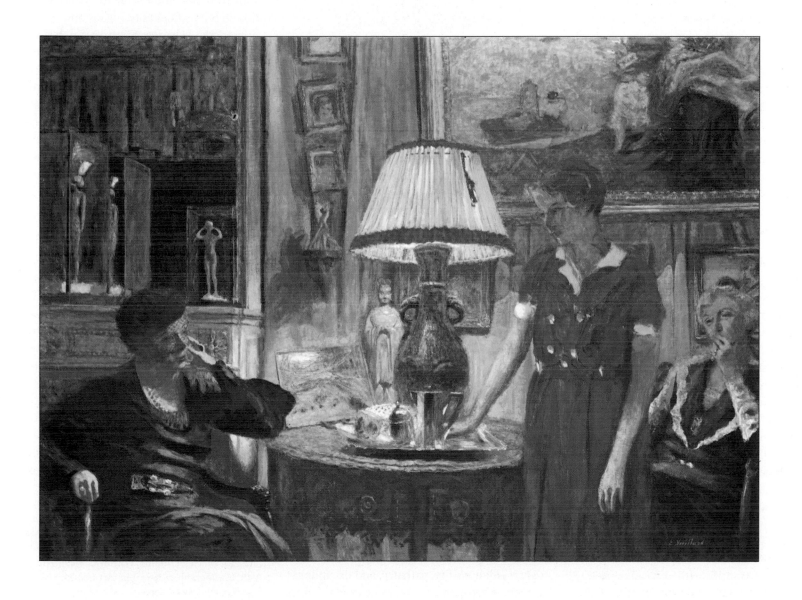

PAUL CÉZANNE

Madame Cézanne in a Yellow Armchair

Hortense Fiquet met Paul Cézanne (1839-1906) sometime around 1869 in Paris, when she was 19 and he was 30. Three years later, Mlle Fiquet bore their only child, a son who was christened Paul Cézanne. Though the couple apparently did not get on well, the liaison continued until 1886, when Paul and Hortense were finally married in both civil and religious ceremonies in the presence of his family in Aix-en-Provence. The regularization of their status did little to improve their relationship, however, and Hortense, now Mme Cézanne, continued to spend most of her time in Paris with their son Paul, now 14, while Cézanne continued to live mostly in Aix with his aged mother and spinster sister. Of Hortense he said, "My wife likes only Switzerland [she had been born in the Jura] and lemonade." Nevertheless, in spite of their temperamental incompatibilities, Hortense was her husband's most faithful model; some 41 sketches and paintings of her are known. Some of her heroic devotion and fidelity can be surmised from a remark of Ambroise Vollard, whose portrait Cézanne did in 1899. Vollard says that no fewer than 140 sittings were required for the one portrait. Moreover, Cézanne demanded that his sitters remain still "as an apple," remaining so for long periods of time while he meditated, brush in hand, before every stroke.

Madame Cézanne in a Yellow Armchair is one of three similar paintings, the other two being in New York, one in The Metropolitan Museum of Art and the other in a private collection. As with all of his portraits, Cézanne had no desire to reproduce

> *"Everything is locked within the picture rectangle, yet wishes to explode."*

a photographic likeness, nor even to make a psychological interpretation. Rather, as in his still lifes and landscapes, he is searching out the essential truth of nature and presenting it, to those who can see, in the wordless language of color. The colors are simple—blues, reds, yellows—but he harmonizes them, much as the composer harmonizes the simple notes of the scale, and shifts from key to key so subtly that the result is not a portrait of Mme Cézanne but rather one of certain, abstract, qualities: strength, repose, and above all, presence. But if the colors are subtle, the structure, on the other hand, is bold and direct. The sitter is almost in the middle of the canvas and almost faces us directly. Rectangles are prominent: picture frame, chair, dado, which is refracted as it passes behind the chair. The result is a tension, but a controlled tension, one which, as one writer has noted, pulls all the colored surfaces into a state of dynamic equilibrium. "Everything is locked within the picture rectangle, yet wishes to explode."

In terms of his painting Cézanne had three qualities that allowed his genius to be expressed: humility, patience, and discipline. He stood before his motif, as he called it, not as its master but as its servant; he did not force its secrets, but he waited until they were revealed; and he set them down, not as his romantic and impulsive nature often wished, but as fidelity to his vision demanded. He had, as Simone Weil has so aptly expressed (though in another context), that "special way of waiting upon truth, setting our hearts on it, yet not allowing ourselves to go out in search of it." He had what she called "a way of giving our attention to the…problem…without trying to find the solution…a way of waiting, when we are writing, for the right word to come of itself at the end of our pen, while we merely reject all inadequate words."

Cézanne has been dead more than 70 years, and yet the analysis of his paintings remains unexhausted. Today's artists still mine the lode and bring up new riches each time. Still, as Cézanne knew when he stood before his motif, truth cannot be forced. In a classic essay some 50 years ago Fry warned thus: "…analysis halts before the ultimate concrete reality of the work of art…in proportion to the greatness of the work it must leave untouched a greater part of its objective. For Cézanne…we cannot in the least explain why the smallest product of his hand arouses the impression of being a revelation of the highest importance, or what exactly it is that gives it its grave authority."

JAMA

THE JOURNAL OF the American Medical Association

January 30, 1978

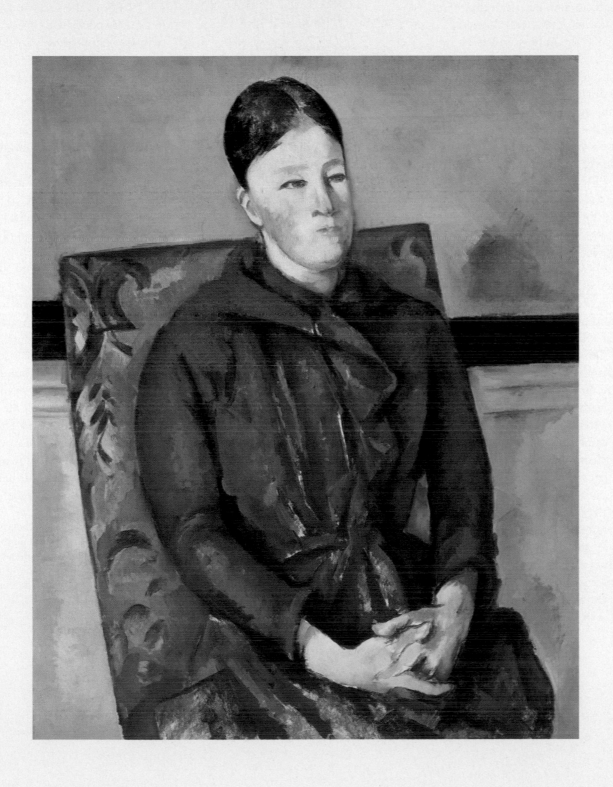

ALFRED SISLEY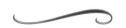

Boulevard Héloîse, Argenteuil

The year 1872 seems to have been a decisive one for the group of painters who were later to be known as the Impressionists. The Franco-Prussian War had ended. Monet and Pissarro had returned from London, where they had gone during the war, and they had seen the paintings of Constable and Turner. Bazille, one of the most promising members of their group, was dead, having been killed while fighting for France. Pissarro had lost nearly all his paintings to the Prussian army. Alfred Sisley's (1839-1899) well-to-do English family had lost its fortune as a result of the war and his father had died, leaving him, at the age of 32, a penniless painter with a wife and two children. But now, once more united, the group gathered in the Île-de-France, in the villages along the Seine close to Paris, and began to apply some of their theories. Often Monet and Sisley or Cézanne and Pissarro or some of the others would set up their easels side by side. Winter scenes are numerous during the season 1871-1872. In such settings—under an overcast sky, before shadowless motifs, in the gray world of "neutral" light—they could test their developing theory that black and white do not exist—that even the most "neutral" monotone vibrates with color.

Boulevard Héloîse, Argenteuil was painted during this postwar winter. (Monet has a strikingly similar scene, and it is known that the two worked together during that year.) It is the muddy midwinter spring, T. S. Eliot's season, "sempiternal, though sodden towards

> *…where the gray world has become stuck on its axis.*

sundown," the time of the thaw, where the gray world has become stuck on its axis. Only the briefest accents relieve the monotone—a slash of blue, a lesser one of red, and a few dabs of green, all in the foreground. For the rest, the painting is a taupeish monochrome of muddy roads, opaque skies, and shuttered houses. The pedestrians—even the liverymen—are indifferent to all except the cold and the damp. They hurry away from us, or are occupied with their horses.

Like his own character, Sisley's paintings are gentle, understated, and subtle. Indeed, just as during his lifetime when Sisley was perhaps the least noticed and least appreciated of the Impressionist painters, today one runs the risk of passing right by a Sisley painting without a second glance if it should happen to be hung near another's whose colors are more aggressive. And yet there is something that holds us, though ever so gently, and bids us look again. Soft and subtle colors are contrasted with a strong and solid design. Grays and browns, while holding the painting to its delicate and muted tone, nevertheless vibrate with

every color of the spectrum. The monotone, in fact, resonates with overtones whose richness is limited only by the perception of the viewer.

While others of the Impressionists went on to other experiments, Sisley remained a landscape painter, surpassing all other French painters in that category, even Corot, according to John Canaday. It can be said that Sisley did for the French countryside what Constable did for the English countryside. Still, Sisley died unrecognized and virtually penniless in January 1899, of cancer of the throat. His wife had died just four months earlier.

This painting has been called, variously, *Street at Sévres* or *Boulevard Héloîse, Argenteuil*. Although Sévres is famous enough for its porcelain and treaty, Argenteuil, which was also the home of Monet at the time, has by far the more romantic associations. It was here that Charlemagne founded a nunnery in 656, which became even more famous in the 12th century through the adventures of its abbess, Héloîse, and Abélard. It is tempting to imagine that it was on the same kind of winter day and down the same boulevard now named for her that Héloîse rushed to her Abélard's side.

JAMA

February 20, 1978

THE JOURNAL of the American Medical Association

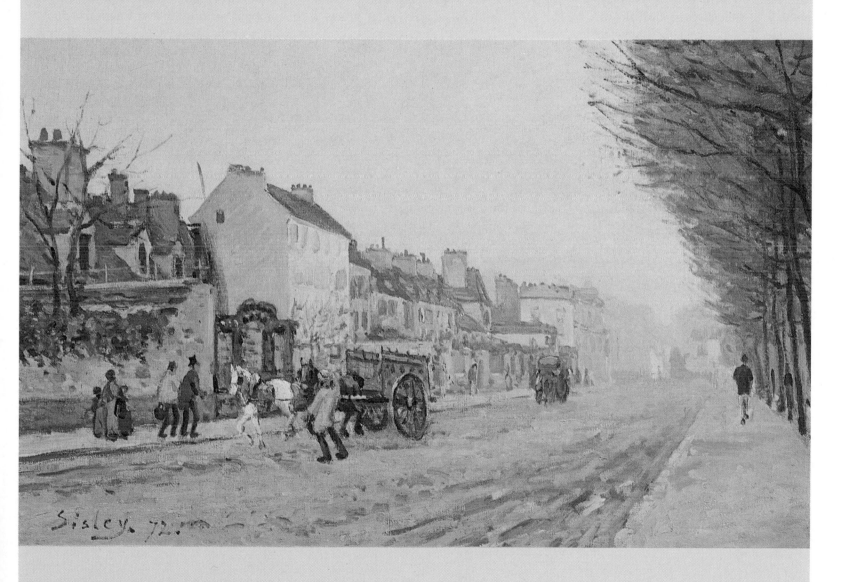

FRANS HALS

The Rommel Pot Player

Of the 20 or so versions of Frans Hals' (1581-1666) lost painting *The Rommel Pot Player*, the version at the Kimbell Art Museum in Fort Worth, Texas, is generally thought to follow the original most closely. Another fine, though considerably smaller, version hangs at the Art Institute of Chicago. The latter, attributed to Hals' brilliant student, Judith Leyster, is also most certainly based on the original. The painter of the Kimbell version is as yet not identified but was probably, like Leyster, a Hals student.

In *The Rommel Pot Player*, Hals gives us the group portrait, wherein each of the members must be distinctive and yet none can dominate. In the center foreground is the rommel pot (Dutch *rommelen*, "to rumble"), a noisemaker used at spring carnival time that emits a sound not unlike the squeal of a pig. In the lower left a young boy holding a coin in his left hand is completely absorbed in the rommel pot. His credulous expression is tinged with just a bit of wonder at how such a small pot can contain a pig. Behind him, two wiser boys watch the "musician's" face and try to get his attention. The two adults peering from the door behind them could be householders aroused from sleep by the noise. At any rate, they do not share the general merriment. To the right, the neighborhood bully reaches an enormous hand around the back of the

> *...the cause of all this hilarity, the rommel pot player, gazes directly at us with his toothless smile...*

rommel pot player, perhaps to trick the youngest boy into dropping the coin into his hand. Meanwhile, the cause of all this hilarity, the rommel pot player, gazes directly at us with his toothless smile and bids us share in the sheer delight of the children. And though the foxtail that trails from his hat is the symbol of the fool, something says this man is no fool at all, especially when it comes to the rowdy behind him. But the entire scene is stolen by the little girl at the left, who, alone of the children, is absorbed, not in the rommel pot but in us. Clearly, she already understands the art of coquetry.

Of Hals himself we would know little were it not for the court records of Haarlem, for he is frequently mentioned. He was married twice and had two children by his first wife and at least eight by his second wife, some of whom are perhaps shown in *The Rommel Pot Player*. One son, Pieter, was committed to an institution because he was *innocente* (feeble-minded), and a daughter, Sara, was sent to a work house because of "lax morals." Most of the court records, however, concern the numerous lawsuits brought against him over a period of 50 years by the small tradesmen of Haarlem for his failure to pay for food and painting materials. Although his sitters were prosperous and his commissions generous, he was either a heavy spender, a poor manager, or, as in at least one case, too stubborn to yield to his clients' requests. To the end of his life he was more often in debt than out of it.

Both Hals and his younger countryman, Rembrandt, are masters nonpareil of the portrait, whether solo or group. But each excelled in his own vision. Whereas Rembrandt could give us a glimpse into the private man, the man as he knows himself, Hals gives us the public man, the man as he is seen by others.

Hals' services were in great demand among the prosperous burghers of the newly independent Holland. His most famous subject was not a countryman at all, however, but a French refugee: René Descartes.

Frans Hals (1581-1666), *The Rommel Pot Player*, c 1618-1622, Dutch. Oil on canvas. 106 × 80.3 cm. Courtesy of the Kimbell Art Museum, Fort Worth, Texas.

JAMA

THE JOURNAL of the American Medical Association

February 27, 1978

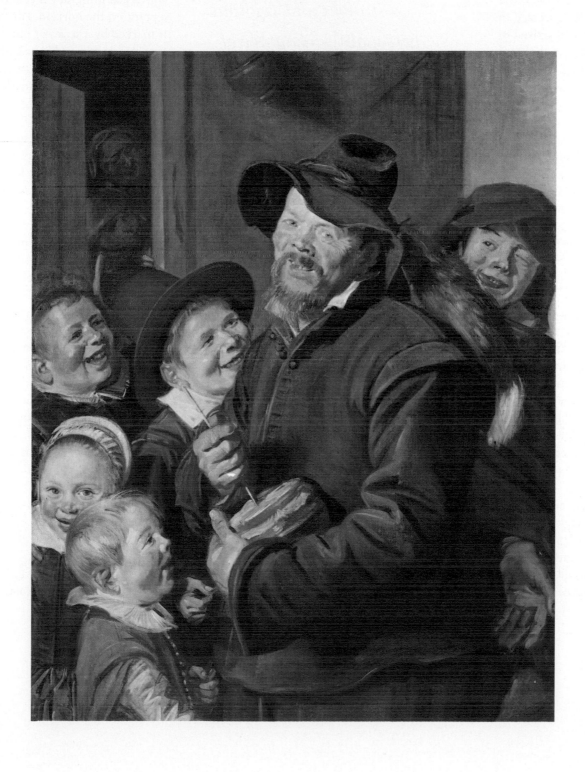

CAMILLE PISSARRO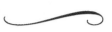

Near Sydenham Hill

For Camille Pissarro (1830-1903) the winter of 1871 must have seemed the nadir of life and hope. He had arrived in Paris some 15 years earlier from his native West Indies to study painting. There he became a beloved member of a group of artists—among them Monet, Sisley, and Renoir—who were experimenting with new ways to define light and color. Then, in 1870, came the Franco-Prussian War, and Pissarro was forced to flee to England. Although later he was to recall that he and Monet (who had also fled to London) were enthusiastic over the English landscapes, and that Lower Norwood, the suburb in which he lived, was charming, during that English winter he was near despair. "Here there is no such thing as art; everything is treated as a matter of business…My painting does not catch on, not in the least, a fate that pursues me more or less everywhere," he wrote to his friend and art critic Théodore Duret. Moreover, toward the end of the same winter he learned that he had lost to the war almost everything he had painted in France. "About 40 pictures are left to me out of 1500," he wrote to Duret. Yet in that same winter soil there germinated the seeds that were eventually to open into the full flower of Impressionism.

Two circumstances peculiar to England coincided to fertilize the work that Monet and Pissarro had begun in France: the instability of the English weather, with the perpetually shifting lights and changing shadows, and the paintings of the English

> *"…a straight and vigorous personality, incapable of falsehood, making of art a pure and eternal truth."*

landscapists Constable and Turner. But while Pissarro freely admits their debt to these two English painters, he also notes that they had "no understanding of the *analysis of shadow*…it is simply used as…a mere absence of light." It is this treatment of shadow *as color* and not as the mere absence of light (black) that advances the work of Constable and Turner. Renoir says it well: "A tree…has the same local color on the side where the sun shines as on the side where the shadow is…The color of the object is the same, only with a veil thrown over it. Sometimes the veil is thin, sometimes thick, but always it remains a veil…No shadow is black. It always has color."

Near Sydenham Hill, painted near the London suburb where Pissarro lived during 1870 and 1871, is Pissarro's winter and Impressionism's spring. The strongly shadowed tree trunks, like the pilasters of a Renaissance painting, support an arch that opens onto a vista that disappears finally into infinity. For the Renaissance painters infinity was marked by a set of lines that

converged until they met and vanished at a point on the horizon. For Pissarro infinity is marked by a series of horizontal planes that also merge and vanish at the horizon, but in color rather than in line. For example, the first plane is boldly marked by the foreground fence cutting across the lower portion of the painting. Behind, the second plane is indicated by slightly paler green tones; it ends sharply at the railroad line just beyond the figure at left center. Beyond are the houses of Lower Norwood, their colors already muted by distance, and finally, on a hill are the cemetery and church tower, where the ground mists merge with and disappear into the infinity of the cloudy sky.

Still, Pissarro remained the realist. "He never composes a picture," said Duret, "and in his landscapes, never arranges nature. For him a landscape on canvas must be the exact reproduction of a natural scene and the portrait of some spot in the world that really exists." Émile Zola, the literary realist, had another kind of praise for Pissarro: "One hears…the deep voice of the soil, the powerful life of the trees…There is a man hidden here, a straight and vigorous personality, incapable of falsehood, making of art a pure and eternal truth."

Camille Pissarro (1830-1903), *Near Sydenham Hill*, 1871, French. Oil on canvas. 43.5 × 53.5 cm. Courtesy of the Kimbell Art Museum, Fort Worth, Texas.

JAMA

THE JOURNAL of the American Medical Association

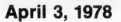

April 3, 1978

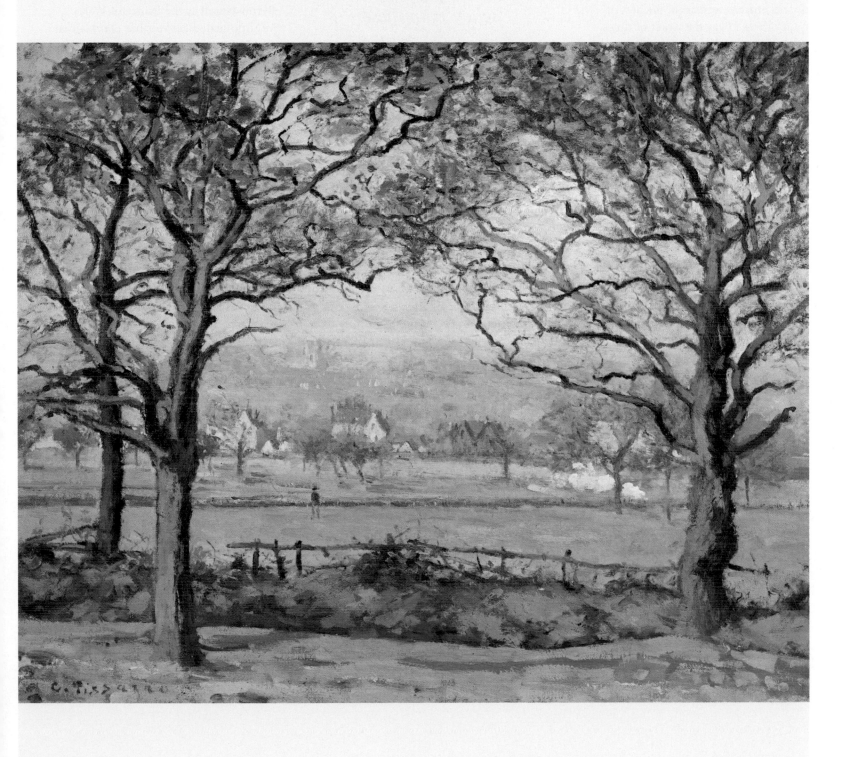

MARIE LOUISE ÉLISABETH VIGÉE-LEBRUN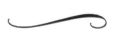

Self-portrait

For some "the dear old year one thousand seven hundred and seventy-five" was, as Dickens has termed it, the best of times; for others it was the worst of times. In England sat a king with a large jaw and a queen with a plain face. In France the king also had a large jaw, but the queen was a fair-faced beauty. All of which would have mattered little to Marie Louise Élisabeth Vigée-Lebrun (1755-1842) except that shortly thereafter the fair-faced queen would summon her to Versailles to do her portrait. To Vigée-Lebrun, the daughter of a painter as well as the wife of a painter, and already, by the age of 20, an accomplished painter herself, it meant her reputation was now established and her future secured. Between 1779 and 1789 she would paint more than 20 portraits of Marie Antoinette, a distinction that gave her entrée to all the fashionable cities and courts of Europe—a privilege whose real worth was only to become evident several years later.

First, however, she would paint her own portrait, one of nearly two dozen she did throughout the years. In *Self-portrait*, Vigée-Lebrun is barely into her 20s, the same age, give a few months, as Marie Antoinette. The pose she gives herself and the mien she

It is tempting to wonder whether in these self-portraits she did not sometimes see herself as the beautiful French queen.

adopts—the ingenue in three-quarter turn with slightly parted lips—is betrayed by the gaze that, while perhaps intended to be merely direct, has instead become bold. It is tempting to wonder whether in these self-portraits she did not sometimes see herself as the beautiful French queen. The style, though perhaps too sentimental and sweet, even saccharine, for our taste, was that of the 18th-century French court, and therefore the taste also of much of the Western world, including Russia. Indeed, when it became expedient for Vigée-Lebrun to leave France, she was able to travel throughout Italy, Austria, Germany, Russia, and England doing portraits of the aristocracy and other

notables. Mostly the portraits were of women and children, but in London she did Lord Byron as well as the Prince of Wales.

Simone de Beauvoir has complained that "Mme Vigée-Lebrun never wearied of putting her smiling maternity on her canvases." Still, of the more than 660 portraits she did over a lifetime, plus a small number of other works and a volume of memoirs, some 20-odd does not seem an excessive number of self-portraits—especially when one considers that the model for such (though not a commission) is always available and always cooperative.

When Vigée-Lebrun died in 1842, in Paris whence she had started 87 years earlier, her life had spanned two revolutions, the fall of the French aristocracy, and the exile of Napoleon. On the throne of England the queen still sat, but she was Victoria, not Charlotte. Meanwhile, because of Mme Vigée-Lebrun's extensive travels, the faces that chronicled those years are to be found in museums throughout the world.

Marie Louise Élisabeth Vigée-Lebrun (1755-1842), *Self-portrait*, c 1776, French. Oil on canvas. 64.8 × 54 cm. Courtesy of the Kimbell Art Museum, Fort Worth, Texas.

JAMA

May 19, 1978

THE JOURNAL of the American Medical Association

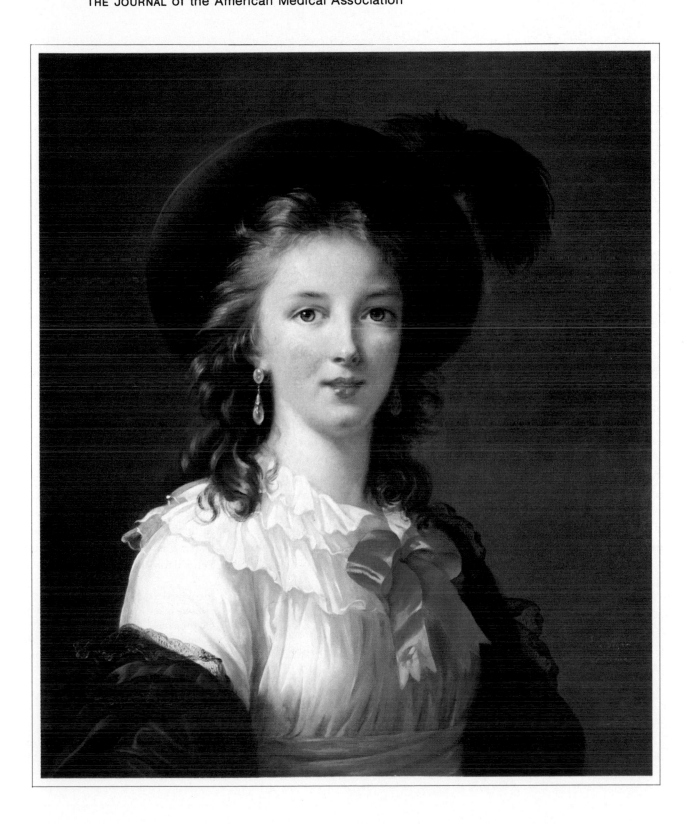

JAN VAN HEMESSEN (ATTRIBUTED TO)

The Healing of the Paralytic

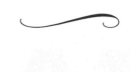

The Renaissance came late to The Netherlands, and when it did arrive it came as a crossbreed that bore little resemblance to either its northern or its Italian forebears. "For a generation or so the north... 'simply could not get its Renaissance on straight,'" recalled art historian Helen Gardner.

At the beginning of this period stands Jan van Hemessen (c 1500-1566), whose uncertain history is typical of many artists of that period. He was born about 1500, in the village of Hemixen, near Antwerp, and died sometime after 1556 but before 1566, perhaps in Haarlem. He married before 1528, had a daughter, Katharina (who herself became a painter of note), was a master by 1524, and dean of the guild in 1548. He sold a house in Antwerp in 1550; after that he disappears from the public records. His last dated painting is in 1556. Further, he was also known as Jan Sanders (son of Alexander), and he may also have been called Jan de Meyere or Jan Voet. Considerable evidence exists to suggest that van Hemessen was also the Brunswick Monogrammatist (so-called from a painting in the Brunswick Museum signed with a monogram made up of the letters *J*, *S*, *M*, and *v* and done in a style suggestive of van Hemessen's youthful works).

The Healing of the Paralytic (formerly "Arise, and Take Up Thy Bed, and Walk") demonstrates this ambivalent northern dawn. True to the Netherlandish style, the subject is biblical—Christ healing the paralytic man—and its depiction is literal, even

> *...one can in imagination paint out the bed-bundle and paint in a cross...*

to the four men lowering the pallet through a hole in the roof. Similarly, the landscape is typically local and contemporary, except for the sheer vertical rock in the right background; small-scale figures on the left blend into the landscape in a muted harmony. But then van Hemessen suddenly declares his Italian influence. The same tiny figure who lay paralyzed at the feet of Christ in the background grouping has now literally picked up his bed, bundled it on his back, and strides past us in the monumental stature and heroic proportions of the Italian figure. Van Hemessen demonstrates his virtuosity in the sharply modeled figure and enamel-like brushwork, in the detail of the drapery, especially in the rolling of the sleeves about the arms, in the heavy musculature of the arms and legs, which attests to the weight the man carries on his back, and in the position and foreshortening of the arms. Indeed, one can in imagination paint out the bed-bundle and paint in a cross without altering the arms or figure position at all and have another popular subject of the time: *Christ Carrying His Cross*.

What is most curious about the painting, however, is a certain incongruity of elements. For example, if one removes the large figure and the rock on which he stands, it can be imagined that the road on the right is a continuation of that on the left, the bottom of the curve passing in the center foreground, where the rock is now painted. Second, the painting styles are quite different, with the landscape, background figures, and foliage typically small and soft, the foreground figure large, sharply modeled, and vivid. Finally, even the pigments are different: Contrast the muted reds of the barn and background figures with the vibrant tunic of the Italianate figure. It would be easier to believe that this painting is the work of two different artists or at best, a work of van Hemessen, who, once he had come into contact with the Italians, was so influenced that he went back and painted over some of his youthful work.

Like the adolescent who lacks the experience and maturity to know in which direction he will "make it," early 16th-century Netherlandish art tried all directions simultaneously. Eventually this ambivalence—shown so clearly by van Hemessen—was to settle down in the robust and fleshy figures of the Flemish painters Jacob Jordaens and Peter Paul Rubens.

Attributed to Jan van Hemessen (c 1500-1566), *The Healing of the Paralytic*, 16th century, Netherlandish. Oil on panel. 107.8 × 76 cm. Courtesy of the National Gallery of Art, Washington, DC; Chester Dale Collection. © 1995 The Board of Trustees of the National Gallery of Art.

JAMA

August 25, 1978

THE JOURNAL of the American Medical Association

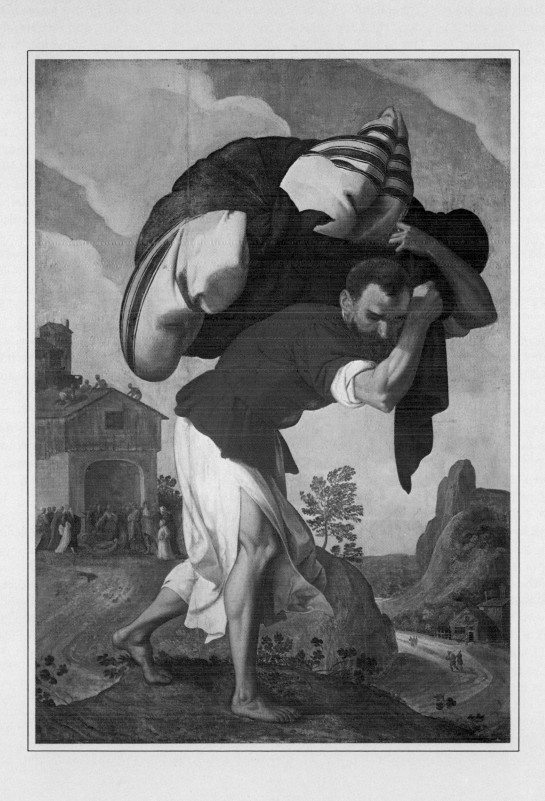

EASTMAN JOHNSON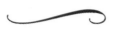

The Early Scholar

Genre painting—the realistic portrayal of ordinary people in ordinary activities of everyday life—has always been one of the most popular forms of painting. Often moralistic, sentimental, even humorous, genre does not necessarily demand a high level of sophistication for enjoyment. It speaks immediately and directly to the viewer. In America, genre developed rapidly in the mid-19th century. Portrait painting was being replaced by the daguerreotype, especially when the portrait was to be a mere likeness; the rending of the nation by the Civil War was followed by a demand for paintings that showed people in their commonality; and the large migration of peoples from Europe created a need for paintings that would serve as models of American life.

Into these circumstances came (Jonathan) Eastman Johnson (1824-1906), son of Maine's secretary of state, and now, at just past age 30, newly returned from six years abroad where he had studied genre at Düsseldorf and the Old Masters at The Hague. So thorough were his studies of Rembrandt that he earned the nickname of the "American Rembrandt" and was even offered the position of court painter at The Hague. Fortunately, he returned to the United States where, in 1859, he was elected to the National Academy of Design and called "the most talented young painter of American domestic life." By the end of the 1860s he was "unquestionably the first name among American genre painters."

The Early Scholar belongs to this immediate postwar period of Johnson's genre scenes. It is typical of its time in that it extols children, the hope of the future to this war-devastated nation, and romanticizes hardship. In the "sad and luminous faces we see that life is serious to the American from

his childhood," wrote a contemporary. The lone child drying his wet feet and warming his hands before the schoolroom's stove, his ears meanwhile still red from his long, cold walk, was enough to ensure the critics' praise, for subject matter rather than style was still the primary criterion for determining "good art." But a closer examination is immensely rewarding. The somber painting is simple, even understated, with only three principal elements: a boy, a stove, and a rocking chair. The rest of the scene lies in shadow—a monotone of browns—

> *"...life is serious to the American from his childhood..."*

but at the same time browns that are warm and almost transparent. The source of the light that plays on the boy's cheeks and hands is one of Eastman's favorites: fire. He used it often, and almost always it is a suprise to realize how essential it is to the composition; it appears as fire on a hearth, as fire under a cauldron of boiling maple sap, as fire in a smithy's forge, even as the flame from a match as an old man lights his pipe. Here, the fire shows as a mere sliver around the door of the stove, but it gives life to the boy and pulls together the rocker and the stove. There is action as well, for so delicately balanced is the boy on the edge of the rocker that the slightest shift of his weight will set it in motion, and, it can be imagined, in violent motion if he were suddenly to rise.

But it is in the composition of the painting, in the display of Eastman's drafts-

manship, that we see best his European training and what it is that makes him different from other American genre painters of the same period. If one can imagine an isosceles triangle, the base of which is the lower edge of the painting and the apex of which is the tip of the boy's ear, it can then be seen that within this triangle lie all the important elements of the painting: the face, the hands, the feet of the boy, the light source, and even the potential motion in the chair implied by the boy's precarious perch. Similar triangles can be constructed as one moves outward, but the subjects are progressively less detailed and less important. At first almost unnoticed in this simple and understated scene, it is the boy's nearly frozen ear that is actually the center of the painting.

For all his popularity during his lifetime, Eastman Johnson has been curiously neglected since his death. Yet it was he and his contemporary, Winslow Homer, who finally gave an American expression to painting. Perhaps it is that Johnson lived too long past his best work, which, it is generally acknowledged, ended with his last genre painting, dated 1887. From then on, for nearly two decades, he did portraits that, while excellent likenesses of the sitters and lucrative as well, were often merely dull. Life itself in his later years was also dull, he said, and he felt shackled by work. Finally, on an April evening in 1906 he rose from dinner to go into the library for a smoke. As he was filling his pipe he died, just a few months short of his 82nd birthday.

JAMA

THE JOURNAL of the American Medical Association

September 1, 1978

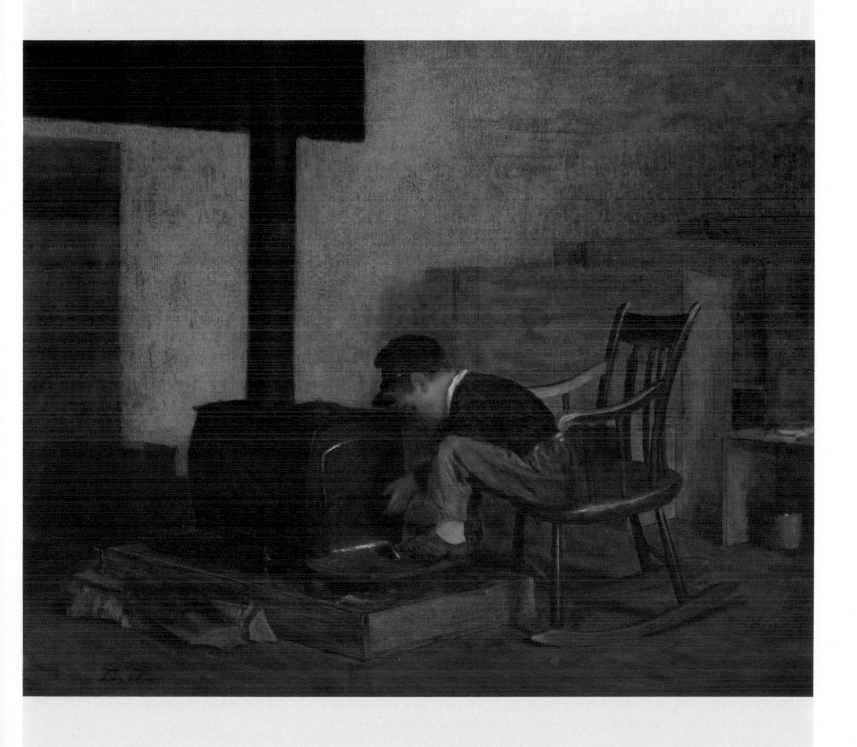

PAUL CÉZANNE

Mont Sainte-Victoire

The year 1886 was pivotal in the life of Paul Cézanne (1839-1906). At best a shy, solitary, suspicious person who was becoming increasingly difficult to get along with, he had few friends left save for the novelist Émile Zola and the Impressionist painter Camille Pissarro. Zola he had grown up with in Aix-en-Provence; Pissarro, alone among his fellow painters, had early recognized Cézanne's genius and continued to encourage him. Still, although Cézanne was now nearing 50, the Paris critics continued to reject his work and even publicly ridiculed it. Cézanne responded by withdrawing; he seldom went to Paris anymore. He also remained financially dependent on his father, who, though 88 years old, was able to keep his tyrannical grasp. And, finally, Cézanne himself was a father; his illegitimate son was 14 years old and although Cézanne supported the boy and his mother financially, he still had managed to keep the secret from his father for many years—but not without the connivance of his mother and sister.

Then, early in 1886, the foundations for even these tenuous supports began to shift. The cruelest blow came first. In March Zola published a novel, *L'Oeuvre*, in which the protagonist, Claude Lantier, is a brilliant and doggedly persistent but overly ambitious painter who finally learns what everyone else had known right along: genius he may well possess, but he is incapable of giving birth to it. In despair, he kills himself in front of the unfinished canvas that was to have been his masterpiece. To Cézanne, not without cause, it was obvious who the model for Lantier was. He felt betrayed, but his bitterness lay not so much in the thought that he was the model for Lantier, but rather in the utter misunderstanding he felt Zola had of his painting. The two men never spoke to or even saw each other again.

On a different note—and probably in acquiescence to demands by his father—Cézanne shortly thereafter married Marie-Hortense Fiquet, his son's mother. Finally,

toward the end of the year, the old man died, and Cézanne was left with a sizable income as well as the family home in Aix. For much of the rest of his life he lived in Aix with his mother and sister, while Hortense and young Paul lived in Paris. Although this meant even greater seclusion, Cézanne also entered into one of the most fruitful periods of his life. It was as though the seed that had lain so long in the ground had germinated finally as the result of these upheavals and was now beginning to yield its harvest. There began a remarkable outpouring of his mature work—landscapes, portraits, still lifes—

> *"The landscape becomes human, becomes a thinking, living being within me."*

each worthy to be called the masterpiece Zola's Lantier never completed. To this period belongs *Mont Sainte-Victoire*.

The Montagne de Ste-Victoire is a steep limestone ridge in southeastern France. Nearly 1000 meters high, it lies some 7 kilometers to the northeast of Aix. For Cézanne, it was his laboratory. He painted it hundreds of times, always hoping for it to tell him something new. His method was first to observe, to wait, to contemplate; only then did he pick up the brush. He was looking, as Roger Fry notes, for an underlying principle of geometric harmony in nature. Cézanne saw the landscape as a series of planes, each of them in turn broken into a series of smaller and smaller facets. As he worked his canvas he would indicate changes in orientation of major facets by touches of color or "nodal points," as Kenneth Clark calls them. Fry likens the process to the phenomenon of crystallization in a saturated

solution, with the nodal points being the nuclei on which the crystals would be built. Fry's apt description is especially evident in the unfinished *Mont Sainte-Victoire*.

Some painters, especially Rembrandt and van Gogh, left behind a large number of self-portraits, through which one can trace not only their artistic but also their psychological development over an entire lifetime. In a sense the *Mont Sainte-Victoire* paintings have served this purpose for Cézanne. Knowing the mountain as he had since boyhood, watching its moods, aging as it aged, it had become his stability, the rock of his life. Its visage as it appears on canvas after canvas is really that of the maturing Cézanne. The mountain was also the one thing he could never alienate; it was always there to come back to. He could part with Zola, with his wife, with his father, but his mountain had become his self: "The landscape becomes human, becomes a thinking, living being within me. I become one with my picture… We merge in an iridescent chaos."

Toward the end of his life Cézanne began to receive some recognition, but he was no longer interested. He had become a recluse; few people in Aix even knew who he was. He died in October 1906 of complications of diabetes and exposure, a few days after a storm had overtaken him while he was working on a landscape. His last letter, written from his sickbed and dated October 17, concerned neither family nor friends. It was to his color dealer: "It is now eight days since I asked you to send me ten burnt lakes and I have had no reply," he wrote. "What is the matter? A reply, and a quick one, I beg of you…Paul Cézanne." Whether or when a reply was made is not known. Five days later, on October 22, Cézanne died.

JAMA

THE JOURNAL of the American Medical Association

September 8, 1978

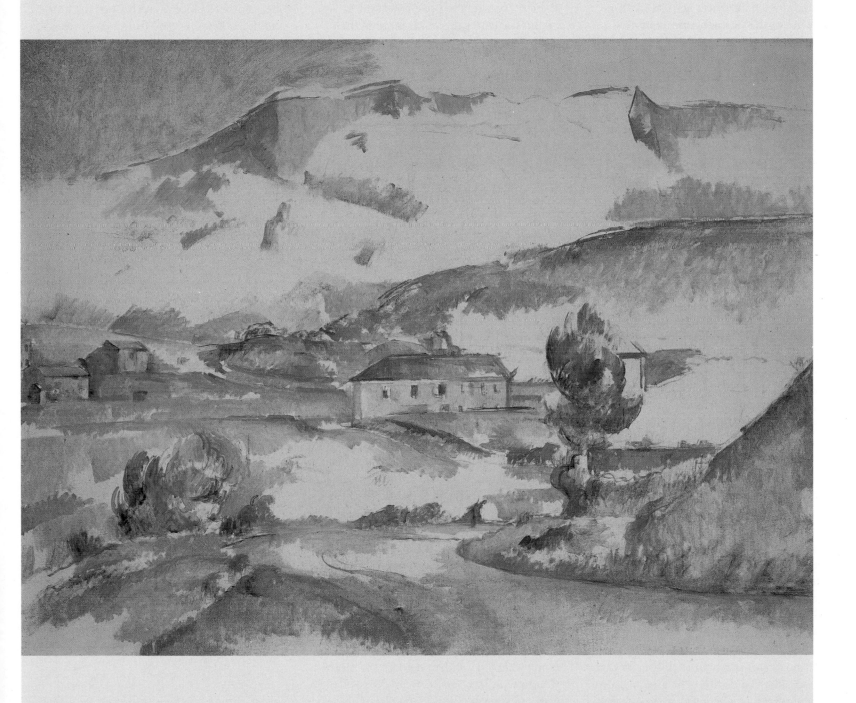

ALBRECHT DÜRER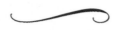

Lot and His Daughters

In an outline of what he apparently envisioned would be a general treatise on painting, the German painter and engraver Albrecht Dürer (1471-1528) noted that the world goes without an "artistic painter" for 200 or 300 years, mainly, as he explained, because the artist's early talent is not recognized and therefore not nurtured. That he knew himself to be just this occasionally appearing artist, however, is evident from his first self-portrait, expertly done in silverpoint when he was only 13 years old. But the decisive moment came some ten years later, when he visited Venice for the first time. Previously trained in the Gothic style of the north, he was dazzled by what the Italians were doing. He returned to his native Nüremberg determined to bring the Renaissance north.

Although Dürer is best known for his large output of woodcuts and copper engravings (*The Four Horsemen of the Apocalypse* and *Melencolia I* being probably the most widely known), he also did a number of paintings. *Lot and His Daughters* is the reverse of a wood panel entitled *Madonna and Child*, which was done for the Haller family in Nüremberg. The Old Testament scene of the destruction of Sodom and Gomorrah was a popular one in Dürer's time. For the artist it was an opportunity to show off his virtuosity in handling the difficult problems of fire and water; for the illiterate viewer it was a graphic representation of the divine judgment, which will not only rain down wrath on the unrepentant sinner in the very tangible form of fire and brimstone but will condemn the unbeliever (here seen in the left background in the form of Lot's wife) to remain behind forever as part of the desolate landscape. The virtuous, on the other hand, will be led away to safety in new lands, as were Lot and his daughters, there presumably to prosper as well.

But for Dürer there was more to the scene. It was an opportunity for him to test some of the theories of art he was developing as the result of his Italian journeys: the juxtaposition of fantasy and naturalism in the same landscape; the creation of three-

> *...the juxtaposition of fantasy and naturalism in the same landscape...*

dimensional space on a flat surface; and a demonstration of his studies on the ideal proportions of the human figure. Beyond that, he was able to display the fruits of his travels in the rich Turkish costume of Lot, drawn no doubt from the Constantinople merchants who at that time still came through Venice, and the sumptuous fabrics and Italian design of the daughters' gowns. Moreover, despite the small surface area of the panel, he managed to give full treatment to the biblical story by attention to even the smallest detail of symbolism and allegory.

Lot, for instance, in addition to his obvious wealth as manifested by his clothing (which, in turn, attests to his righteousness) carries wine and bread, symbols of hospitality. The daughter on the left carries the household needs bundled on her head; the other daughter, in her right hand, carries the family valuables and, in her left, the distaff wound with flax; over her shoulder is the yarn already spun. While the distaff alone would signify that this daughter has assumed her mother's place as mistress of the household, the keys hanging from her girdle ratify this new authority. Most interesting is her obvious pregnant state, the heavy draping of her costume notwithstanding.

In *Lot and His Daughters* Dürer has retained some of the features of the older, Byzantine style of painting in which past, present, and future events are shown as happening simultaneously. For example, although Lot's daughters left Sodom as maidens, they each later became pregnant by their father (after plying him with wine) and gave birth to sons from which the countries of Moab and Ammon are said to have descended. Again, Dürer retains some of the older, 14th-century influences in the sharply outlined or "graspable" figures and the near absence of shadow, but he also places these figures in a carefully constructed design, demonstrating some of the new principles of composition he had learned in Italy.

Dürer has earned the title of both gentleman and Renaissance man. In addition to the some 1000 woodcuts, engravings, drawings, and etchings, and the more than 100 paintings that comprise his graphic work, Dürer also left treatises on painting and on ideal human proportions, a large body of correspondence that reflected some of the newest humanist thinking of the day, and a detailed diary of his travels. He is often called the "Leonardo of the North," justly so.

JAMA

THE JOURNAL of the American Medical Association

September 15, 1978

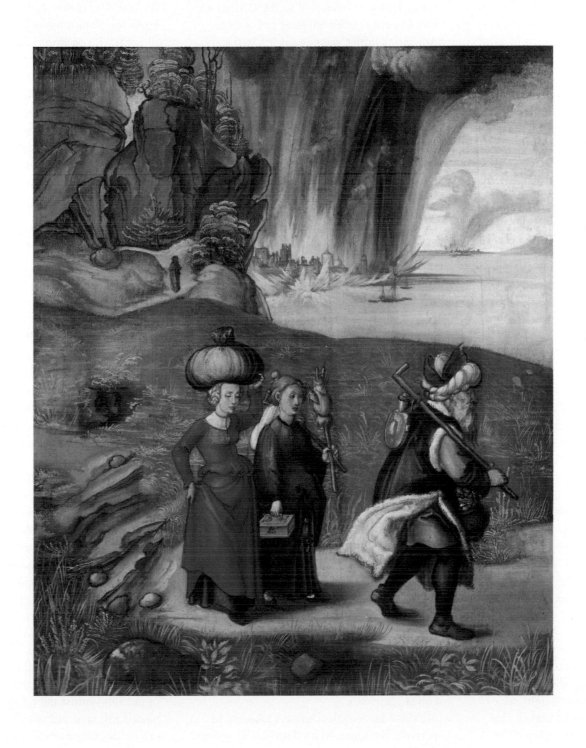

FREDERICK LEIGHTON

Miss May Sartoris

I f one concurs with John Henry Cardinal Newman's definition of "gentleman," then Frederick Leighton (1830-1896) was the quintessential gentleman, the beau ideal of Victorian society in mid-19th century England. Urbane, charming, witty, handsome, he was early dubbed "the Admirable Crichton." Not only did he seem to succeed at whatever was appropriate to his station in life, but he succeeded with little visible effort. So impressive was he, even in physical appearance, that he appears only thinly disguised in works of fiction by Adelaide Sartoris, Benjamin Disraeli, Henry James, and William Makepeace Thackeray.

Leighton's grandfather, Sir James, had been court physician to the Czar. His father, Frederick Septimus, also practiced medicine in Russia, and his older sister, Alexandra, was named for her godmother, the Czarina. Frederick Septimus, however, had more inclination toward travel and study than to the practice of medicine, and the family returned to England, where young Frederick was born. They continued to travel throughout Europe, however, and young Frederick's education continued apace in whatever city the family happened to be. He learned his Latin in Rome from a priest, and by the time he was 14 years old he was fluent in French, Italian, and German. Meanwhile, his art studies, begun casually in Rome, took him to Frankfurt, where he studied with a quasireligious group of painters called the Nazarenes; like a similar group in London, the Pre-Raphaelite Brotherhood, or PRB as it was first called, they sought a simpler way of life, as well as a simpler form of art, which they believed had existed prior to the time of Raphael.

But it was his return to Rome in 1852 as an accomplished young man of 22 that was to be decisive for young Leighton. Quickly he became the social lion of that group of peripatetic Victorians which included the Brownings, Elizabeth and Robert, and Thackeray. But most important was Adelaide Sartoris, part of the Kemble clan, whose fortunes (and misfortunes) had for generations been tied to the Drury Lane and Covent Garden theaters in London. Adelaide's father was the actor Charles Kemble, her sister Fanny was a well-known writer, and her aunt was Sarah Siddons. Adelaide herself, before her marriage, had sung *Norma* to great acclaim. Later, Leighton's social circle intersected that of the Prince of Wales, and it became more or less expected that Leighton would one day occupy the pinnacle of English art, President of the Royal Academy—most likely at the expense of the then heir-apparent, John Millais. It

> *...the lips are too brilliant and the eyes too guarded to suit the girlhood innocence...*

did not harm matters any that Leighton had already acquired the royal patina when Queen Victoria, at the urging of Prince Albert, purchased Leighton's first major work, completed when he was only 25. Nevertheless, it is with the Sartoris circle that Leighton is most closely identified; unlike some of his fellow Victorians such as Millais and John Ruskin, there were no major scandals associated with his name, but it is interesting to speculate that there were undoubtedly some delicious bits of private gossip from time to time—whether substantiated or not. No one could be as public and as polished as Leighton without someone scratching for the tarnish. It never did appear, however.

Miss May Sartoris shows Adelaide's 15-year-old daughter, Mary Theodosia, against the landscape of the Sartoris Hampshire home. The painting is immediately arresting, as befits a portrait of the daughter, niece, and granddaughter of the Kemble family, for its dramatic contrasts, but it is also disquieting for certain incongruities. The brilliant red scarf, for example, contrasts strongly with the deep midnight blue of the rest of the girl's costume. On the other hand, the girl is young, vulnerable, and full of promise, but she has been placed in a decaying landscape. The tree has been cut down; its leaves have browned. To the right, in the gully of the middle ground, stands a ruined building, perhaps a church. Beyond that stands a field of corn stooks full of crows picking at the leavings of the harvest. The girl herself, little more than a child, is dressed as an adult, swathed in a heavy and voluminous riding dress as elaborate as a costume worn on the stage by her mother or aunt. Only the small triangle of her face identifies her, but even so, the lips are too brilliant and the eyes too guarded to suit the girlhood innocence suggested by the delicate lace collar. A certain feyness causes us to fear for her. Most mysterious, however, is Leighton's repetition of the colors of the girl's plumage on a tiny cock (hardly visible in the reproduction except with a glass) that struts in the yard of the thatched cottage at the right: its comb is brilliant red, its tail feathers midnight blue, and its body feathers the brown of the girl's riding gloves. One is uncertain whether to draw a moral or to smile. Throughout the painting Leighton has maintained a strict classical design, with diagonals paralleling and crossing in harmonious proportions. The riding crop in the girl's left hand, for example, quietly continues the vivid diagonal of the scarf, the two meanwhile intersecting the fallen trunk, which itself parallels the green rise of the hill and is crossed in turn by the leafy branch at the left. The girl's figure fills almost the entire frame. She is placed full face and wholly vertical, the otherwise uncompromising severity relieved only by the softness of her face. Balance is achieved by the verticals of the building at the right and the windmill at the left.

Continued on p. 202

JAMA

THE JOURNAL of the American Medical Association

September 29, 1978

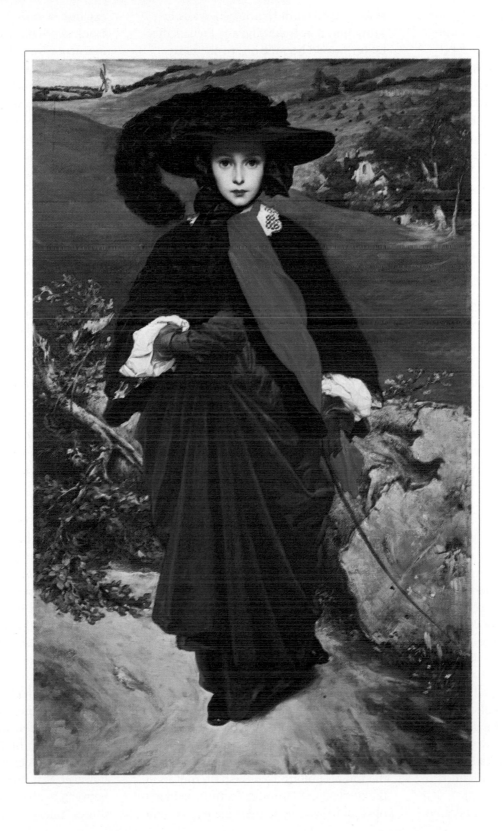

ROBERT HENRI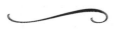

Snow in New York

Robert Henry Cozad (1865-1929) was the second of five sons born to John and Theresa Gatewood Cozad. The three youngest boys died in infancy. The eldest, John A., became a physician and Robert became an artist. One of the most influential painters in the United States, he founded "The Eight," a group of radical painters in New York City, and was leader of a group of five Philadelphia painters dubbed "The Ashcan School." He helped organize the Armory Show, an exhibit of some 1300 American and European paintings that was held in New York in 1913 and decisively changed the course of American art. And he is the author of *The Art Spirit*, a small, unprepossessing volume, which between 1923 and 1969 sold in excess of 76,000 copies and is still in print. But as Robert Henry Cozad, he is virtually unknown.

The elder Cozad, father of John and Robert, had been a professional gambler, a trade he had learned as a boy on the riverboats out of Cincinnati. So skillful was he that many casinos reportedly banned him. After his marriage to Theresa Gatewood, however, he turned to real estate and the family began an odyssey that led from Cincinnati to the Platte River in Nebraska, to Denver and Leadville, Colorado, to New York City, and finally, in 1883, to Atlantic City, New Jersey, where the family settled permanently. By 1886 both boys were in Philadelphia, embarked finally on their professional careers, John at Jefferson Medical College and Robert Henry at the Pennsylvania Academy of Fine Arts. Later, Robert Henry would spend several years at the Académie Julian in Paris.

Meanwhile, however, the Cozad family name had disappeared from public record. After an incident in Nebraska in 1882 in which a man shot in self-defense by the elder Cozad had died, each of the Cozads took a new name: The father became Richard H. Lee; John A. Cozad became Frank L. Southrn; and Robert Henry Cozad became Robert Earl Henri. Henri (hen-rye as he pronounced it, eschewing any French affectation) would become one of the most familiar names in American art.

Snow in New York belongs to Henri's best and most productive period, the years between 1900 and 1904. Newly returned from Paris, he became a master of the streetscape, catching its mood just at the point of deepest mystery, the "moment the artificial lights are turned on," as Whistler has called it. The compositional lines follow the pattern he had developed in Paris:

> *...behind the facade of every human person always lies a surprise.*

prominent center diagonals lead into the distance, where they are limited at either side by strong, solid verticals. Within the limits of this stage he sets his people along the sides and across the distance, each engaged in some mundane activity.

As Henri advised his students, the painting is simple. But like the work of a master, it is deceptively so. The lines are straight and strong, the angles unmistakable. The balustrades of the brownstone echo each other at exactly 45-degree angles, and each is capped with a lintel of snow. The wagon is solid in the white foreground, expressing its "carrying power," as Henri says it must. Touches of red on an otherwise somber palette are a technique he had admired in Corot. The rutted snow, meanwhile, contains the history of the day. Arrested motion—the turn of the foreground horse's head, the sweep of the girl's arm at the left, and the slightly slanted fall of the snow—pull us from the past, root us in the present, and promise a future. As in a musical composition, there are pauses—the

expanse of snow between the horses, the blank sky behind—where the eye may rest momentarily while the rest of the composition forms itself in the consciousness. "Places of silence," Henri called them.

Meanwhile, there are other echoes, this time, curves: wagon wheels, the arc of the lamppost, the rightward sweep of the street, the hazy dome of the building in the background. But, as Henri says, curves cannot exist in their full power unless contrasted with straight lines, so he provides an abundance of triangles and rectangles, some prominent, others less so. Paradoxically, the dominant line—the line Henri says must be in every painting whether or not it is actually drawn—is hardly visible. If the arm of the girl in yellow at the left is extended horizontally it will cross just at the base of the vertical lamppost, forming a perfect perpendicular. This lamppost is the final touch, that "small" touch that Henri said expands its influence over all the area of the painting. At dusk, unnoticed at first, "at the moment of its lighting," the lamp becomes the appoggiatura of the composition. Quickly played, hardly noticed, it is nonetheless the measure and harmony of the music. Block it out and there remains a skillful painting; put it back and the work is art.

But for all his paintings, it is perhaps Henri's teaching and his book, *The Art Spirit*, that is his most loved work. In his writing he confesses to his idols: Whitman, Emerson, and Isadora Duncan, among them. He regretted that he came to Wagner's music late for, as he said, its rhythms would have affected his paintings; but he did have Beethoven, Ibsen, Strindberg, and Rodin. Above all, he had Rembrandt, El Greco, Whistler, Homer, Velázquez, Daumier, and his greatest idol, Thomas Eakins.

What effect his family may have had on him is impossible to say. One can note, however, that there is little difference between the basic qualities needed for the professional gambler, such as Henri's father,

Continued on p. 202

JAMA

January 5, 1979

THE JOURNAL of the American Medical Association

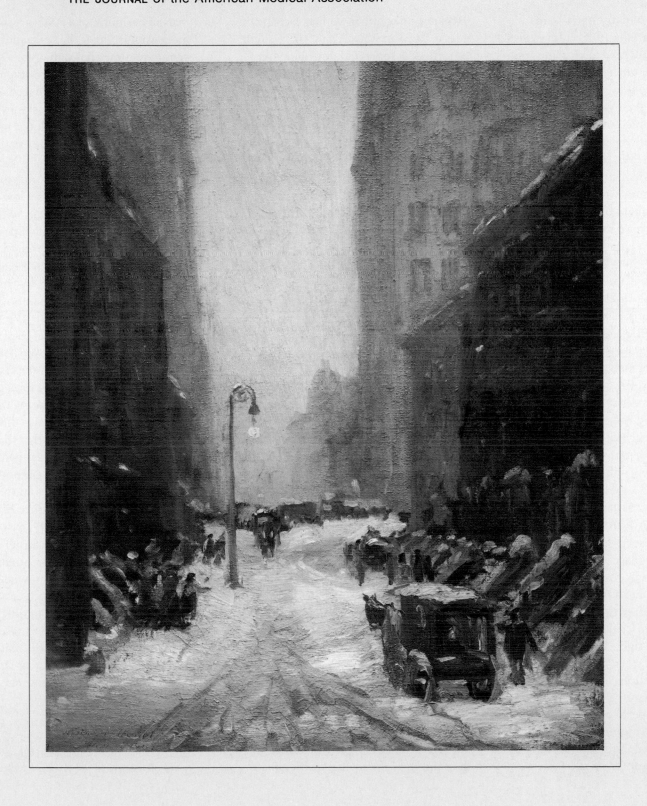

ADRIANUS EVERSEN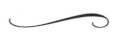

Amsterdam Street Scene

In the literature of painting, it seems almost as though the 19th century existed nowhere but in France. Though some countries—United States, Britain, Germany—managed a penumbra in varying degrees, the Dutch, despite their own 17th century of genius, were eclipsed totally by the French and especially by the brilliance of the Impressionists. Even the two Dutch names that appear with any regularity during the 19th century—Jongkind and van Gogh—are thought of more often in terms of France than of their native Netherlands. They stand at either end of the Impressionist movement like two avenging angels: Jongkind its herald, van Gogh its knell, and both, tragically, quite mad.

But there were other Dutch painters working in the Netherlands during this time. Largely unnoticed, they were producing the quiet, tranquil, predictable scenes of Dutch daily life so reminiscent of the 17th-century townscapes of Vermeer and de Hooch. Among them was Adrianus Eversen (1818-1897). Not suprisingly, we know little of his personal life, only that he was born in Amsterdam, worked there and in Rotterdam, and died in Delft.

Amsterdam Street Scene manifests Eversen's debt to his 17th-century countrymen. Even a cursory glance shows that every brick is in its place, every leaf is on its tree, every tile is on its roof. The work is as neat, as orderly, and as tidy as a Dutchwoman's kitchen. Likewise, the lines are sure and certain. The artist knows that every line he places is exactly right. The scene itself arouses no particular passion, no stirring thoughts, no aspirations after great deeds. It is simply what it seems: a glimpse of an Amsterdam street, perhaps one that is a filled-in canal, on a midmorning in May, with people involved in the restful routine of daily chores. A woman markets, men exchange news, other women exchange gossip. The sun waits. The scene is solid, unruffled, as sober and untroubled as a burgher's conscience on a Sunday morning.

More than anything, however, *Amsterdam Street Scene* is a lesson in solid geometry, a study covering the complete repertoire of shapes and lines, from the rectilinear doors, windows, and chimneys, the horizontal lintels, sills, and hoist supports, the equal-angled gables, the cylindrical roof tiles, right down to the asymptotic curves of the roofs.

> *The scene is solid, unruffled, as sober and untroubled as a burgher's conscience on a Sunday morning.*

Even the human figures are stuck-together ovals and cylinders of featureless faces and ragdoll joints—and indeed, Eversen did use stuffed dolls as models for his people. But while there are clouds and sunlight and shade to soften the angles, the effect is still almost too architectural, too structured—almost dogmatic, one could say. There is no mystery here; things really are what they seem to be. One is not pushed to ask questions. A brick is a brick, a tile is a tile, and a cobblestone is a cobblestone. Nothing more and nothing less.

And still there is a charm that seduces us. Besides the obvious shapes and lines, there are hidden horizontals, verticals, and a profusion of isosceles triangles that bear searching out—even other, complete paintings within the painting—all moving in strict, mathematical harmony, like a Mozart sonata. Even more astonishing is the realization of the painting's dimensions: they are less than those of an ordinary sheet of typing paper. Still, the detail Eversen managed to include in such a tiny space is not as astonishing when one remembers that he belongs to the same people who first opened the micro-universe with a magnifying lens.

In the hierarchy of painting, townscapes have traditionally occupied a low order, since they are concerned only with man's earthly existence. Even landscapes, because they can lift the heart and mind to things divine, are placed higher than townscapes, though still considerably below history, mythology, and religious painting. But because the Dutch made the townscape so popular does not mean that they were less religious than landscape lovers, only that they preferred to deal with the visible and the tangible, not surprising for a people who could build a city by separating the dry land from the sea. Townscapes also differ from landscapes in another element that is essential: a townscape must always contain people. Even if the figures are not visible, their presence is felt—there, at that window, behind the ever so slight movement of the curtain. Their footsteps echo down the sidestreet, just beyond the corner turned. Their voices hang in the air, caught like beams in the sunlight. Thus, while a correctly placed tree, or a brook, or a cow may enhance a landscape, only in the townscape are people the essence. The landscape is primeval. Only at the end of creation, after man has been created, is townscape possible; this is what the Dutch discovered.

JAMA

THE JOURNAL of the American Medical Association

May 18, 1979

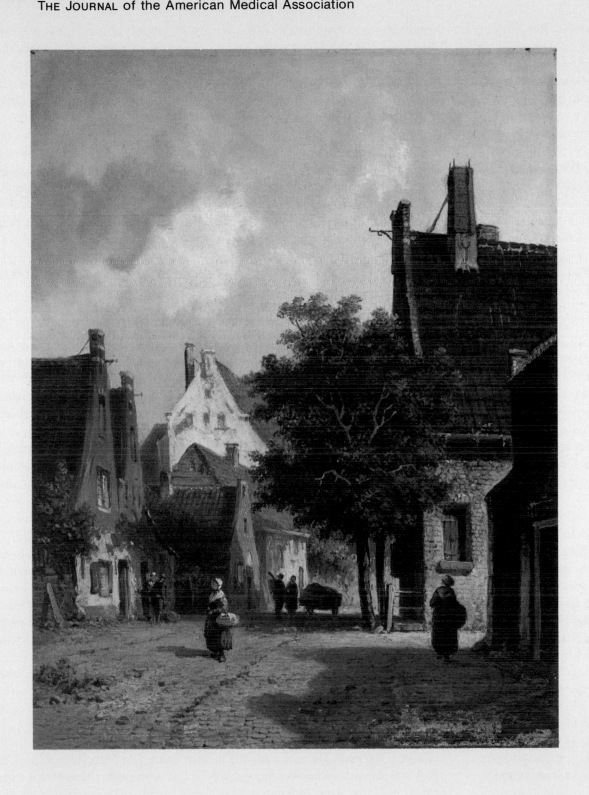

EDVARD MUNCH

Girls on the Jetty

In one of the "prose-poems" for which he was noted, the Norwegian painter Edvard Munch (1863-1944) described the Christmas that occurred just after his fifth birthday. "Huge snowflakes fell, endlessly, endlessly… We could follow them with our eyes until they were almost on the ground…There were so many white candles all the way to the top of the trees…The light shone… mostly in red and yellow and green…She sat in the middle of the sofa in her heavy black dress which seemed even blacker in that sea of light, silent and black. All around her we five either stood or sat. Father walked back and forth, and then sat down next to her…It was so silent and light everywhere. And then [Sophie] sang 'Silent night, holy night, angels float to earth unseen.' The woman on the sofa…stroked our cheeks… We had to leave…It was dark in the room now…We had on our coats and the girl who was going with us stood in the doorway and waited. And so we had to go up to the bed one by one, and she looked at us so strangely and kissed us. And then we left, and the girl took us to some strangers. They were all so good to us…They woke us in the middle of the night…We understood…We got dressed."

The place was the Munch home in Kristiania (now Oslo). "She" was Munch's mother, Laura, fatally ill with tuberculosis. "We five" were the Munch children, from the oldest, Sophie, age 6, who was also Edvard's favorite and almost "alter ego," to the youngest, Inger, born just a few months earlier. "Father" was a physician who had devoted his life to Kristiania's poor and who now, with the death of the wife, doubled the children's privation by withdrawing into a life of religious preoccupation that sometimes seemed to touch on insanity. Late in his life the painter would say to his own physician, "Disease, insanity and death were the angels which attended my cradle, and since have followed me throughout my life." He did not exaggerate. Edvard himself was ill with tuberculosis during childhood, but his

greatest blow came at the age of 14 when his beloved Sophie, like their mother, died of tuberculosis. His father died in 1889 when Munch was 26 years old, and in 1895 his only brother Andreas, a physician and newly married, died, again, of tuberculosis. A sister and a grandfather died in asylums.

In the meantime, at age 17, Munch had begun art studies. Three years later he became part of the Kristiania "Bohemian set" and began a frenetic round of study, work, travel, exhibits, unhappy love affairs, drinking, and public brawling that was to

Munch painted in the lean line of poetry.

end finally, 25 years later, in Professor Jacobson's psychiatric clinic in Copenhagen where he remained for eight months. But always Munch painted, and always his themes were love, death, and women, themes that in his life and in his emotions were so inextricably linked as to be one and the same.

Girls on the Jetty is one of at least five similar paintings Munch did with this title and is probably the last. It is dated 1904, during the last turbulent years before his breakdown. Yet the viewer's first impression is one of simplicity and straightforwardness. The place is a jetty in Aagaardstrand, a town some 60 kilometers south of Oslo that Munch was especially fond of. The time is that tranquil twilight time when everything pauses for the moment that exists between day and evening. Three girls, perhaps on the way home after an outing, pause on the jetty leading from the town dock. Two gaze into the water at the reflected linden trees, or perhaps at the midnight sun, while the third gazes back toward the sea. The houses are neat, walled, and silent, with everyone safely returned from the day's work. The colors are strong, but pleasing, and the line sweeping,

almost lyrical, as it curves into the right upper distance. It is a sentimental, almost sticky, pink and blue world of little girls.

But first impressions can be deceiving. Almost as we watch, the scene takes on a menacing, unpleasant tone. Now the houses are inhospitable and look out at us through vertical slits, which are distorted in the water. Now the railings of the bridge are gashed with red. Even the road itself runs red, while the harbor water is nearly black. The green trees are sinister for what they might conceal. The girls are ill-proportioned and portrayed with as few strokes as possible. The first has no face, the yellow hat of the second is askew, while the third is painted so sketchily as to remain almost as a guess. The sun—it could be called a moon—is ambiguous; the water sends back no reflection. And over all is a sky done with angry, almost violent jabs of a sharp-bristled brush. Most of all, there remains an unfinished quality to the painting, a haste, an agitation, an inner tension, controlled, but just barely.

Yet although this painting was done at a time of great turmoil in Munch's life, it still retains those qualities of coherence, unity, and order that characterize a work of art. In spite of the anger, in spite of the haste, there is not a syllable out of place, nor a line too many. Some artists paint in the voluminous cloth of prose; Munch painted in the lean line of poetry. And like poetry, his statements compress a meaning waiting to explode.

In the context of his other work, the three girls on the bridge are not three separate girls at all, but rather three aspects of a single woman. The first is the woman of innocence. Her face has nothing written on it. She is vulnerable, and as she looks directly at us with her sightless eyes, we are drawn into her world and perhaps the experience of her first sensual stirrings. The woman in red, on the other hand, is the experienced woman, the woman of erotic love. She is, as Munch sees her, the seducer, the initiator, the woman of all-engulfing passion; her love will

Continued on p. 202

JAMA

THE JOURNAL OF the American Medical Association

June 8, 1979

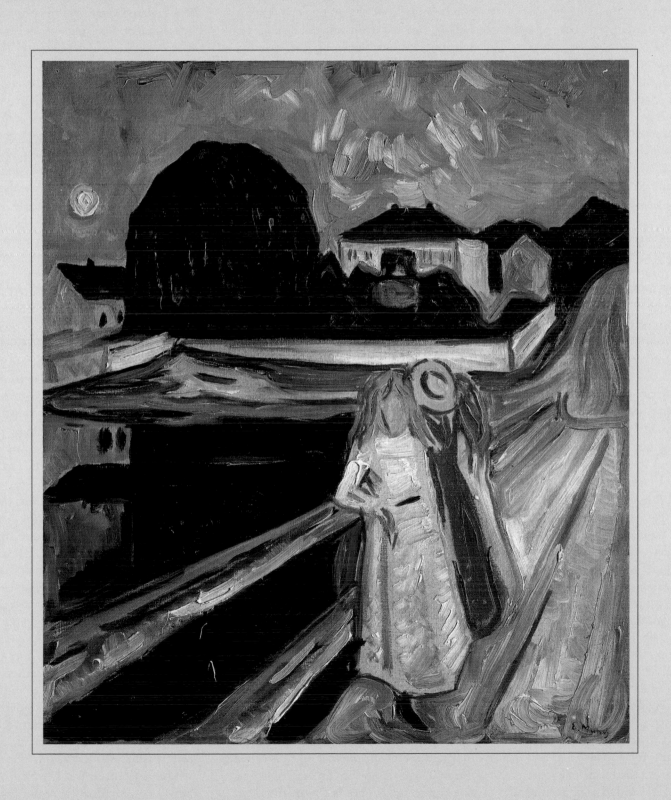

FRANK WESTON BENSON

Portrait in White

As though by some strange alchemy of period and place, the Philadelphia Centennial Exposition of 1876 became both the coffin and the cradle of American art. The old romanticism of the earlier part of the century died, while the next quarter of a century saw a profusion of styles and repeated beginnings that climaxed in 1893 at the World's Columbian Exposition in Chicago. The drift was generally eastward, to New York and Boston, but especially to Paris where a kind of "prep" school existed for those young talented Americans who wished to enter the profession of art. After a couple of years at the Académie Julian under the tutelage of Boulanger and Lefebvre and a vacation trip or two around Europe sketching and painting, most of these young would-be artists returned home to set up shop. Some were disillusioned, others had both social success and handsome incomes, but, regardless, most contributed to the development of a new American art. It was to become art no longer native nor yet European, but like America itself, an art formed by many individuals striving to amalgamate various influences while they themselves remained unique.

Such was the training of Frank Weston Benson (1862-1951). He was born in Salem, Massachusetts, that best sort of New England city of pure Puritan dwellers, as one early 20th-century writer termed it, where any furnishing but ancestral mahogany gave rise to the unpleasant suspicion of being parvenu. On his return from the Académie Julian in 1885, Benson painted portraits in Salem, taught briefly in Maine, and finally, in 1889, began a longtime association with the Museum of Fine Arts in Boston, teaching in the Department of Drawing and Painting From the Nude Figure. He became Boston's best-selling artist, and his annual income often reached six figures. During this time he was best known for portraits and for outdoor figure paintings, done in a loosely Impressionistic style and usually portraying his wife and daughters walking through sunny landscapes, or standing on a bluff looking out to sea, or sitting half shaded by a tree, but always with wind-blown hair and in wind-billowed white dresses. Benson's world was the genteel world, the stable world, the world of the well-regulated life lived on the sunny side of the street in an ancestral house whose windows looked out on a perpetually blooming garden. And like the gentleman, whose tastes are always moderate, Benson was not obsessed with painting. "He wisely limits his hours of work in the studio and classroom," wrote William Howe Downes in

> "'...such was the fashion of painting her grace and firmness, her delicacy and strength of character...'"

1900, "...works with all his heart while he works, then quits, locks the studio door, and makes for the woods and fields." He exercised systematically in the open air year round, and, moreover, he was a "canny hunter and a braw golfer."

Portrait in White was painted in 1889, four years after Benson had returned from Paris and also the year he began teaching in Boston. At first glance the painting may seem merely conventional in its beauty and competent in its technique—the portrait of Anywoman posing for her posterity in her favorite gown. The simple cut of the gown emphasizes a trim waist that rises to a full bosom, set off by a deep V, which in turn sets off the slender neck and soft angularity of the face with its exquisitely set cheekbones. The dress itself could well have been the occasion for the portrait, for it is expensive in its very simplicity, an undergown of fine French muslin overlaid by a froth of tulle, which is striped with satin ribbon. The ribbon is bowed at the elbows and left shoulder. The single jewel is a cameo discreetly placed on the bodice. The portrait is sentimental, it could have been saccharine, but restraint has saved it. Instead, the painting, from pose, to model, to technique, is disarming because of these very qualities of reserve combined with honesty.

The sitter is Benson's young bride, serene and pensive, obviously posed, though with a natural grace that overcomes the stiffness, especially of the hands. Still, she betrays a certain self-consciousness and even a lack of ease in the set of her lips, but it is this shyness that charms the viewer. Most important, however, is the restraint that exists between sitter and painter, for while we are permitted a hint of their intimacy in the sitter's gaze, the artist has withdrawn the brush just short of a full statement.

Instead, the "public" artist takes over and certain "painterly" qualities become evident. There is, for example, a dialogue between the sitter and the chair. She leans to the left; the chairback answers by angling right. The single cameo, so importantly placed, is twinned in the knobs of the chairback. The delicate ribbon stripes of the sleeves are set off against the thick slats of the chair, which then are themselves continued downward to end in the graceful and rhythmic arcs of the folds of the skirt. Benson has also taken a lesson from the French Impressionists, who had been at the height of their popularity during Benson's Paris study; even more so, he is probably indebted to Whistler's famous portrait, *The Woman in White*, that had caused such a scandal in London and Paris 20 years earlier. Surely, Benson would have known about it, perhaps even studied it. As in the Whistler work, Benson has also chosen to paint a figure dressed entirely in white, playing off white against white, shadow against shadow, and texture against texture. The similarity of the ribbon stripe and fabric of the sleeves in the

Continued on p. 202

JAMA

THE JOURNAL of the American Medical Association

June 22, 1979

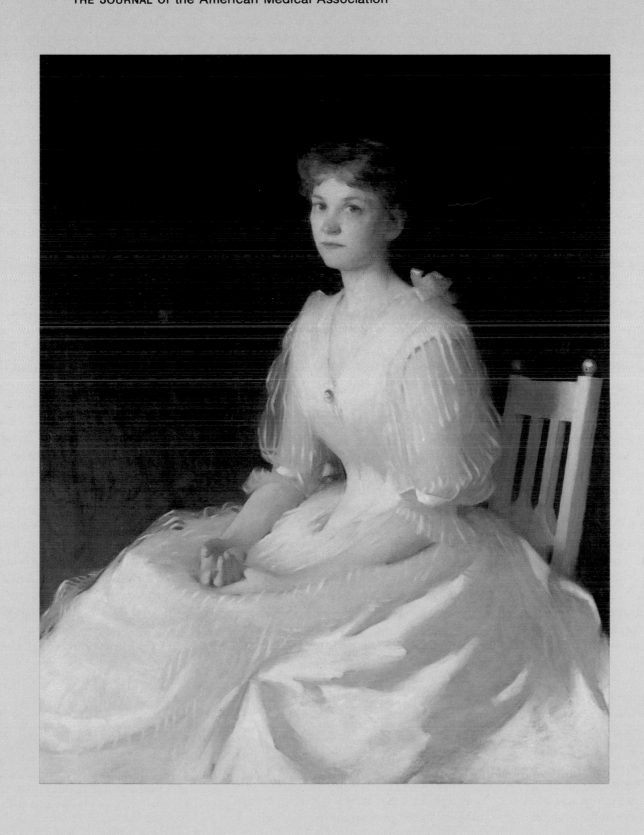

PIERRE AUGUSTE RENOIR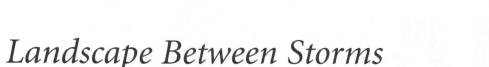

Landscape Between Storms

Often in the early days of their acquaintance, the Impressionists (though they did not yet know themselves as such) worked closely together in the environs of Paris, even to setting up their easels side by side and painting from the same motive. The results in some cases were so similar that it was almost impossible to distinguish, for example, a painting by Renoir from one by Monet, or a Monet from a Sisley, or even Sisley from Pissarro. The story is told that when a painting of water, foliage, and ducks turned up in an art dealer's shop in 1913, a scene that both Renoir and Monet had painted some 40 years earlier at Argenteuil, the artists themselves had to be consulted for identification—and even then neither could at first identify his own work.

But back in the 1870s attribution was unimportant. What was important was technique, and technique consisted largely in attempts to catch light in its quick passage across a landscape or, as one contemporary writer put it, to paint air, for which no color existed on the palette. Nevertheless, the signature on *Landscape Between Storms* still comes as somewhat of a surprise when we consider that this Impressionist is more often thought of in terms of his paintings of fussily dressed children with golden hair and rosy cheeks or of women whose complexions are the color and texture of commingled ivory, heavy cream, and rose petals. Even more familiar perhaps are his paintings of dappled nudes beneath leafy trees or his frequent use of brilliant reds. But always his paintings convey, like his life, an overall, general air of gaiety, even joyfulness.

Pierre Auguste Renoir (1841-1919) was born in Limoges, the son of a tailor, but moved to Paris with his family at age 4. At age 13, he went to work in a china factory and spent several years painting roses and silhouettes of Marie Antoinette on porcelain pieces. In 1861 he began the serious study of painting at the Gleyre studio in Paris.

Here he met Monet, Bazille (who would be killed in 1870, a casualty of the Franco-Prussian War), and Sisley. Their mutual aims and aspirations were to culminate in 1874 in the movement labeled "Impressionism." Monet and Renoir, who so often worked together, were to give the movement its chief impetus before each went on, in the late 1870s, to his own particular style. Only Sisley remained the true Impressionist, painting in the same manner long after the style had climaxed and died.

Landscape Between Storms belongs to the period of High Impressionism, just after the

> *...not the smooth passage of light from dawn to noon to evening, but rather a light that is whipped about like a roller coaster...*

group had held its first independent exhibit in 1874. The motif is especially apt for Renoir the Impressionist because a stormy sky is a rapidly changing sky. It is a sky that reflects not the smooth passage of light from dawn to noon to evening, but rather a light that is whipped about like a roller coaster—a superb challenge to one who wishes to catch its motion in paint. It is perhaps this rapid change of light that also accounts for the haste of the artist as evidenced in the broad comma strokes and coarse brush strokes (not to mention his wish, perhaps, to avoid being drenched by the oncoming storm). Yet, true to the teaching he was to give to a young artist many years later, Renoir obeys his ideas of color and light. Though many of the strokes are barely discernible, he still is careful to put the blue of the sky in the green of the grass as well as in

the mud of the road. Over it all, there is a veil: invisible droplets of moisture in the air soften the outlines of discrete objects by reflecting neighboring colors.

Renoir was subject to the same criticism, often coarsely stated, as were his colleagues. When he exhibited a painting of a nude woman seated under a tree at the group's second exhibit in 1876, with her skin dappled by sunlight filtering through the leaves, a critic wrote in *Le Figaro*, "Try to explain to M. Renoir that a woman's torso is not a mass of flesh in the process of decomposition with green and violet spots which denote the state of complete putrefaction of a corpse!" A contemporary cartoon shows a painter speaking to his model: would she mind spending another couple of days at the bottom of the river? Her skin still lacks a few of the tones he needs.

Late in his life Renoir was asked for the key to his painting. "I have no secrets," he said. When he looked at a nude, for example, he saw "myriads of tiny tints." All he had to do was to find the tints that would make that flesh "live and quiver" on his canvas. Nor, he said, could a picture ever be explained. To be art the work must be not only "indescribable" but "inimitable" as well. One wonders what Renoir would have said had he known that well before the first centennial of Impressionism workers would be spending entire lives making imitable products: screwing identical bolts into identical chassis to make identical automobiles, cloning fried potatoes into symmetrical chips so that they could be stacked neatly in their cans, and that even art would consist of rows and rows of red and white tomato soup labels, identically painted.

Pierre Auguste Renoir (1841-1919), *Landscape Between Storms*, c 1874-1875, French. Oil on canvas. 24.4 × 32.7 cm. Courtesy of the National Gallery of Art, Washington, DC; Ailsa Mellon Bruce Collection, 1970. © 1995 The Board of Trustees of the National Gallery of Art.

JAMA

THE JOURNAL of the American Medical Association

July 6, 1979

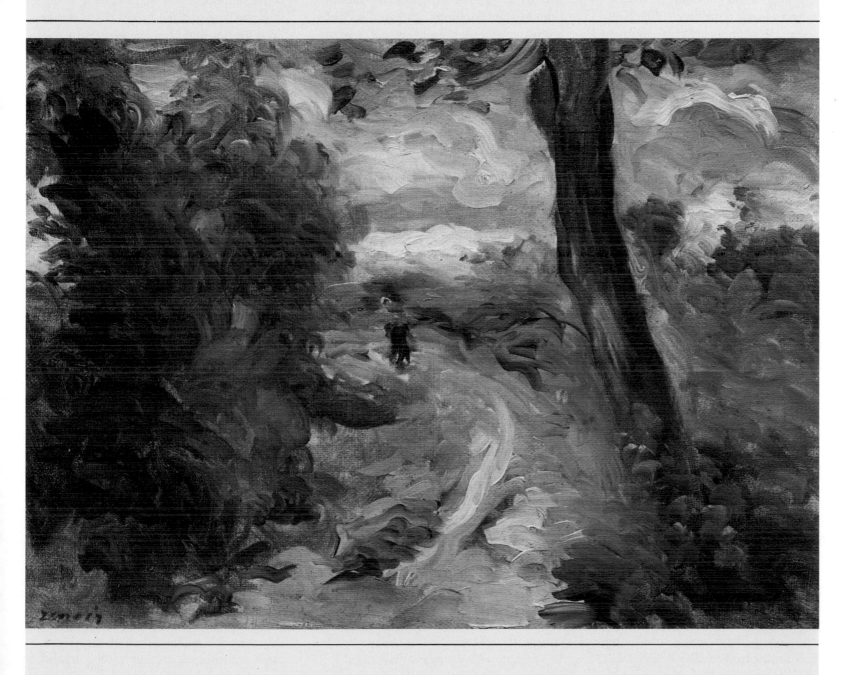

THEODORE WORES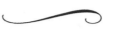

The Chinese Fishmonger

In the spring of 1875 Mrs Joseph Wores, herself a German expatriate and the wife of a Hungarian revolutionary now established as a merchant in San Francisco, traveled with her 16-year-old son Theodore (1859-1939) across the newly completed Transcontinental Railroad from Oakland, California, to St Louis. Here Mrs Wores remained to visit relatives, while Theodore continued alone by train to New York, by steamer to Hamburg, and finally again by train to Munich. He had come to study art, a talent evident already in his early teens, at one of the major art centers in the Europe of the 1870s, the Royal Bavarian Art Academy in Munich.

Theodore was not to see San Francisco again for some six years, and when he did return he was no "local boy made good," but a conquering hero, an artist made good on his own, internationally known, with exhibits behind him in the major cities of Europe and the United States. The much matured 23-year-old Wores arrived home short of paintings, but long on talent, ambition, discipline, and, fortunately, number of years ahead as well.

Less than three months after his return to San Francisco, Wores painted *The Chinese Fishmonger*. An actual scene, it is perhaps one that first took root in young Wores' mind when he had so often walked up Washington Steet from his father's wholesale hat business at No. 609 to his home on McAllister Street. But besides these nostalgic qualities, the subject was also exotic, much to the public's taste at the time, and finally, it gave the young artist a chance to prove himself, something like the triumphant Roman warrior returned home who must earn his laurels all over again, or more to the times, like a well-trained concert pianist returned from a lion's tour abroad who must now play for the home folks a composition that will display every skill he has stowed away in the luggage of his virtuosity.

That Wores was a critical, and not merely a popular, success in his native city is attested by the fact that many critics consider this one of his finest paintings. Moreover, the painting has an immediacy to it that we, a century removed, can easily miss. In 1865, with the Union Pacific advancing westward from Missouri to meet the Central Pacific advancing eastward from Oakland in what was to become the Transcontinental Railroad (the very railroad that took Wores to St Louis on his way to Munich), it became evident that the Pacific portion may not advance beyond Cape Horn, a rock cliff in the Sierras that rose 400 meters above the American River at an almost 90-degree angle. But the builders had not reckoned on

> *…both are dislocated creatures, except that it is the man who knows, remembers, and feels.*

the ingenuity of the recently hired Chinese workers. From reed baskets they wove themselves and attached to cables secured from above, the men swung out from the perpendicular cliff, attached powder charges, set them off, and scurried up the cable to safety; little by little, with infinite patience, Cape Horn was conquered. Is it not tempting, then, to speculate that perhaps this very fishmonger who served as Wores' model once helped to build the Transcontinental Railroad, or if not him, one of his family, or certainly a friend who blasted the rock that connected East and West. With the railroad completed, the Chinese were to become fishermen, much like the young man pictured.

There are as many ways of looking at a painting as there are ways of looking at a blackbird. But when all is said and done, it is no one element of the painting that holds us, but rather the entire work. It is a banquet of line, color, and texture combined as subtly as the flavors, colors, and textures of a 3-star Michelin menu. First, the viewer's eye finds itself drawn almost irresistibly to the head of the salmon, then is swept along its white underbelly and up the S of its tail where the fin splits neatly to carry the attention across the hand of the fishmonger, where even the thumb conspires to make sure we follow the oval rim of the basket to the young man's face. Then, following the focus of his eyes we meet the beady eye of the flounder, which is in fact the right angle of the triangle of fish being dumped from the basket. From there we are swept down the upper slope of the triangle, around the bottom of the copper pot, up its left side, around and over the top of the pot once again, and then clockwise around a circle that encompasses the mussels and crawfish, then up along the left side of the pot still again, and across on a diagonal to meet the netting hanging above. From there we travel to the left in a figure eight around the hanging catfish and smelts and end at the head of the salmon whence we began. But the eye cannot yet rest; so compelling is the S-curve of the hapless salmon that we must again follow it to the face of the fishmonger.

Still, just as in the Wallace Stevens poem, where "The only moving thing/Was the eye of the blackbird," it is the eye of the flounder that transfixes our attention, even as it transfixes the gaze of the fishmonger, perhaps in one last unfelt, prehuman plea that it be returned to the icy waters of the Bay whence it came. And there is in the fishmonger's gaze the slightest flicker of a pain, which hints that he recognizes a certain kindred with the fish: he is as much, and even more, out of his milieu as is the flounder. Though it is the man who caught the fish and the man who will sell the fish, both are dislocated creatures, except that it is the man who knows, remembers, and feels.

Theodore Wores (1859-1939), *The Chinese Fishmonger*, 1881, American. Oil on canvas. 88.9 × 116.8 cm. Courtesy of the National Museum of American Art, Smithsonian Institution, Washington, DC.

JAMA

July 27, 1979

THE JOURNAL of the American Medical Association

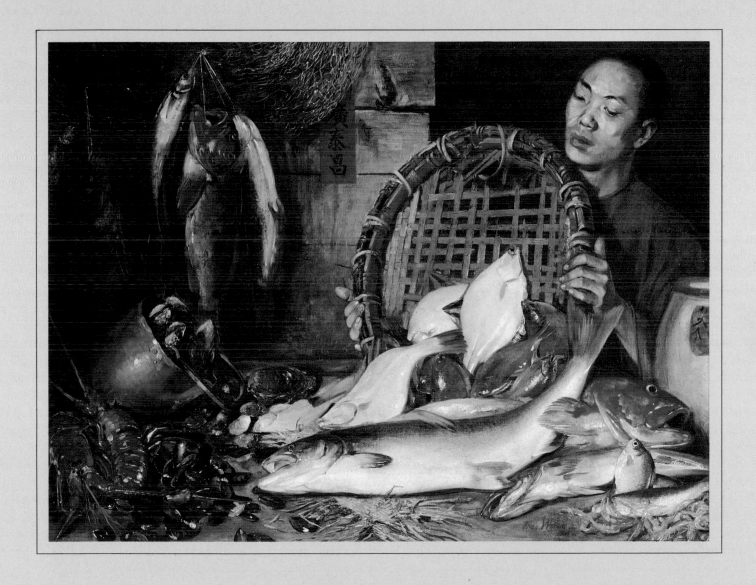

FREDERICK CARL FRIESEKE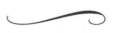

The Garden Parasol

In a delicious heading to a chapter on some of the lesser-known American Impressionists, Richard Boyle allows Gully Jimson, Joyce Cary's broken-down but still expugnable painter, to speak about some of his own old Impressionist works. It is straight from *The Horse's Mouth*: "Tea cakes. And when they showed me a room full of my own confections I felt quite sick." But Gully's creator allowed the ex-Impressionist even unkinder words: "People like impressionism…because it hasn't any idea in it… it doesn't ask anything from them…like grandpa brought to a nursery tea."

One of these lesser-known—though not necessarily "lesser Impressionists"—is the American expatriate Frederick Carl Frieseke (1874-1939). Born in Owosso, Michigan, his life span symbolizes, perhaps, an era now gone. Born just a week before the French Impressionists held their first group exhibition in Paris, he died in France just days before the outbreak of World War II. Frieseke studied briefly at the Art Institute of Chicago (so briefly, apparently, that it is difficult to find anyone at the museum who has heard of him; even his three paintings there are in storage) and then at the Art Students League in New York City. In 1896, he went to Paris to study where most Americans of that period did: the Académie Julian. Although he would return to the United States from time to time for exhibits of his works, from 1898 on Paris was his home.

In 1906, a year after his marriage to Sadie O'Bryan, he settled even closer to the heart of French painting when he moved to Giverny. There, in a village halfway between Paris and Rouen on the Seine, he bought the property immediately adjacent to Monet's. The marriage—to Sadie and to Giverny— was happy on both counts: he now had not only the family life so important to him, but even the setting he desired. The generosity of Monet's Giverny garden, so familiar to today's viewers from his many flower-laden canvases, extended also to the Frieseke garden, sepa-rated as they were by only a wall. Even the lazy Epte, which bore on its surface the water lilies and irises so often painted by Monet in his later years, flowed through Frieseke's garden as well. Still, it was Renoir that Frieseke most admired, especially his canvases of dappled nudes. Frieseke mastered Renoir's technique well enough to be called, at least for a time, the best American painter of nudes. Frieseke, in fact, often protested that the only reason he remained in France was that only in France was he free to paint nude models in his garden and by his stream. America, he claimed, was still too Puritan to

> *It is as though the sun has been shattered into a million shards…*

accept his nudes. On the other hand, his grandson, in a recollection written some years later, does admit that his grandfather found the trout fishing rather good in France.

The Garden Parasol was painted at Giverny sometime around 1913, perhaps during the last summer days before Europe would erupt into war. Ignoring for a moment the brilliant color and trying rather to see the painting as a monotone of grays, one can tease out a rather strict compositional structure, something not always so easily discovered in the works of the French Impressionists. For example, the right third of the painting is composed almost entirely of verticals—the most prominent of them being not only upright but properly hatted and corseted as well. In contrast, the left two-thirds of the painting is made up almost entirely of more relaxed curves and recumbent diagonals, suggesting the languor of an August day. The sense of relaxation is even more enhanced by the seated lady, perhaps the artist's wife, who spreads just a little too comfortably, even under her loose gown, to be much corseted. Also in keeping with what seems to be her easygoing nature is the fact that the tea things have not yet been cleared. And why should they be? Is it all that important on a hot day, after all, if a bit of leftover milk sours in its jug?

Still, there is tension. It can be spotted along a triangle that could be formed by drawing lines between the eyes of the two women and the small yellow book. Scarcely noticed by virtue of its shape, size, or color, the book becomes very important when the viewer realizes that Frieseke has placed it deliberately in nearly the center of the painting, equidistant from all corners. Whatever may be actually transpiring between the two women is hardly important, no more so than the forgotten milk. But what is important is how Frieseke contrasts physical postures to point out mental attitudes: Which is better, the thinker or the doer, the listener or the actor, Mary or Martha? For an August afternoon, it should not be difficult for the viewer to decide who has chosen the better part. Yet simply because the visually stronger verticals are compressed into only a third of the space does not make them subordinate elements. On the contrary, it is as the Greeks have said: Without the vertical, the oblique does not exist. But Frieseke refuses to war one against the other. Instead, he unites them by means of horizontal and vertical ovals—the chair arms, the flowered hat, the rise of the chair backs—and then uses the same oval shapes to call attention to the near perfection of the circle of the face of the seated woman.

Frieseke has not yet finished, however. With a courage that could come only from a confidence in his own artistic judgment, he adds to this balanced, peaceful, and subdued composition a large, garish, overpowering parasol that fills an entire quarter of the canvas. It is a device learned from the Japanese prints imported into Europe in the previous century and used often by the

Continued on p. 202

JAMA

THE JOURNAL of the American Medical Association

August 3, 1979

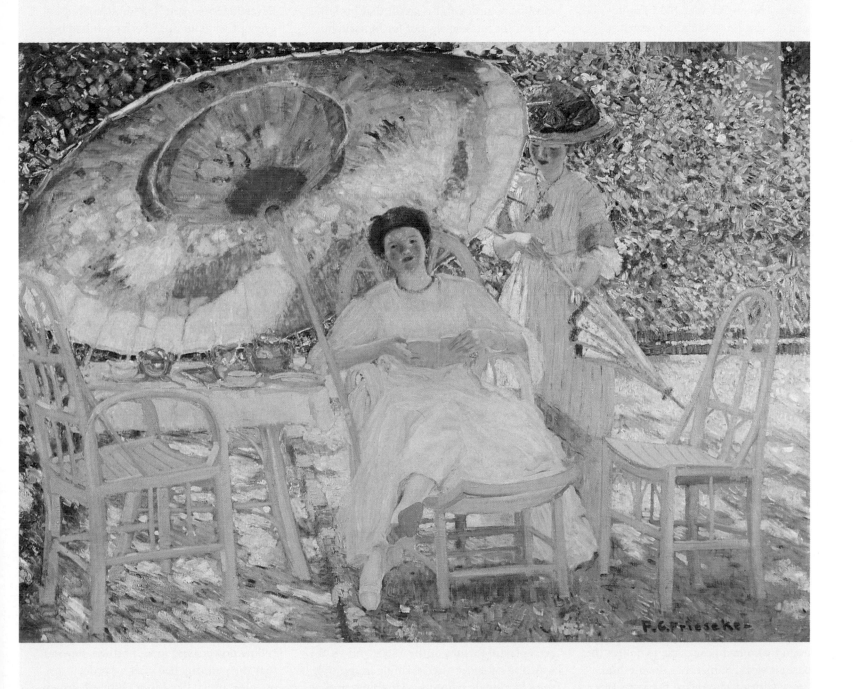

F.C.Frieseke

CLAUDE MONET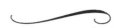

The Artist's Garden at Vétheuil

For Oscar Claude (as his family called him) Monet (1840-1926) the year 1879 was his time of crisis, both personally and artistically. Thirty-two-year-old Camille (née Doncieux), who since 1865 had served successively as his model, mistress, mother of their two sons, and wife, died in late summer, not long after they had left Paris and moved to Vétheuil, a small village on a loop of the Seine. Michel, their second son, was still an infant; Jean, their first son, had been born in 1867. Claude and Camille had been married since 1870, shortly before Monet had gone to London (alone) to escape the Franco-Prussian War.

All of this was not without effect, either on the lives of these "star-crost" lovers or even on the future of Impressionism itself. Monet had been disinherited by his family when he chose the study of "nonofficial" painting in place of his family's hopes for Academy training. Camille had received only a portion of her dowry because of her obvious liaison with Monet before their marriage. Furthermore, modest as the young couple's expenditures were, their finances seem to have swung like a pendulum between having some money and having none. Not only was Camille's dowry gone soon after the marriage, but an inheritance she received after her father's death in 1873 was gone by 1876. By 1878, with Camille mortally ill, the young couple's destitution was matched only by the eloquence with which Monet tried to extract money from friends and acquaintances. It mattered little what method he used. Sometimes he tried to force the sale of a canvas on an acquaintance; other times he would upbraid a friend who had already paid Monet for a "future" canvas and who had now come to collect the nonexistent work. Sometimes the method was heavy with psychological pressure. On the move from Paris to Vétheuil with the mortally ill Camille, infant Michel, and 11-year-old Jean, Monet begged his friend Charpentier for money because, as he said,

all their furniture had been loaded on the wagon and he had nothing "with which to pay the moving man, not a penny." But it must be recorded to his credit that his last request for money was not for himself, but for the dead Camille: He wanted to retrieve her favorite locket, which he had pawned, so that she might be buried wearing it.

With Camille's death Monet changed greatly. So did his painting. It is almost as though, during the 14 years of their association, Monet had used Camille's soul as his own, just as he had used up her dowry and her inheritance; now that she

> "What does the subject matter!…One instant, one aspect of nature contains it all."

was dead, Monet had returned her soul, just as he had retrieved her favorite locket and placed it in her grave on the hilltop in Vétheuil near the church.

Camille died in September; Monet spent that winter at Vétheuil in utter desolation, although he never stopped painting. Some of his famous gray and white ice floe scenes of the Seine belong to this winter. But then, with the mourning period passing and the summer upon him, both Monet's mood and painting changed dramatically. As profligate as he once had been with money, so he now became with color. His style and content also changed. Gone were the cheerful, gay, even playful themes of the 1860s and 1870s, which so often featured Camille in multiple roles in a single painting—laughing, smiling, hiding from herself behind a tree, as though she were the sun itself playing on earth for the joy of man. Now, rather, Monet began to concentrate less on images of figures and

more on color for color's sake, on acquiring that technical proficiency that was to occasion Cézanne's remark, so well known, but nevertheless so apt: "He's nothing but an eye, but what an eye!" Perhaps it had been a trade-off: Monet lost Camille's soul; he gained an eye.

In his personal life, too, there were changes. His somewhat irregular liaison with Mme Hoschedé, the wife of a once wealthy merchant who had helped Monet financially, but who was now himself bankrupt, became open. The two families, Monet and his two sons and Mme Hoschedé and the five youngest of her six children lived at Vétheuil (although they had been living there even before Camille's death). Monet ceased writing begging letters. He gained a new assurance.

The Artist's Garden at Vétheuil, although dated 1880, was actually painted in 1881, according to Wildenstein. Michel Monet stands in the foreground on the walk. Jean-Pierre Hoschedé, Mme Hoschedé's youngest child, stands on the stairs. Thus, this painting belongs to the first critical year after Camille's death (in the house shown on the right), or perhaps to the second summer. At any rate, it is the beginning of decisive changes in Monet's painting. Characteristically, he paints the shapes, and especially the vertical lines, he loves—the stairway, the chimneys, the small figures, the rectangles of roofs and walls. Also characteristic of much of French painting in general at that time is the Japanese influence, the large open space in the foreground and the chinoiserie—blue and white jars that flank the path. The tall, sweeping strokes of their flowers accentuate the converging diagonals of the path and the steps and contrast nicely with the daubs of yellow flowers and jots of brown. Beyond that the painting becomes a prodigal son of color, much like Monet himself, growing wild, luxuriant, and extravagantly in the present moment. Such extravagance is perhaps how one sees the world when the shade in the room of one's grief is first lifted.

Continued on p. 203

JAMA

THE JOURNAL of the American Medical Association

August 17, 1979

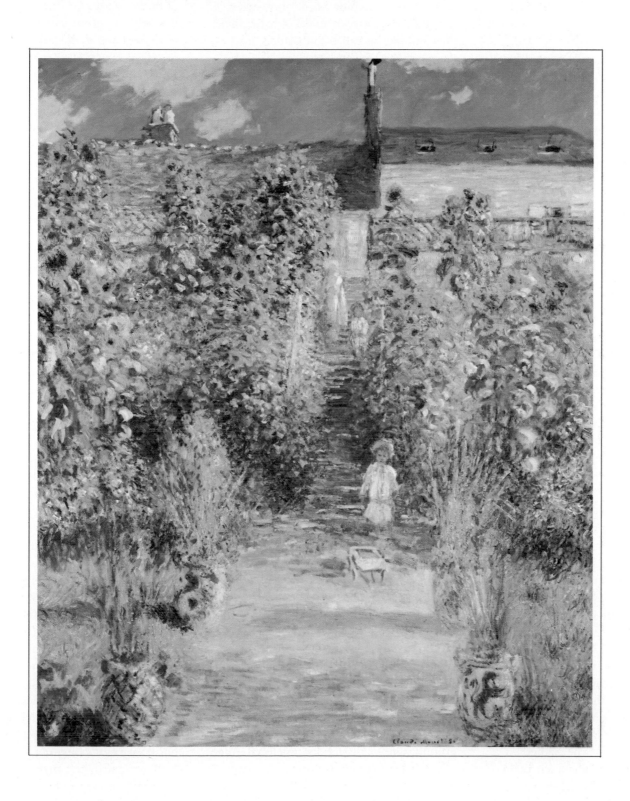

WINSLOW HOMER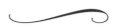

Beach Scene

Shortly before he quit the United States for good in 1875, Henry James reviewed the current American art scene: "A frank, absolute, sincere expression of any tendency is always interesting, even when the tendency is not elevated or the individual not distinguished," he wrote of one artist in particular; "…to see, and to reproduce what he sees, is his only care…to think, to imagine, to select, to refine, to compose…all this [he] triumphantly avoids. He not only has no imagination, but he contrives to elevate this rather blighting negative into a blooming and honorable positive. He is almost barbarously simple, and, to our eye, he is horribly ugly…" James was discussing no less than the 39-year-old Boston-born painter Winslow Homer (1836-1910).

Descended from almost two centuries of Yankee stock (the first American Homer had sailed his own ship from England to Boston in the mid-1600s, while his mother's people were from Maine), Winslow was the middle child of three sons. His father was a hardware merchant and his mother an amateur painter. At age 19 he was apprenticed to a lithographer, and on his 21st birthday he set up his own studio, becoming known for his illustrations in *Harper's Weekly*. He covered Lincoln's inauguration as well as the Civil War. About this time he added oil painting to his repertoire.

One of the first American paintings to be exhibited in Europe was his well-known oil *Prisoners From the Front* (1866). In 1867, like most other American artists, Homer made the obligatory trip to France and returned within ten months, apparently unimpressed. He continued as he had, largely self-taught, progressing at an agonizingly slow pace, but maturing solidly. Until the mid-1870s his subjects were children, young women in fashionable dress, or, as James phrased it in his 1875 review, subjects he (James) detested—"his big barren plank fences, his glaring, bold blue skies, his big, dreary vacant lots of meadows, freckled, straight-

haired Yankee urchins, his flat-breasted maidens, suggestive of a dish of rural doughnuts and pie, his calico sunbonnets, his flannel shirts, his cowhide boots."

Beach Scene probably belongs, at least generally, to James' parting blast at Homer's painting, for it was done most likely between 1870 and 1874. The locale is not known for certain, but it could well have been Gloucester, Massachusetts, or a nearby town on Cape Ann; it was about 1873 that Homer first began painting there. *Beach Scene* is also probably one of Homer's last oils, for in his Gloucester trips he began turning increas-

> *Truly, Homer has left eternal children at a perfect beach on an endless day.*

ingly to watercolor as the method of best expressing the brilliance and spontaneity he wanted.

Ugly or not, Homer's painting of children playing in the surf can hardly bring more pleasure. It is evocative of everyone's childhood, if not in fact, at least in essence. The mood is a composite of *Tom Sawyer*, *Huckleberry Finn*, *Little Women*, and even Tenniel's *Alice in Wonderland* illustrations for Lewis Carroll. A group of boys (one of them still wearing his blue-ribboned boater) rush headlong into the water, heedless of anything except to embrace the wet, wonderful surf and to taste its salty dangers to the fullest. In contrast, a group of calico-sunbonnetted girls, their feet barely touching the spent surf, search for shells; in the foreground stands a mysterious pinafored "Alice," still wearing her high-buttoned shoes and long white stockings. Two sailing ships, as unmindful of the children as the children are

of them, pass in the distance. Meanwhile, in the right midground two more breakers are imminent and to the left several others are promised. Truly, Homer has left eternal children at a perfect beach on an endless day.

If one can liken the painting to music, then the composition of the work resembles the strong harmonic stability of a simple inverted triad whose thirds are the rectangles of sky, sea, and sand. The strength of the rectangles is measured by the sailing ships on the horizon and by the horizontal line in the foreground that passes through the bare feet of the girls. The harmony has been enhanced by adding a seventh to the chord—the dissonance of a wide diagonal band whose lower edge cuts across the foreground in a blue streak and whose upper edge is formed by the heads of the boys, framed by the girl at the extreme left and punctuated by the girl in red. It is this strong, vertical figure that also resolves the tension created by the diagonal back to harmonic stability.

But colored music, as painting has indeed been called, is more than a chord; it must also have rhythm such as that shown by the balanced repetition of color: specks of red in the clothing of the girls on the extreme right and left match the obvious central red; the tiny blue line of the band on the boy's boater is repeated in the sash of the girl's dress to his right, and is also repeated by the blue of the sky reflected in the foreground—this latter being a silent part of the rhythm, like a rest, for the portion of the sky that is reflected is not visible to the viewer. There is also the obvious rhythmic repetition of each child's figure in the wet sand, akin perhaps to modulation into a secondary key. (It should be noted here that the sand contains an extra pair of feet and a body, a source of almost unending speculation once one begins thinking about it.)

But the strongest rhythm is in the sea, prophetic of the work to come. For example, on the right, the breakers repeat themselves,

Continued on p. 203

JAMA

August 24/31, 1979

THE JOURNAL of the American Medical Association

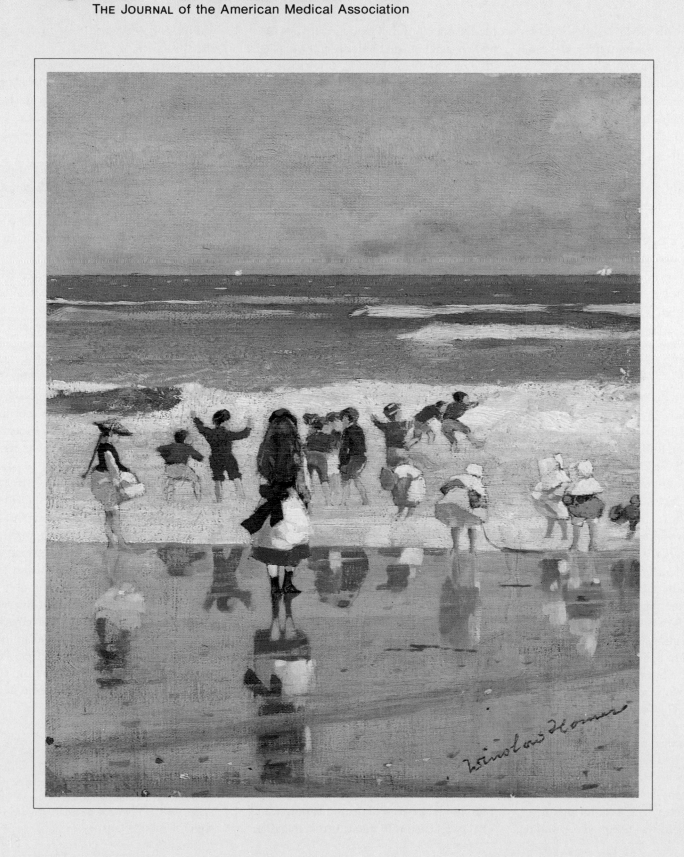

PETER PAUL RUBENS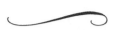

Lion

Peter Paul Rubens (1577-1640) is one of those rare souls to whom the gods seem to give their entire bounty. It is as though the gods, nearing the end of the day's work and discovering that not only do they have a surplus of gifts, but that what remains is also the choicest of the lot, solve the matter simply by emptying all that is left over on the next person along.

In an age already great for its painters and sculptors, Rubens fathered a style that was truly new, the Baroque. Mostly for lack of proper study, it is a style that in our own century is often dismissed as "ugly," is misunderstood, or, worse, is overlooked. Yet in Rubens' century, it brought persons of taste from all over Europe to watch him at work in his studio in Antwerp. With its exuberance and extravagance of color and line, the Baroque is an expression of Rubens' joie de vivre; it is also as tightly disciplined in its composition as were his life and his work habits.

A devout Catholic living in the southern Netherlands, which had remained loyal to the Spanish crown, Rubens rose each morning at four, heard Mass, breakfasted lightly, and then went to his studio, where he worked until the evening meal, sketching, drawing, designing, painting, receiving visitors, dictating correspondence, listening to the Classical writers read aloud, and even directing the work of others. He took exercise each evening by riding a favorite horse or walking, and ate sparingly, at least by the Flemish standards of the day. He was also a shrewd and careful businessman, a talent often considered to be incompatible with that of creativity. Not only did he handle the sales of his own works, but he was a collector as well. That he was fair in his prices is often attested to by his contemporaries, but he was also noted to be as inflexible once he had set the price, as were "the laws of the Medes and the Persians"—as one contemporary complained.

But talent begets talent, and during his own lifetime Rubens was regarded even more highly as a court diplomat, greatly trusted, and engaged in what today might be called a kind of "shuttle diplomacy" among the major countries of Europe. He was thus able in 1630 to achieve peace between England and Spain, but to the end of his life was never able to achieve that which lay closest to his heart, the reunification of the northern and southern Netherlands. He was here perhaps too close emotionally to recognize and tackle the problems with the same dispassionate judgment he brought to the sale of his paintings.

> *...the German novelist Heinse called Rubens the Homer and the Aristophanes of painting.*

Nor were the gods stingy with Rubens in his personal life. His brother was one of the most promising Classical scholars of Europe, and Rubens benefited from his work and from his friends. Moreover, Rubens married a woman he deeply loved, and they were blessed with a daughter and two sons. But some of the gifts had to be returned. In the space of just a few years, Rubens lost his brother just as he stood on the brink of recognition as the leading scholar of Europe, he lost his wife of 17 years, and he lost his daughter just as she reached the threshold of womanhood. But again, the gods were merely exchanging gifts. In 1630, when Rubens was 53 years old, he married a second time, a girl of 16 years. Once again was he blessed with deep love and even a second family a generation away from the first. It was almost as though he had lived twice. Rubens died suddenly in May 1640, but even in death his power and vitality reached into the future. A daughter was born in February 1641, eight months after his death.

In his painting, Rubens excelled at nudes, being especially adept at the rendering of the nuances of color reflected by skin. He is also known for his animal paintings, most often painting horses or lions. The latter were especially apt subjects for a painter who might himself be called the king of painters and who dealt as diplomat with countries whose symbol was the lion.

Lion is a study for one of a denful of animals Rubens sketched for his painting, *Daniel in the Lion's Den*. With his hind feet in a slightly different pose, this is the lion that stands closest to Daniel in the final painting. The lion's facial expression is almost human and surely shows more compassion and generosity, both leonine attributes, than did the faces of the humans who had thrown Daniel to him. But the lion can afford to be generous. By sparing Daniel for a single night he will in the morning have all of Daniel's accusers as a meal: scores of satraps and a pair of presidents, along with their wives and children.

Two hundred years ago the German novelist Heinse called Rubens the Homer and the Aristophanes of painting. An expression of the new favor Rubens is finding in this century is voiced by the contemporary American artist Raphael Soyer, who compares him with Shakespeare. But even more telling of Rubens' extraordinary vitality and influence is Soyer's remark, made when he viewed his works in the Alte Pinakothek in Munich in 1963: "Often I found myself copying details from Rubens. It was like drawing from life, from living models in action."

JAMA

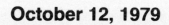

THE JOURNAL of the American Medical Association

October 12, 1979

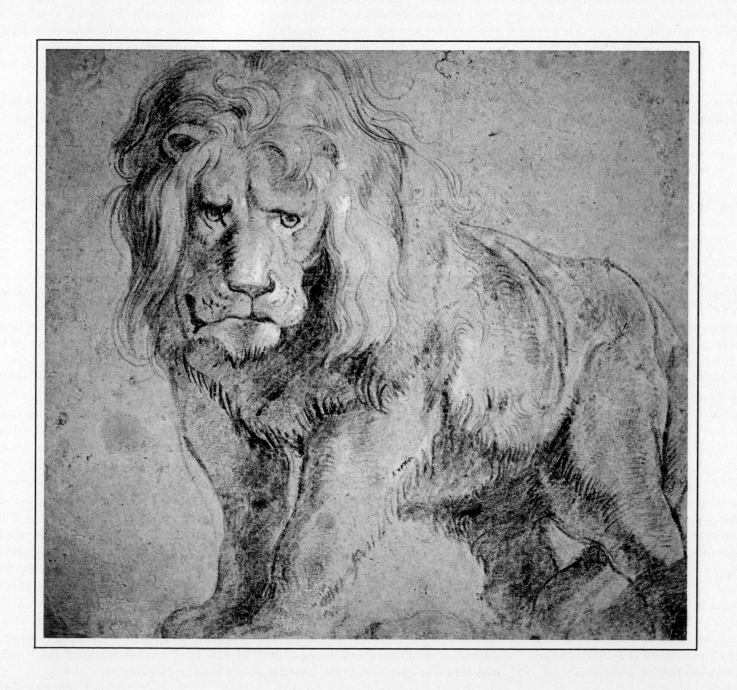

WALT KUHN ⌒

Pumpkins

In the beginning was The Eight. After that there was Club 291. Then came the Armory Show, and American art has never since been the same.

Variously dubbed the Revolutionary Gang, the Apostles of Ugliness, and the Ashcan School, The Eight were the first to revolt against the juried system of exhibitions at the National Academy of Design. Under the leadership of Robert Henri and at the invitation of Arthur B. Davies, they held the first major independent exhibition of American art. It took place in 1908 at the Macbeth Gallery in New York. In 1910 the second no-jury show of contemporary American art took place at Club 291, so called because it was the address of Alfred Steiglitz's gallery on Fifth Avenue. But this was only warm-up. In 1913 the Association of American Painters and Sculptors held an International Exhibition of Modern Art at the 69th Regiment Armory located at Lexington Avenue and 25th Street in New York, the so-called Armory show.

The purpose of the Armory Show was to bring together European and American contemporary art, marking for the American public, as well as for the American artist who could not travel abroad, the "starting point of a new spirit in art, at least as far as American is concerned." Again Davies was one of the leaders, but this time he had the enthusiastic support and inexhaustible legwork of Walt Kuhn (1877-1949), who was not only responsible for garnering and shipping the European pieces, but who also plotted the advance publicity for the show with the professionalism of an impresario.

When the show was finally hung, more than 300 American artists, including all but one of The Eight, as well as Bellows, du Bois, Myers, and Kuhn himself, had contributed between 1200 and 1600 works. How successful was Kuhn's part in organizing the European portion of the show can be measured by the fact that despite the great number of Americans represented, it was the international section (largely French) that was the sensation. Included in retrospective were Cézanne, Gauguin, and van Gogh, seen until then by few Americans. Also included were the living artists, variously labeled Fauves, Cubists, and Moderns, and a painting that became immediately notorious: Marcel Duchamp's *Nude Descending a Staircase*.

How well the show met Kuhn's wish for a "new spirit in art" is still being discussed. Kuhn wrote at the time of making "the big wheel turn over both hemispheres." As for the spectators and viewers, one of the more

> *It is, in fact, not a static painting at all, but one in which the fruits have only paused in their tumbling…*

tolerant ones said: "The Cubists are entitled to the serious attention of all who find enjoyment in the colored puzzle pictures of Sunday Newspapers…There is no reason why people should not call themselves Cubists, or Octagonists, Parallelopipedonists, or Knights of the Isosceles Triangle, or Brothers of the Cosine, if they so desire" (Theodore Roosevelt, March 9, 1913). A professional critic, Kenyon Cox, commenting also on the international section, was sorry only that no Futurists had been included, so "that the whole thing might be done once for all. In a case of necessity," he continued, "one may be willing to take a drastic emetic and may even humbly thank the medical man for the efficacy of the dose…To have looked at it [the show] is to have passed through a pathological museum where the layman has no right to go. One feels that one has seen not an exhibition, but an exposure." Both Roosevelt and Cox, however, found the American artists far superior to the Europeans. As for the art-buying public, they did the expected: They began buying the Europeans, especially the French moderns. The French were "in"; American art was "out."

Meanwhile, Kuhn was undaunted. Nearing 40, with few sales, and with his wife Vera and daughter Brenda to support, he remained faithful to his painting, constantly studying, seeking, trying always to do "one fine painting." Not until 1929, when he was already past 50, did he write to Vera that he thought he had one, *The White Clown*. He did. In 1931 he painted *The Blue Clown*. It was another "fine painting." By now his many portrayals of clowns, acrobats, blowzy, tired show girls, and other circus people were not only becoming a kind of trademark, but were also finally winning him critical notice (but few sales), even causing him to be called "the American Toulouse-Lautrec."

But always Kuhn kept searching. During the 1930s, after a visit with Picasso in Paris, he wrote Vera that he had learned that Picasso "is just the opposite [way] for me to go." On the other hand, although he had not liked Cézanne's work when first he had seen it, he now began painting similar subjects in similar settings: apples on a cloth, a tub of potatoes, a loaf of bread and a knife. In another departure from his usual style, he also did a number of small paintings, perhaps as a matter of discipline, for, like the performing musician, the painter interprets with his muscles as well as with his intellect and emotions, and periodically muscles must be retrained. It was at the end of this period of small paintings that he did *Pumpkins*, a larger than 3 × 4-foot canvas. What a relief it was, he wrote to Vera, to return to the large canvases where he could "swing his arms" as he painted.

Kuhn was 64 years old when he did *Pumpkins*. Perhaps he chose the subject matter because pumpkins are more patient posers than acrobats. Or perhaps it was for the challenge of rendering the tonal values

Continued on p. 204

JAMA

THE JOURNAL of the American Medical Association

November 2, 1979

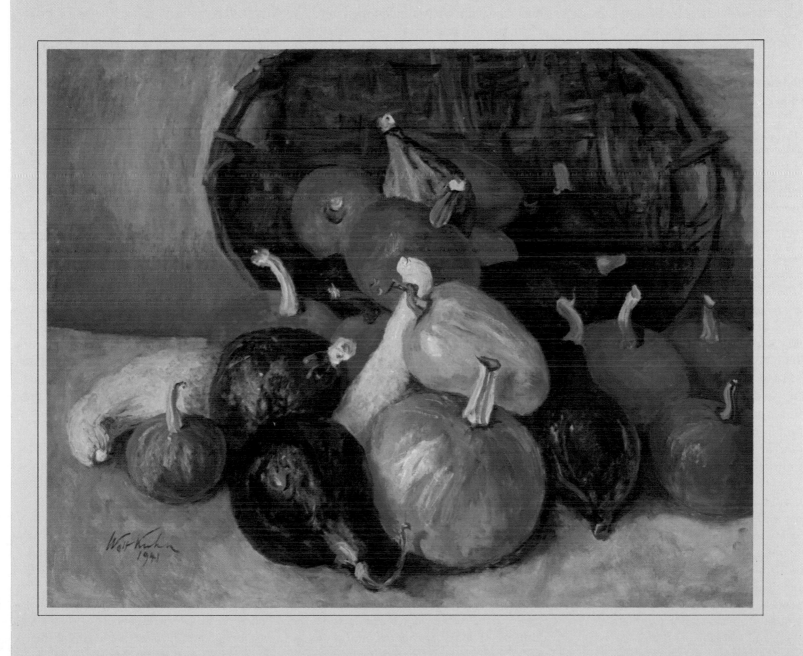

ALFRED SISLEY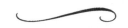

Early Snow at Louveciennes

For the people of Paris, the autumn of 1870 was a difficult time and but a prelude to an even more difficult winter and spring. France and Prussia were at war. Napoleon III had been taken prisoner at Sedan, and Paris was under siege. Not until May 1871 was a peace treaty signed, only to be followed by an insurrection that left 30,000 dead in a single "bloody week," as it was put down by Versailles government troops. Yet, if anything, this bloody birth of the Third Republic was in proportion to the new hope in the nation. "It is our reign coming," Zola wrote. Correct as he was, Zola's prophecy had at least another generation to wait for its fulfillment, even though the artists of whom he spoke had already been at least a decade on the scene.

Among the students at the studio of Gleyre in Paris in 1862 had been four young men, each studying there for vastly different reasons, ranging from parental rebellion to casual interest to avocation (one was studying medicine), but passionately united in a common reason: their refusal to go along with the "official" Salon style of painting. At 23, Alfred Sisley (1839-1899) was the oldest. Monet, Renoir, and Bazille were all 21 or 22 years old. These four may be said to be the earliest Impressionists, though it was to be some years before the style was fully developed and before they would call themselves such.

Meanwhile, however, the 1870-1871 war was having more immediate, physical effects on the group. Of the four who had entered the studio of Gleyre together, Monet fled to England, Renoir was drafted and nearly died of dysentery, and Bazille, often thought to be the most promising painter of them all, joined up, and was killed at Beaune-la-Rolande. Only Sisley, who was a British subject (his family was from the Romney Marsh area of Kent, but lived in Paris, where he had been born) was not affected by conscription. Ironically, it was into his life that the war brought the most sustained hardship.

Sisley was a serious painter, but as the son of a prosperous family, he had never been concerned about income from his work. The war, however, ruined the family finances, his father died, and Sisley found himself not only in need, but unschooled in any method of making a living, even to that of selling his paintings. Moreover, he had a wife and two children. Never again was he to be financially untroubled. When his work sold at all, it sold for less than that of his colleagues. Even today Sisley remains the least known, the least French, and among the lowest paid of the Impressionists.

> *Sisley's painting stops and even compresses time: past, present, and even future are seen as a single instant.*

Early Snow at Louveciennes is thought to have been painted in 1870. If so, then it corresponds to the autumn of the siege of Paris, which lay only some 15 kilometers away. Yet, except for the lone man in the center of the road (one of the Prussian soldiers billeted here?), and the snow, which portends a cruel winter for the Parisians, there could be no scene more innocent, more gentle, more commonplace—nor more reassuring. The town has been surprised by an overnight early snow, perhaps even the first snow. It is perhaps only mid-October, for the trees have been caught still wearing green and the women still in shawls. It is a little past midday, four hours until sunset, maybe. Two women are returning from town, where they have been marketing. They walk on the sunny side of the street, where the overnight snow has already melted. Farther on, other people in pairs disappear down the hill, toward the center of town.

Only the soldier has no companion. In the midground are the village houses, their roofs arranged in an intricate pattern of color determined by how the sun has touched them during the morning. The single, barely visible house surrounded by trees just beyond the fence on the right effectively balances the entire weight of the other houses in the left half of the painting. In the right foreground is a mosaic of earth, stone, snow, and grass—a cold corner where no sun either has or will reach that day. Meanwhile, the two halves of the painting are spanned by a bridge of trees whose tops are just touched by light. Not only do these trees unite the two halves of the painting; they also add length, steepness, and even mystery to the curving road, which would otherwise simply be cut off in midground. Above all is the sky, properly called a Sisley sky.

The Impressionists were often criticized for concentrating on color at the expense of composition. Not so Sisley. His color, subtle and understated, is only the skin of his painting. Beneath it lies a skeleton of curves and angles at once as graceful and as strong as one of Degas' ballet dancers. Remove the color, tease away the flesh, and *Early Snow at Louveciennes* is immediately seen as a skeleton of strong verticals (the women, the soldier, the facades of the houses, the chimneys, the poplars, the fence slats) crossed by less prominent horizontals (the fence top, the tops of the poplars, the eaves of the roofs, the flat-bottomed clouds, the soldier's belt). Stacked one against the other are the triangles of roofs and rectangles of shutters. From the lower right corner, above and below Sisley's signature, diagonal lines radiate to the opposite side, while superposed over all is a long, graceful curve that begins at the lower left, carries along the edge of the gutter, touches the soldier's head and the two figures just behind him, sweeps across the distant houses, cuts through the base of the chimney and the peak of the roof of the two centerground houses, and, finally,

Continued on p. 204

JAMA

THE JOURNAL of the American Medical Association

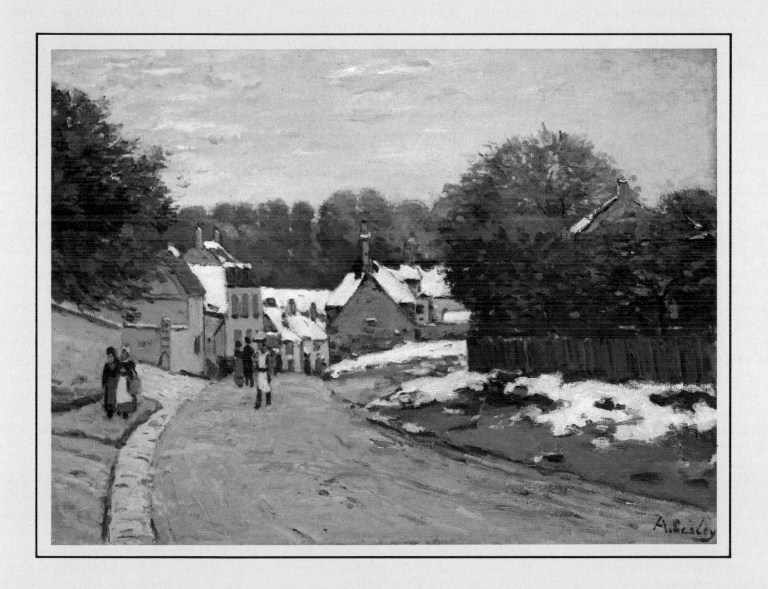

ÉDOUARD MANET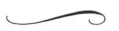

Flowers in a Crystal Vase

For the French painter of the 19th century success had but a single track, and that track passed unswervingly through the Salon. So called because the exhibitions had been originally held at the Salon Carré of the Louvre, this annual Exhibition of Living Artists, as it was officially known, soon grew to gigantic proportions. By the 1850s, the Salon had to be moved to the Champs-Elysées, where it was housed in the Palais de l'Industrie, a huge building that served as well for horse shows as for art shows.

Without question, the Salon was the event of the year. Thousands of paintings were viewed by tens of thousands of visitors. Newspaper coverage was extensive, critical, and often cruel. Careers, and fortunes, could be made. Old scores could be settled. Once each year, Parisians—rich, poor, or bour-geoise—could officially look at paintings and at each other. For the artist the Salon was a kind of annual olympiad, with strict entrance requirements, prizes consisting of various class medals, including the Grand Medal, the Grand Medal of Honor, and, not the least, sales, commissions, and, with a little help from the journalists, enough crit-ical acclaim and coverage for a financially assured future.

But the Salon could cut both ways. It was important, for example, that the paintings not jar the taste of the public, "None but true connoisseurs—all 60,000 of them!" said Daumier of the 1857 Salon. Further-more, the Salon was under the aegis of the French Academy, the "officialdom" of French painting, and the jury that selected the works for exhibition at the Salon each year was drawn from the Academy members. It was only realistic, therefore, to recognize that the Salon would suffer from all of the stigmas of such inbreeding, including the exclusion and even the ridicule of anything not in its own image. (Of the judges of the Salon of 1866 Zola said that his countrymen were so prudent that even to make a somer-sault in public, a man first must have been

examined and approved by the proper authorities. He also called the Salon an "*immense ragout*," prepared by 28 cooks and served up to a public with a delicate stomach in consideration of whom the pepper had been withheld and the wine watered.) Thus it was that a group of painters who were to be ridiculed (and immortalized) by the term "Impressionists" held their own separate independent exhibitions from 1874 to 1886. And thus it was that Édouard Manet (1832-1883), while also ridiculed by "officialdom," refused the invitation to exhibit with his Impressionist friends, instead stubbornly

> ## They do nothing; they simply are.

persisting in his belief that true success could come only from approval by the Salon. Annually, he died the death of public ridicule.

In a sense, this divided passion—to be true to his art and yet to be recognized by the Establishment—was Manet's private tragedy. Degas remarked that Manet had only one ambition, to be famous and to earn money, whereas he ought to have been satis-fied that he already had the appreciation of the elite, his fellow artists. (Ironically, at the Salon of 1865 Manet did finally hear himself being congratulated on two seascapes. Knowing that he had not submitted any seascapes, he rushed to the "M" room only to find that there were indeed two seascapes hung next to his own two entries, but that the artist was Claude Monet. His rage spent itself in depression when the critics con-tinued to praise Monet on these seascapes, which were his first entries to the Salon.) Still, Manet persisted. "The Salon is the real field of battle," he said. "It's there that one must take one's measure." Actually, Manet's ambition extended beyond Salon awards. He even entertained the possibility that one day

the French government might award him the Legion of Honor.

It was to be so. In 1882, when he was 51 years old, and when his lifelong friend Antonin Proust had become Minister of Fine Arts, Manet was finally named a Knight of the Legion of Honor. But for Manet it was 20 years too late. As far as he was concerned, it was a case of justice delayed being justice denied. Less than a year later, he died.

Flowers in a Crystal Vase (formerly *Still Life With Flowers*) is one of many similar paintings Manet did during that last year or so of his life. No longer wanting honors, or needing them, he turned, in a marked change of style, to painting the simple arrangements of roses, pinks, pansies, marigolds, bachelor buttons, and stock, often brought to him by his maid from the summer garden. Like their painter, who could conceal a great hurt beneath his dapper, almost dandified appearance, debonair manner, and witty speech (he is said to have been a master of the bon mot, as was Degas), these crystal vases of flowers also conceal much. Sometime in his mid-40s Manet began to have sharp, jabbing pains in his left foot. As they worsened over the next few years, Manet's illness was finally diag-nosed as "locomotor ataxia" (almost at the same time Fournier was publishing his work in Paris on the syphilitic origin of the disease, *l'ataxie locomotrice*).

But, as with the coveted red ribbon of the Legion, it was already many years too late. Manet's own physicians could do little more than advise him to rest and to take the waters. No longer able to stand before the large canvas, he turned increasingly to these small flower paintings for which he could remain seated. And where once he had painted elegant models in his studio, he now moved outdoors to the garden or painted the casual bouquets brought in by his maid.

Whatever his feelings may have been, or whatever pain Manet may have had, he kept to the discipline of his art. These last paint-

Continued on p. 204

JAMA

THE JOURNAL of the American Medical Association

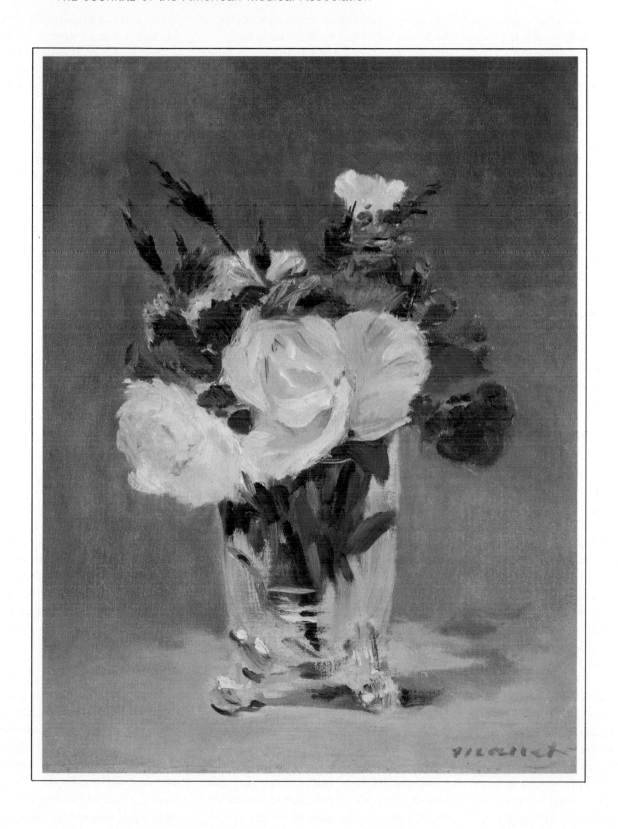

CAMILLE PISSARRO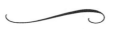

Orchard in Bloom, Louveciennes

The decade of the 1870s was the seed-time of Impressionism. Past were the chilly years of the 1860s when this small group of rebel painters had not only to survive public opinion, but had also to struggle to establish an identity. Then came the war of 1870, and the soil lay fallow for a while as the group dispersed, some to military duty and others to avoidance of conscription, either by traveling abroad or by hiding in the provinces. By 1872 most were back again, their ideas fertilized no doubt by the experiences just past. It is perhaps then that Impressionism first took recognizable form, although the movement was to receive its name only in 1874. By the end of the decade, the movement was already fading, and by the end of the 1880s, perhaps even as early as the mid-1880s, it had disappeared, having burst as suddenly as a blossom in spring and falling as soon, but leaving behind a fruit as sturdy as a chestnut.

Camille Pissarro (1830-1903) was born in the Danish West Indies of a Creole mother and a Sephardic father, studied briefly in Paris as a boy, and then, after unsuccessful attempts to accommodate himself to his father's hardware business in St Thomas, returned for good to Paris to pursue his first love, painting. He arrived in 1855, when the city, in the first flush of its intoxication with the new Empire, was celebrating its huge *Exposition Universelle*, a combined international show devoted to industry, commerce, and, for the first time, art. Even Victoria came, crossing the Channel to tour the exposition with Napoleon III as her escort. Pissarro was 25 years old.

Over the next 15 years, Pissarro was to study with Corot, to exhibit occasionally at the Salon, but more important, to begin painting with Monet, Cézanne, Renoir, Sisley, Bazille, and other future Impressionists. Like his colleagues, he had little commercial success or critical acclaim and, in 1869 to live more cheaply, moved to Louveciennes, a small village some 10 kilometers

from Paris noted chiefly for its aqueduct, which Louis XIV had built to carry water from nearby Marley to the fountains of his palace at Versailles. Renoir and Monet were also working in the area. Pissarro brought to Louveciennes a stock of some 1500 paintings done in the 15 years since his arrival in Paris and a son and a daughter, aged 6 and 4 years, the fruit of his liaison with Julie Vellay, who at one time had been his mother's maid.

In 1870 the Prussians occupied Louveciennes (see Sisley, *Early Snow at Louveciennes*), and Pissarro was forced to flee with his family to London. Although he was in

> *The year was at the morn;*
> *their world was*
> *dew-pearled.*

London for only ten months, returning to Louveciennes in June 1871, these months were decisive in his career and in Impressionism. It was here that he again met Monet, who had also fled, and together they saw for the first time the great landscapes of Turner and, more important, Constable. Furthermore, when Pissarro returned to his home that summer of 1871, he found not only that it was a shambles, but also that most of his oeuvre of 1500 paintings had been destroyed by the occupying army or were otherwise missing. A few days shy of his 41st birthday, with Julie now legally his wife and with the birth of a third child approaching, Pissarro had little choice but to begin again, and this he did. He did it, however, not in the sense of trying to replace what was lost, but with a sense of freedom from the past and an opportunity to try out new ideas.

Orchard in Bloom, Louveciennes was most likely done in 1872, a year that is considered pivotal in the development of Impressionism.

It was the end of Pissarro's first winter after his return from England. His tones are considerably lightened, and he has assimilated into his own experience what he had learned from the English, for whom landscape, as has been said, was a religion. The compositional format retains some of the classical elements, and the subject, some of the romanticism, even sentimentalism, of earlier French paintings; the execution, on the other hand, is unmistakably Impressionist.

The time is an early morn of early spring. Winter's chill rises from the freshly turned soil, but the sun, its reflection caught in the mauve at the horizon, has surprised this day in an April gown of blossoms. Two peasants, their blue, brown, and white clothes marking their kinship with the earth, till the soil. Their backs are bent to the earth, the woman to prepare the furrow, the man to sow the seed. Only a bird looks up to see the trees stretching their limbs in the sun as they offer blossoms to the sky.

The motif of the French peasant in a rustic landscape is a remnant of romanticism, even sentimentalism; so is the composition traditional. At the lower edge of the painting a path decisively marks off the right third from the left two-thirds of the painting. The eye travels into the picture along this path until it is stopped just short of the horizon by the hint of a curve to the right. From here we are directed to the figure of the man, then pulled by the strong horizontal shadow to the tree across the path and to the figure of the woman. Her globular form directs us to the globular tree above her, whence the eye travels across the top of the branches and down, as the line ends in the mauve haze of the sky directly above the path where we entered. Strong vertical lines are matched by equally strong horizontals, tempered by obliques. On the left these obliques lean from the vertical, whereas on the right they rise from the horizontal. More interesting, however, is the balance of weight and shapes on either side

Continued on p. 204

JAMA

THE JOURNAL of the American Medical Association

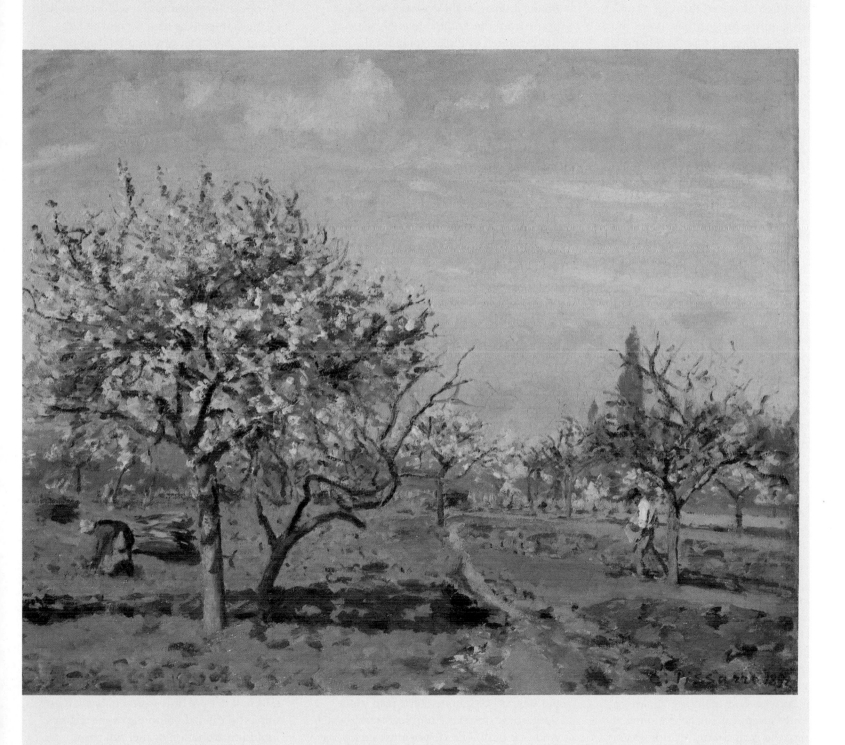

HENRY BACON

On Shipboard

The development of a young country can often be traced through its artists. The new country, for example, is not much given to art at all, except as the functional can also be beautiful. It is only later that the new people have time or inclination for paintings, and then they will want portraits, first of their country's heroes, later of its history. In time, the well-to-do will come to order portraits of themselves to leave to their descendants. Increased leisure time will parallel an increased appreciation of the land and a rise in painters who show its rivers, its seas, its waterfalls, its forests. Finally, when the country is prosperous, secure, and self-satisfied, we will see an increase in genre—paintings of fairly common, everyday scenes undistinguished by anything but the more or less personal interest of the artist, a kind of "painted snapshot." So it was with the Dutch of the 17th century, who perhaps brought genre to its peak. And so it was with the Americans of the 19th century as they neared their Centennial.

The latter half of 19th-century America abounded with genre painters, some well known—Eakins, Johnson, and Homer, and others lesser known—Quidor, Durrie, and Woodville. But the taste for native art developed far less slowly than did the number of painters, and many went abroad, not only to learn technique in Düsseldorf, Munich, and Paris, but to stay there permanently, as true expatriates. To this last group belongs Henry Bacon (1837-1912). A contemporary of Winslow Homer, he, too, was born in Massachusetts. Like Homer he also served at the front during the Civil War as an illustrator, but whereas Homer worked for *Harper's Weekly*, Bacon worked for *Leslie's Weekly*. Bacon was wounded in battle and in 1864 left for Paris to study painting. He was apparently successful, for he exhibited at several of the Paris Salons over the years from 1868 to 1895 (where, it has been noted, his paintings received favored hanging "on the line," ie, at eye level). A painting of a

Revolutionary War scene, *The Boys from Boston and General Gage*, won him high praise from the *Atlantic Monthly* when it was exhibited in Philadelphia for the nation's Centennial. Bacon, however, never returned home for any length of time, preferring to make Paris his base. From here he traveled widely, to Greece, Sicily, Ceylon, and Italy. The last ten years or so of his life were spent in Egypt, where, like Homer, who turned to watercolor in the last years of his life to capture the luminosity of the Maine sea, he turned to watercolor to capture the transparency of the Arabian desert.

> *For here is a moment in history, not only of the United States, but of the world: the passing from sail to steam…*

On Shipboard was painted in 1877, when Bacon was 40, perhaps from sketches made while he was on his way to Philadelphia for the Centennial, or perhaps on his way back to Paris or London. Whatever, he has graciously left the painting, as a genre painting should, to speak for itself. Some of what it has to say is obvious: A group of passengers pass the time on the afterdeck of an ocean liner. The sea is calm. Thick black smoke pours from the ship's funnels. The deck awning has been removed to allow whatever sun there may be to shine through. Tea, or morning bouillon, is just over. Some of the passengers play quoits, some read, some sleep, some observe. An officer stands watch. And that is all. The viewer must supply the rest. Are the passengers going to or coming from Europe? Or elsewhere? If they are going to America, will any one of them be

numbered among the more than 100,000 European immigrants that will pass through Castle Garden (the then version of Ellis Island)? And if any are immigrating to America, why? Who have they left behind? Are some well-to-do people returning from the Grand Tour? Where are their maids or other servants? Is the young woman on the bench ill or merely asleep, or could she be pregnant and the couple hoping to have their child in America? Who is the man with the red beard, and who are the two women with him? What is the relationship of the two women pitching quoits and the two men behind them? What are the two men in the background whispering about? And what of the woman in the deck chair? Is she ill, or asleep? Is the little girl waking her to ask permission for something, or is she anxious over her mother's health? Where is the husband or father? And what of the little boy? With whom is he traveling?

In these matters, Bacon has been deliberately provocative. But in his choice of subject, he has been less deliberative, perhaps even intuitive. Like the good journalist, he has chosen the significant moment, the one that contains history, much as he probably chose those battle scenes of the Civil War that best condensed the current situation. For here is a moment in history, not only of the United States, but of the world: the passing from sail to steam, from the inexhaustible but temperamental wind power to the dependable but limited resources of coal power. Even though by the 1870s transatlantic steamships had become fairly fast and relatively common (in the 1840s Samuel Cunard's steamships could cross the Atlantic in less than 15 days, while by the mid-1870s, improved technology in the form of ship design and building materials had cut the time to seven days), many ships still carried sail in the event engines should malfunction or fuel run short. Although it is doubtful that Bacon had the prescience to see the transatlantic crossings of 100 years hence and the power problems,

90

Continued on p. 205

JAMA

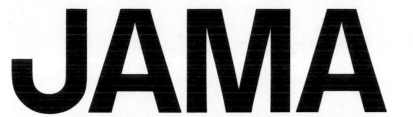

THE JOURNAL of the American Medical Association

April 11, 1980

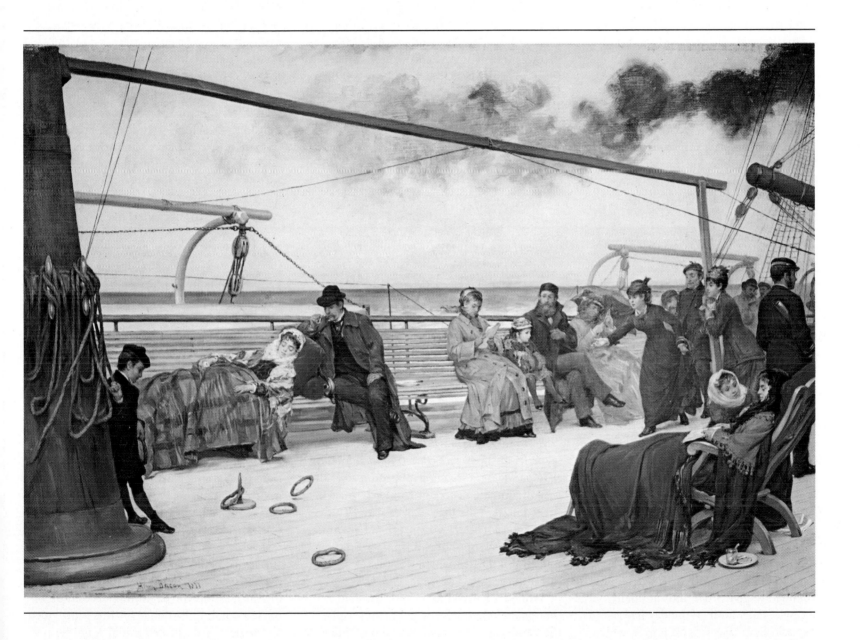

ARTIST UNKNOWN

Saint John Dictating to the Venerable Bede

The years between 400 and 1400 AD have been known commonly as the Dark Ages, so called because with the decline of the Roman Empire, Western civilization seemed to enter into a deep slumber that was to remain undisturbed for a thousand years. They have also been called the Middle Ages because these years represent the period between the two Roman civilizations: the disappearance of the first at the end of the fourth century and its renascence in a second great Roman period a millennium later. The latter is perhaps the more accurate of the two designations, for the period was anything but intellectually or artistically stagnant. It was, in fact, prelude to the Renaissance.

One of the most important developments in the intellectual life of the Middle Ages occurred at the beginning of the era: The scroll, or long continuous roll of papyrus, was replaced by the codex, which was made up of separate sheets of uniform size that could be bound together at one side, much as a present-day book. In addition, the delicate papyrus was replaced by sheets of veal skin (vellum) or sheepskin (parchment). Not only were these animal materials more durable, thus ensuring dissemination and preservation of the manuscripts, but the skin surfaces were more suitable for painting.

At the same time, in a quite separate development, there arose the great monastic systems, the first among them in the West being the Benedictines, founded in the early sixth century. The instructions or "Rule" formulated by St Benedict for these groups of monks living in community was strict and was intended to give order and rationality to their lives. Each hour of the day had its specific task. Emphasis was on prayer, which included reading, study, meditation, contemplation (and by extension, writing), and manual work, which included not only agriculture and building, but arts, handicrafts, and the copying of manuscripts. The last was done usually by many monks, working in large communal writing rooms, or scriptoria. Often, the manuscripts were illuminated, ie, decorated with intricate patterns that filled the border or formed an initial letter. Sometimes the entire page was carpeted with design. The colors were often rich, with gold and silver freely used. Small pictures (miniatures), which could range from an elaborately drawn and colored life history to a simple, often even crudely drawn sketch, were also part of the manuscript. Within the scriptorium the division of labor and the duties of each monk were as clearly defined as were the hours of the day and the

> *...it is the writing itself that is important and not Bede, except as an instrument for recording.*

duties proper to each: painting was done by *miniatores*, calligraphy by *antiquarri* (masters) and *scriptores* (assistants), while the *rubricatores* did the initials.

Saint John Dictating to the Venerable Bede is the frontispiece to Bede's *Commentary on the Apocalypse*, a manuscript produced at the Benedictine monastery in Lambach, Austria (near Linz), in the mid-12th century. The Lambach monastery was just then becoming noted for its school of painting, writing, music, and theater, which was to survive into the 17th century.

While far less elaborate and "finished" than many other illuminated manuscripts, the Lambach leaf nevertheless shows many features of its Romanesque period, features that were perhaps even incorporated into a "rule" for scribes. For example, the disparity in the size of the two figures clearly indicates who is on earth and who is speaking from Heaven. St John is also identified by his attribute, the island of Patmos, on which he sits. The letters above his head also identify him: Ioh[anne]s, not to mention the halo and the pointing index finger that signifies his teaching authority. The divine inspiration of John as author of the Apocalypse, or Book of Revelation, is signified by the divinely haloed dove, which represents the Holy Spirit, descending from a cloud. The arch and towers are a primitive rendition of church architecture of the time and signify that John's teaching is under the protection of the Church. Bede and his writings, meanwhile, are also within the Church, but his earthly status is indicated by his smaller size, lower placement, and the word "[B]ed[e]" (partially erased) above his head. Most interesting, however, is the disproportionate size of the instruments for recording the dictation: Bede's hands, the feather quill, the knife, the ink horn. It is clear that it is the writing itself that is important and not Bede, except as an instrument for recording. Thus, while the visual proportion and order we have become accustomed to is not yet known in the 12th century, the artist has nevertheless maintained a definite order and hierarchy of values; it is, however, an inner proportion and not one that the eye can perceive or measure.

The linear style and symmetrical and rigid folds of the garments help place this manuscript at the end of the Romanesque period, just as it begins to merge with the Gothic. According to the catalogue notes from the National Gallery of Art, the clumsily applied green and yellow were most likely added at a later time by another illuminator, as was the beginning decoration of the left column. Evidence for this is provided by the heavily decorated initial A on the reverse (the ornate green pyramidal shape that shows through the vellum), whose style belongs to a later period. The vellum itself is heavily soiled and has many worm holes. Close inspection of the left border will show a series of "pinpricks" along the entire length.

Continued on p. 205

JAMA

THE JOURNAL of the American Medical Association

April 18, 1980

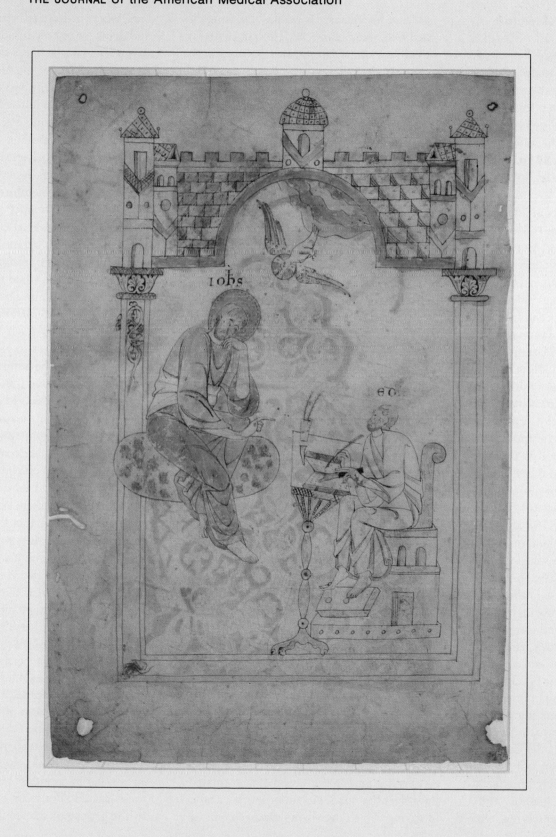

MAURICE UTRILLO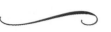

Rue Cortot, Montmartre

Any account of the life of Maurice Utrillo (1883-1955) must perforce be only a sketch, for the verifiable facts are as scarce as the people along the streets of his Montmartre paintings. On the other hand, the legends that have sprouted from the life of this man are as tangled and twisted and as intoxicating as the fruit of the vineyard of *la Butte*, as Montmartre is locally known. One gets the impression that the legends were not left entirely uncultivated.

Be that as it may, the facts are these: Maurice, born December 26, 1883, rue de Poteau, Montmartre. Mother, Marie-Clémentine Valadon, 17-year-old street gamine, one-time circus acrobat, then artist's model, later to be the famous painter, Suzanne Valadon. Father, unknown. Grandmother, Madeleine-Céline Valadon, Limousin peasant turned Montmartre laundress. Grandfather, unknown. Schooling, scant; excelled at arithmetic only. As a boy, highly strung, nervous, uncommunicative; considerably calmed by the *chabrol* (soup laced with wine) given him by his grandmother, after the fashion of the Limousin peasants. By age 10, drinking freely in the Montmartre bistros. At age 18, the first of more than a dozen admissions to psychiatric hospitals, clinics, even lunatic asylums, for alcoholism. At first relapse, physician friend of mother urges occupational therapy; suggests painting because Utrillo's mother paints. For the next 20 years, his life a round of painting, bistros, hospitals, violent scenes, growing fame, and arrests until, after jailing for a morals charge in 1921, he is released into the perpetual custodial care of his mother and a nurse-bodyguard. In 1935, with his popularity at its height, and himself a knight of the Legion of Honor, but his genius bursting into only occasional flickers, he marries the widow Pauwels, who becomes not only his wife, but his keeper, business manager, and Joan of Arc. He is reduced to painting his streets, bistros, and churches from memory and from picture postcards, for he is not allowed

to leave his villa. He is wealthy. Suzanne dies in 1938, Maurice in 1955. He is buried in the Cemetery of St Vincent, after 30 years in the chateaus and villas of his mother and wife, back home on the Butte, in the shadow of the dome of Sacré-Coeur, a stone's throw from his studio in the rue Cortot, across the street from the famous vineyard of Montmartre, and within easy walking distance of all his favorite bistros.

The legends that have grown up around Utrillo, *la légende d'Utrillo*, are less easy to contain. For example, at the time of his birth, his mother was living with a journalist

> *…the painting is brutal in the way it pulls in the viewer's eye and then bounces it from wall to wall…*

named Boissy. She was also an artist's model for Puvis de Chavannes, and later for Toulouse-Lautrec (who gave her the name Suzanne), Renoir, and Degas (who called her "terrific Maria" and was so impressed with her talent that he gave her a few drawing lessons, the only she ever had). All have been mentioned at one time or another as Maurice's father. Suzanne never said. Perhaps she never knew. The man considered least likely is the Spanish architect and art critic, Miguel Utrillo y Molins, who, when Maurice was 7 years old, officially gave him his name. It is interesting that Utrillo signed his canvases in the Spanish fashion, "Maurice Utrillo, Valadon," later simplifying it to "Maurice Utrillo. V." The rest of Utrillo's youth and life until age 40 is lost among the streets of Montmartre, in absinthe mists, violent outbursts, a suicide attempt, in strange living arrangements in

bars, where he bartered paintings for lodging and drink, or in households in the rue Cortot that would consist of his grandmother, his mother, her lover of the moment (who at one time was also his best friend and three years younger than himself), and in behavior that included extreme possessiveness toward his grandmother, mother, the Virgin Mary, and Joan of Arc, with a fear equally extreme of pregnant women (it is reported that he would try to kick them in the belly).

Rue Cortot, Montmartre, which looks up the street where he lived at No. 12, was painted at the very beginning of what is considered Utrillo's "best period," the years from 1909 to 1914, when he was in his late 20s. He had no training beyond that which his mother, herself untrained, gave him, and his palette remains much as the first one she gave him: two reds, two yellows, and zinc white, except for the addition of a blue. Much as his boyhood mind had been at ease only in the defined world of arithmetic, his adult vision is rigidly geometric. He composed his scenes with straightedge, T square, and compass, and he drew his lines with a ruler. He painted on cardboard because canvas was too rigid. And he applied his pigments with a palette knife, building up an impasto so thick that the lumps of paint began to resemble the stones themselves. Sometimes the pigment was so heavy that it looked like he had laid it on with a trowel. Indeed, when he wished a truly realistic effect, he would scrape plaster from the walls of real houses, mix it with a zinc white, and build his palette houses. Some say he was influenced by Sisley, perhaps in the diagonal street that always leads into the distance. Others say he resembles Pissarro, perhaps in the twisted trees. Most often he is considered to have no forebears.

Rue Cortot, Montmartre is unlike the serene, creamy, linear paintings of churches so familiar in countless reproductions. Here there is a seething color, barely constrained by the geometric shapes. The broad strokes

Continued on p. 205

JAMA

THE JOURNAL of the American Medical Association

April 25, 1980

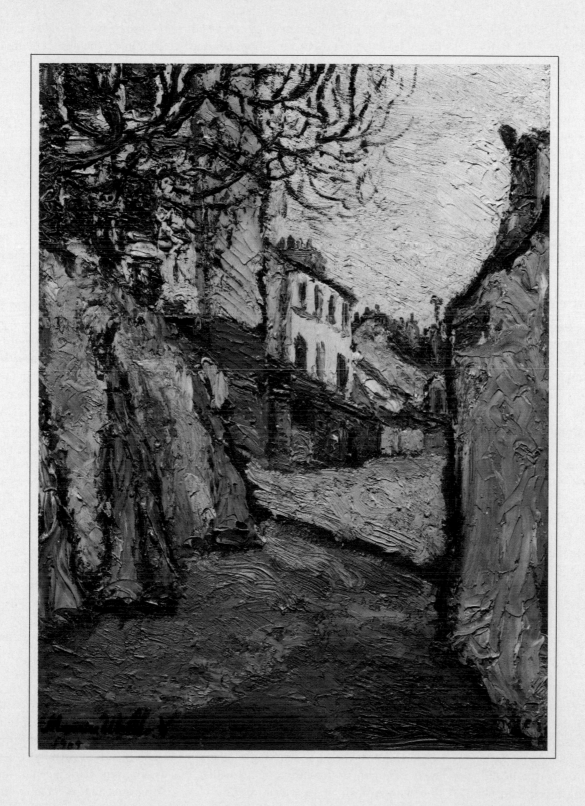

SIR WILLIAM BEECHEY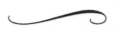

The Oddie Children

Until the 18th century, England was forced to import her portrait painters: Holbein from Basel (for Henry VIII), Gentileschi from Italy, Rubens and Van Dyck from Antwerp (all for Charles I), Lelay from Haarlem (for Charles II). But in the mid-18th century, a trio of painters emerged who themselves were not only native, but also who made the art of portrait painting the English art. These three—Gainsborough, Romney, and Reynolds—so dominated the field that the names of their immediate successors, artists such as Northcote, Opie, and Lawrence, are often overlooked. It is to this second tier of portrait artists, who belong to the last quarter of the 18th century, that Sir William Beechey (1753-1839) also belongs.

Beechey was born in Burford, Oxfordshire. Some accounts have him beginning his career as a house painter, others as being articled to a solicitor in Gloucestershire. However he began, he soon transferred to a solicitor in London, but there discovered the fine arts, was released from his law apprenticeship, and entered the Royal Academy as a student. He was 18 years old. Three years later he exhibited some small portraits. From then on his progress was steadily upward. His first life-sized portraits appeared before he was 30, and he was elected to one of the 20 associate memberships of the Royal Academy before he was 40; the same year, 1793, he was appointed Her Majesty Queen Charlotte's portrait painter after he had done a portrait of her. Five years later when he painted a large equestrian portrait of George III and two of his sons, the prince of Wales and the duke of York, he was knighted and also elected to full membership in the Academy. He was also to do for the king full-length portraits of all the royal family, for the prince of Wales, the portraits of his sisters, and for Queen Charlotte, the complete decoration of a room in the royal lodge at Frogmore. With so distinct a royal favor, he did not want for portrait commissions of other distinguished people during a long career.

Of his personal life there is little of record, except that he was married twice and had at least three sons, two of whom became painters. The art gossip has it, as one biographer notes, that he "did not abstain from the thoughtless use of unmeaning oaths" and that as he grew older, he bemoaned the "increasing sobriety and decreasing conviviality" of the art world, artists and patrons alike. He especially lamented the days when a party did not break up until at least one duke and one painter had drunk themselves under the table.

The Oddie Children, which Beechey did when he was in his mid-30s, shows, in life-size, Henry, Jane, Sara, and Catherine, the

> *…the ageless charm that is a child's by birthright…*

son and daughters of Henry Hoyle Oddie, a London solicitor, and Mrs Oddie. Since this portrait predates his royal commissions, it is interesting to speculate that the commission may have come through ties he still maintained from his early days of law study in London. On the other hand, he did not want for distinguished sitters. His account book for the year 1789 shows 49 commissions, including numerous lords and ladies, dukes, earls, two captains, a bishop, and a "Dr.," along with many untitled sitters. For this, the Oddie entry, which was paid in full, he charged £84 (as against £5 5s for small single subject portraits, £10 10s for large portraits, to a top price of £105 for Dr Strachey).

In *The Oddie Children* Beechey's skillful blending of the many artifices of line, composition, and color demonstrates his prowess at portraiture. The three standing children form a roughly triangular grouping, with the oldest girl widely separated from the other two. Coherence is established by the youngest child, who bridges what could otherwise be two unrelated groups of figures. Moreover, the other children gaze off at something beyond the right of the painting, quite eliminating the viewer from any visual dialogue, but in sharp contrast, the youngest gazes directly at us with frank, open curiosity. There is no resisting her invitation to enter the picture. From here the eye is swept upward around the arch of the bow (which, if extended, would turn the boy-girl figure into a separate three-quarter portrait enclosed in a circular frame), down the left and across the arch of the hem of the little girl's dress, the circle of the boy's hat, to the similar hem of the oldest girl's dress, up to the oval of her hat, and, finally, to her face, which is not only the logical resting place for the viewer's eye, but is in itself arresting in the very detail and strength with which it is finished in comparison with the faces of the other children. This is, in fact, no longer the face of a child. It is the face of a young girl, composed, calm, and already adept at the art of keeping her own counsel, a subtle foil to the open look of the baby. Her separateness from the trio is confirmed by her placement not only apart from the solid group of three at the left, but at the very edge of the pool of light, her dress already entering into shadow.

Beechey demonstrates his virtuosity in other ways as well. Fair heads are placed against dark trees, the dark head against the pale sky. Facial poses pass from three-quarter to full to silhouette. Body postures alike cover the gamut. Curved lines echo and re-echo each other across the canvas, like spreading circles on the surface of a pond; straight lines find parallels or point out perpendiculars. And colors are skillfully chosen to progress across the canvas in the same order they hold in the spectrum. Beginning at the right, the blue of the girl's hat and sash blends in the blue-green of the baby's sash, to the dark green of the boy's suit. The deep green is repeated in his hat, the inside of which is accented by a patch of rose, itself

Continued on p. 205

JAMA

THE JOURNAL of the American Medical Association

May 2, 1980

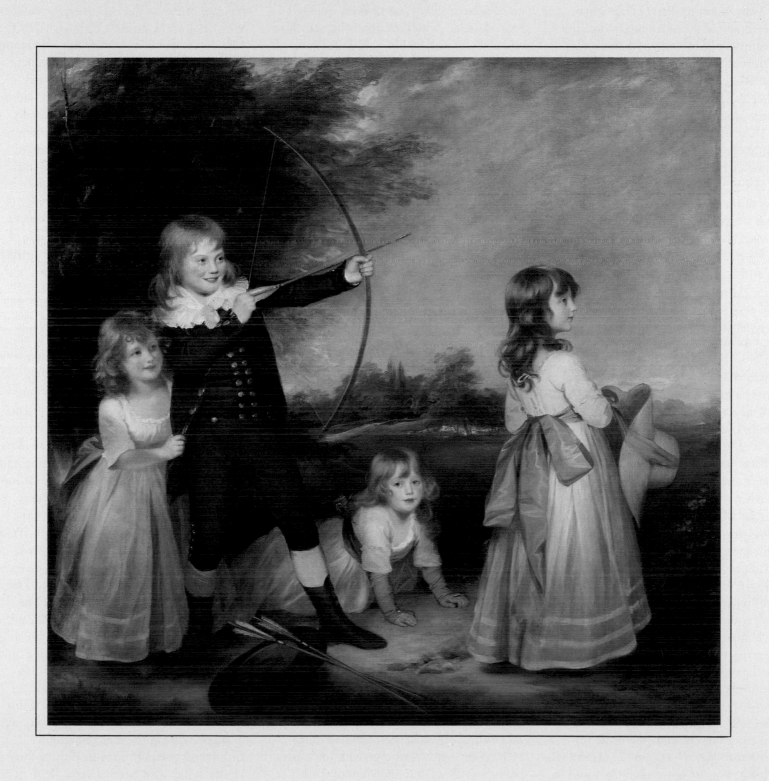

PIERRE AUGUSTE RENOIR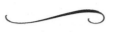

Still Life With Bouquet

For France, and for Paris in particular, the decade of the 1870s began on a less-than-promising note. The 1860s had ended on the upbeat, with the mingling of cultures, East and West, at the Paris World's Fair of 1867. The Salons were still "the" art event of the year, and Paris was prosperous. Then, in July 1870, France "lightheartedly," in the words of its premier, declared war on Prussia. It was not a lengthy war. Less than two months later, Napoleon III had been taken prisoner at the battle of Sedan, and Paris had been laid siege. Only after four months of cold, disease, hunger (Manet wrote that the people were eating not only horse meat and donkey meat, which were very expensive, but also cats, dogs, and rats), and, finally, artillery bombardment, did Paris surrender. But more was to come. Six weeks later, in March 1871, a citizen uprising took place, which was suppressed only during the "bloody week" in May when 30,000 lives were lost. Still, Zola could proclaim to his friend Cézanne that their [own] reign was coming and Puvis de Chavannes could pose a young nude against a scarred landscape, put a flowering branch in her hand, and call the painting *Hope*. Zola and Puvis were not idle dreamers. It was indeed a hope that was to be realized, especially in the world of art, but it came only from lives drastically altered by the war.

Of the group, who were only later to be called "Impressionist," Pissarro, who was 40 years old, and Monet, who was 29, both went to England (although without either knowing at the time about the other), Monet leaving behind the wife he had just married, and Pissarro marrying while in England, each to the mothers of their children. In London they saw the great canvases of Turner, which perhaps deepened their own concepts of light, but, more important, they met the art dealer Durand-Ruel who from then on was to play a large part in obtaining commissions for the group. Pissarro also lost most of his oeuvre of 15 years to the occupying soldiers in France. Cézanne, now 30

years old, was living and working quietly near Marseilles with his future wife, somehow managing to conceal both his draft status and his irregular household arrangements from the military authorities and from his tyrannical father, respectively. Sisley, not a French subject, was exempt from the draft, but remained in France. Heretofore comfortably well-off, with a wife and children, he suddenly found himself, at the age of 31, penniless and without work skills when his inheritance was lost during the war. Bazille, thought by some of his colleagues to be the most promising of all, quickly enlisted in the

> *The color, on the other hand, is a feast, like all of Renoir's work.*

hard-fighting Zouaves at war's outbreak and was killed at Beaune-la-Rolande four months later. He was a few days shy of his 29th birthday. And (Pierre) Auguste Renoir (1841-1919), who, like Monet, was also 29, was offered preferential war duty but waited to be inducted and was sent to the Pyrenees to train horses, a task for which he had never shown any particular aptitude. Here he also apparently acquired near-fatal dysentery, being saved only by the intervention of an uncle who had him moved to Bordeaux.

However, besides the war and its effect on these lives, other influences were shaping French painting. In 1855 at the Paris World's Fair, Japanese colored prints appeared for the first time in Europe, probably brought in by Dutch merchants, who had always remained in the Nagasaki area even after other Europeans had been expelled in the 17th century. Now, however, with the general reopening of Japan to the Western world (Commodore Perry went from the United States in 1853), all things Japanese became

the rage of Paris (and also of England, where Whistler was the greatest enthusiast). By the 1870s French painters commonly kept among their studio props such things as Japanese fans, vases, boxes, even gowns, and they appear frequently in their paintings. "Japonisme" was the word coined in 1872 by art critic Philippe Burty for this phenomenon. Other effects of the Japanese prints manifested themselves in the use of color and line, the flatness of planes, the angle of viewing, and in the organization of space. Degas, for example, often left large, empty spaces of stage in front of or to the side of his ballet dancers. For Renoir, it was perhaps the color and asymmetry that he liked best in Japanese prints: color, because it had always been his first love, asymmetry, because it confirmed his horror of "regularity" in a painting, as he termed it.

Still Life With Bouquet, while showing some of the borrowings from Japanese prints, such as the color, the obvious "props," and even the asymmetry, is not typical of Renoir's usual subjects: nudes, landscapes, dancing parties, flesh, filtered light, sun and shadow. There is a curious "feel" to the painting and the date (1871) suggests that perhaps it was done during the period of convalescence from his dysentery when he did not have access to his usual models and friends. There is about it the atmosphere of a cluttered, stuffy room, too long left unvisited, except for the telltale fresh bouquet of flowers left casually on a table already crowded. The color, on the other hand, is a feast, like all of Renoir's work. The colors of the fan and the bouquet reflect each other: the one bold, vivid, direct, Western; the other delicate, fragile, the colors hinting, rather than stating, Eastern. More curious is the unfinished painting on the wall, meant no doubt to suggest one of the many horizontal regimental portraits done in 17th-century Holland, the most famous being Rembrandt's *Nightwatch*. Perhaps it reflects the Dutch-Japanese connection, perhaps not.

Continued on p. 206

JAMA

THE JOURNAL OF the American Medical Association

July 11, 1980

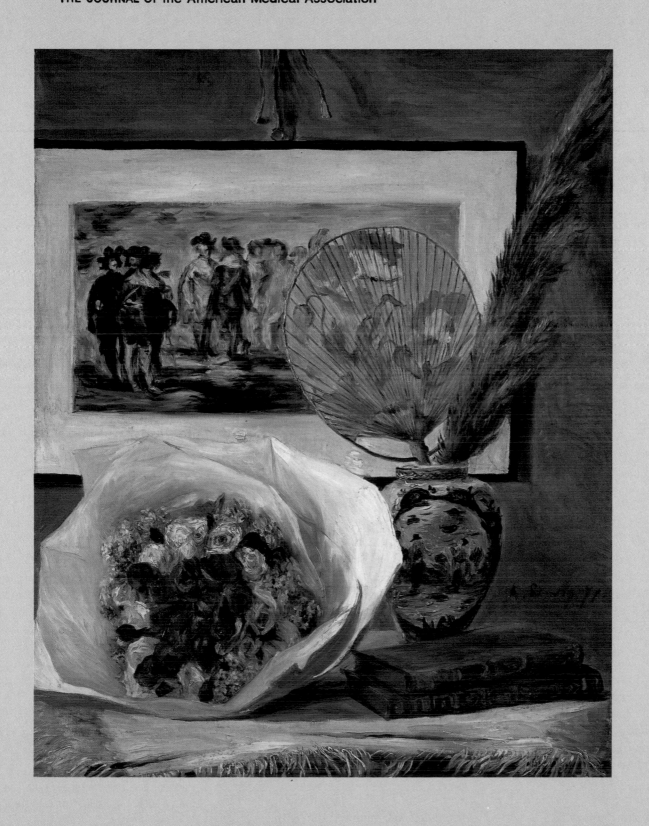

GUSTAV KLIMT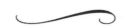

Baby (Cradle)

For all its reputed gaiety, *gemütlichkeit*, and general aura of amiability, turn-of-the-century Vienna was not the most forgiving father for certain of its native sons. Mahler, for example, who had just completed his fourth symphony, had to go outside the country to earn a living; Freud, with publication of *The Interpretation of Dreams* in 1900, and his theories of infant sexuality, met with the greatest resistance from his own colleagues; and Gustav Klimt (1862-1918), who had been commissioned to do the ceiling paintings for the Faculties of Philosophy, Medicine, and Jurisprudence at the University of Vienna, scandalized the burghers when the first, *Philosophy*, was shown in 1900. When *Medicine* was shown the following year, a parliamentary investigation of Klimt was begun, and, finally, in 1905, Klimt bought back the paintings for all three Faculties from the government, and the ceiling commission was withdrawn. (Disastrously, the paintings were lost in 1945, when the retreating armies set fire to the castle in Austria in which the paintings had been stored.)

The second of seven children, son of a goldsmith, Klimt studied art, and later worked, with his younger brother Ernst. Together they did decorative work on important commissions in Vienna, including the spandrels and panels on the stairway of the Kunsthistorisches Museum. In 1892 Ernst, not yet 30 years old, died, and two years later, in 1894, Klimt's father died also. Doubai, Klimt's principal biographer, observes that from the mid-1890s on, male portraits disappear from Klimt's work. His mother, who was the subject of several of his drawings, was mentally ill and died insane. Klimt never married, but lived, apparently happily, with Emilie Flöge, a Viennese couturière and sister of his brother Ernst's wife, for some 27 years. Shy, reticent, and not much given to either reading or expressing himself in writing, Klimt was still often flamboyant and provocative, throwing his colorful behavior over his private life like a protective patchwork comforter.

Like his life, Klimt's work, especially that of his last 20 years, is veiled and hard to get at. Heavily influenced by van Gogh and by the Symbolists, he is called the Viennese master of the Art Nouveau style, a term borrowed from the French to describe the "new art" style that took as its model prodigal nature, in all its profusion of writhing, serpentine forms. Klimt applied the style not only as flat decorations as it was originally intended, but incorporated the ideas into his figure and landscape paintings as well. Thus, his women are characterized by nervous, frizzy hair, his flowers by nervous, serpentine

> *What had begun as a classical symphony switches into ragtime.*

tendrils. At other times he encases his women in rigid gold mosaics of Byzantine design that become an integral part of the background, or he carpets his landscapes with color, obliterating even the horizon line. Sometimes, as in *Baby (Cradle)*, he seems to have begun a painting in the traditional manner but then doodled his way down and across the canvas in a kind of visual stream of consciousness, much like the painted thoughts of a Buck Mulligan—a regular Rorschach of color. Always, however, there is ambivalence, tension, and a powerful sexuality. Some of his work is frankly erotic. Asked once, toward the end of his life, to describe himself, he made a quick sketch of a bearded, balding man and titled it *Self-portrait as Genitalia*.

Baby (Cradle) was one of the paintings Klimt was working on at the time of his sudden death (from apoplexy) in Vienna at age 55. Here again, the "tension of ambivalence" is felt. Certain elements of the painting are traditional, or conventional: the bal-

looning, pyramidal shape, for instance, is almost Renaissance in its stability; the baby is also conventional, its sweet face and raised chubby fist approaching schmaltz. The baby's head rests on a round, pink, ruffled pillow, which is set off against a blue, rectangular, smooth-textured pillow, tipped at the opposite angle. But then everything changes direction and tempo. What had begun as a classical symphony switches into ragtime. The modeled, three-dimensional head of the baby leads into a flat, two-dimensional quilt; the overall pyramidal shape becomes distorted, even grotesque; the delicate tints of baby pink move into vivid, even harsh, patches of color; and what had begun as regular, geometric forms of the baby's head and pillow now become a Gordian design of irregular shapes, curlicues, and twisting Medusoid forms. Even the shape of the canvas contributes to the tension and the ambiguity. The square can imply unlimited potential in all directions. Or the lack of clear dominance of one dimension over the other can mean a paralyzing ambivalence. The subject, too, carries us in more than one direction, for who can read from the painting what the sex of the infant is?

Klimt's paintings are like dreams. They bear endless looking at and analysis. Like dreams, their parts—colors, shapes—are changeable, one form freely becoming another, not as logic or chronology dictate, but according to the context and need of the viewer. The line does not define a shape as much as it suggests another. Looked at, thought about, turned over in the mind, the paintings sometimes, like the dreams of Freud's Vienna, give back quite startling revelations.

JAMA

THE JOURNAL of the American Medical Association

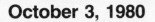

October 3, 1980

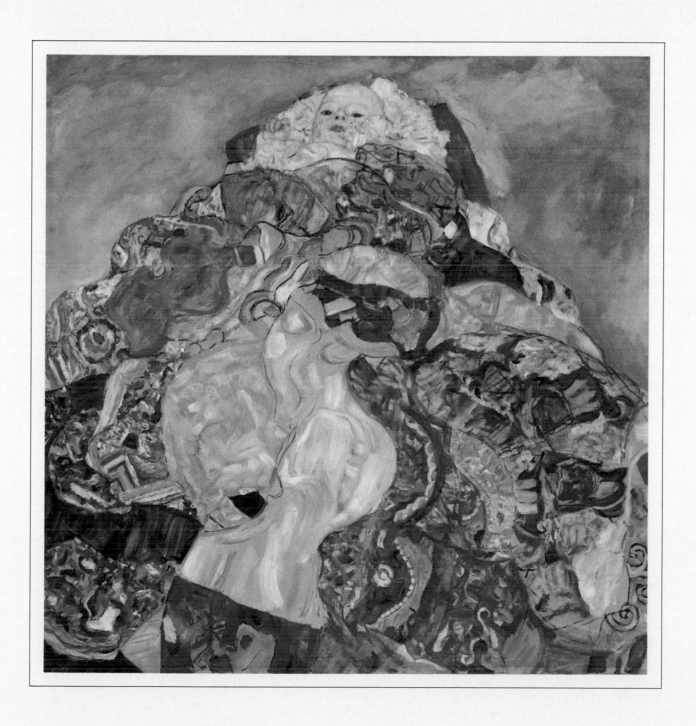

ÉDOUARD MANET

The Plum

A favorite gathering place for the offbeat artists, writers, and intellectuals of 19th-century Paris was the café. Here they could meet for drink, companionship, and warmth, and test new theories, argue, or simply replenish creative stores. In the early 1870s the Café Guerbois on the Grande rue des Batignolles was the favorite of the Impressionists. It was here that Édouard Manet (1832-1883) also came; although not an Impressionist himself, he was the natural leader of the Batignolles group and also a great influence on Impressionism. Later, many of the "Batignolles" moved to the Café de la Nouvelle-Athènes on the quieter place Pigalle, where two of the marble-topped tables in the right-hand corner were reserved for Manet, Degas, Renoir, and others who came less regularly. The chief attraction of the café was a huge dead rat painted on the ceiling.

The Plum shows one of Manet's models at the Café de la Nouvelle-Athènes in the late 1870s. The lines are simple and strong; the mood is powerful. The young woman sits alone, lonely, and forgetful of her brandied plum and her unlit cigarette. But as the poet says:

"...she saw the world as it is—make-shift, full of endless detail."

She was not always so.
In fact, just this morning,
waking up between grey sheets,
she saw the world as it is—
make-shift, full of endless detail.

After the first drink
her blood began to hazard the rapids;
she combed her hair.

After the second drink she could say,
to nobody in particular:
"Shall I wear the bombazine or
peau de soie? And which
of my hundreds of bonnets?"

After the third drink
she chose the black straw
and made her way carefully down the stairs
with their carpet of monstrous roses,
through beveled-glass doors and out
into the street.

It was Paris in the '70s.
There was still too much of everything.
She winced at the light
and turned toward a café.

After the anisette
she will permit us to find her,
dreaming over a plum in a glass dish.

JAMA

December 12, 1980

THE JOURNAL of the American Medical Association

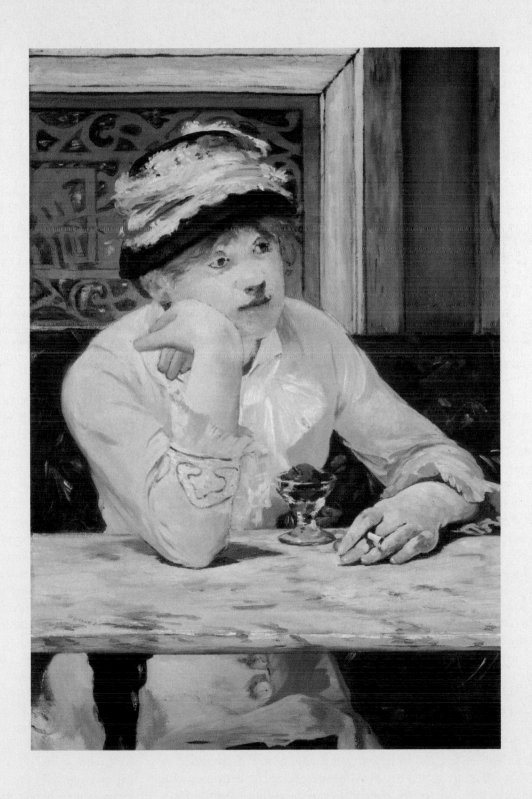

CHARLES DEMUTH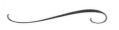

The Figure 5 in Gold

During the years surrounding World War I, William Carlos Williams, newly married and establishing a family, was setting up his medical practice in Rutherford, New Jersey. Three days a week he went into New York City for pediatric clinics, first at Babies' Hospital and, later, at Post Graduate Clinic. He also continued to write plays, poetry, and criticism—even to paint occasionally. One hot day in July, as he relates in his *Autobiography*, he was coming back, exhausted, from the Post Graduate and stopped at the studio of his friend, the painter Marsden Hartley, on 15th Street for some tea and some talk before returning to Rutherford. But as he approached his friend's house, he heard "a great clatter of bells and the roar of a fire engine passing the end of the street down Ninth Avenue." He turned "just in time to see a golden figure 5 on a red background flash by." So forceful was this impression that he was compelled, there, on the spot, to take a piece of paper out of his pocket and write a poem about the event. It was called "The Great Figure," and began, "Among the rain/and lights/I saw the figure 5 in gold." Years later, much as a musician might have set the words to music, another artist friend, Charles Demuth (1883-1935), was to paint this poem. It was one of several *hommages*, or poster portraits, Demuth did of his friends (among them Eugene O'Neill, Gertrude Stein, Georgia O'Keeffe, Arthur Dove, and John Marin) in the late 1920s in which he used abstract design to describe them and their work. For his part, Williams had earlier dedicated one of his collections of poems, *Spring and All*, to Demuth and later was to write the poem "The Crimson Cyclamen" in his memory.

In 1928, when *The Figure 5 in Gold* was painted, Demuth and Williams, both now in their mid-40s, had an established friendship dating back to their student days in 1904. As Williams recalls in his *Autobiography*, their lifelong friendship was formed "on the spot," when Williams, a medical student at the University of Pennsylvania, met "over a dish of prunes at Mrs Chain's boarding house on Locust Street," where both were then living. Demuth was "a wisp of a man: he was lame, tuberculous, with the same sort of chin as Robert Louis Stevenson and long, slender fingers. He had an evasive way of looking aslant at the ground or up at the ceiling when addressing you, followed by short, intense looks of inquiry." As Williams recalled in a later interview, Demuth had a "habit of hiding his thoughts, so that his close friends scarcely knew him."

...the painting has sound and rhythm the same as a poem or a fire engine has sound and rhythm.

Demuth was born in the Plain-sect town of Lancaster, Pennsylvania, the only child of Ferdinand and Augusta. It was the sort of town where "people almost never cross streets against traffic signals." The Demuth household discipline was such that Augusta regularly did her own marketing at the Mennonite market before six in the morning so as to be assured of the freshest greens. The Demuths, a family of tobacconists, had been in Lancaster for five generations and had lived at the same address since 1800. Except for his studies and his later periodic "debauches" when he would go off to Paris, New York, or Provincetown, Charles Demuth lived there with his mother (his father had died in 1911, when Charles was 27) until his own sudden death in 1935.

Like Toulouse-Lautrec, whom he greatly admired, Demuth was lame, possibly from a hip injury at the age of 4, or from tuberculosis, as Williams believed; nevertheless, with the help of his cane, which he carried with such flair that his friends were never sure if it was essential or accessory, he managed to make the infirmity part of his general aura of charm, elegance, gentleness, and mystery. In 1920 Demuth was discovered to have diabetes mellitus. He left for a last trip to Paris, but in less than two months returned, "in bad shape," as Williams says. In 1922 and 1923 Demuth spent two lengthy periods at the Physiatric Institute in Morristown, New Jersey, which specialized in the then-popular Allen starvation treatment for diabetes. On a visit to the Williams' home during this time, he "brought a pair of scales and weighed his food carefully." The Morristown clinic was also the first in the United States to use insulin, and Demuth is reported to be their second patient to receive it, in 1922. Thus, although Demuth was to have frequent and violent hypoglycemic attacks, for which his friends would feed him sugar, orange juice, or saccharin, he was to live another 13 years and to continue his painting until the last year of his life. Whereas the years 1916 to 1921, just before the onset of his illness, are considered to be his best in terms of artistic output, these last "insulin-years" were, for Demuth, a second flowering. It is to these years that the hommages belong.

The Figure 5 in Gold, while being a portrait of Williams, is also a reflection of Demuth's personality: it is correct, aloof, and detached, the kind of painting, as a critic noted about some of his other work, that one might have a martini with. The facts are all in plain view, but it is for us to penetrate their mystery. Some of the meanings come with little teasing, for they are the lines of the Williams poem: The 5 in gold, the rain and the lights, the red firetruck, the dark city, the rumbling wheels, the clanging gong, the howling siren, the movement, the tenseness. Other clues pertain to the author of the poem: The initials "W.C.W.," "Bill," as his friends called him, "Carlos," as Demuth preferred to call him; the "Carlos" in lights like a Broadway marquee, and the black and

Continued on p. 206

JAMA

The Journal of the American Medical Association

January 2, 1981

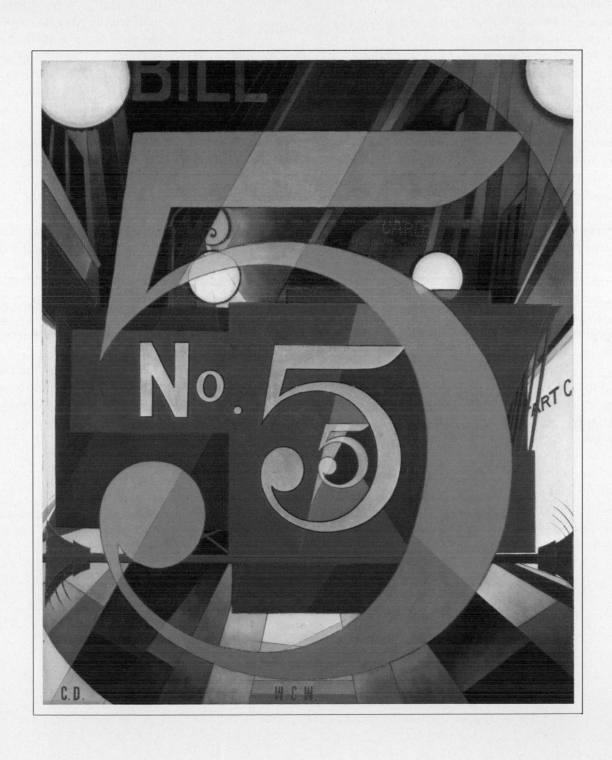

EDGAR DEGAS

Woman Ironing

Although Edgar Degas (1834-1917) was never, properly speaking, an Impressionist, he was one of the regulars at the Café de la Nouvelle-Athènes and he exhibited in all of the Impressionist group shows, from the first, in 1874, to the eighth, in 1886, save one, that of 1882. He was a member of an aristocratic family of bankers, with connections in Italy, and later, through his brother René's marriage, in the United States; as expected, he studied law. However, this he had abandoned by the time he was 20 years old, and from then on he devoted himself exclusively to art. Apparently, this exclusiveness applied even to marriage or other liaisons, for at one point he said: "There is love, and there is work, and we have but a single heart." His closest friend was probably Mary Cassatt.

Temperamentally, Degas was difficult. His clever and incisive mind often led him to argue with those of his colleagues not so graciously endowed. Like Manet, he was also the master of the bon mot, but one suspects he used his wit not so much for pleasure, but to conceal his own sensitivity and hurt. Of this he had much. Not only did he always seem to be in conflict about his work and to have doubts about his abilities, but his eyesight began to concern him as early as 1870. More important, his father died when Degas was 40, leaving the bank's affairs in disastrous shape, a financial burden that

> *…the young woman, completely absorbed in her work, is unaware she is not alone.*

Degas felt obliged to assume. Later, his younger and favored brother René abandoned his young wife, who was blind, in New Orleans; within three years, four of his nieces and nephews died, most victims of yellow fever. Again, his aristocratic sense of family increased his sorrow and he withdrew increasingly from his colleagues.

Woman Ironing comes near the end of this period, as Degas was approaching 50. The theme is one he liked: the working woman, whether she be the ballet dancer, the milliner, or the laundress. Unlike the paintings of his fellow Impressionists, the form is solid, the line is strong, the colors are somber. Degas was not so much interested in capturing light as he was in capturing motion: in arresting the motion already in progress, much like the shutter of the camera records the instant. The young girl's right hand is caught mid-motion as she leans on and pushes the iron, while with the left she pulls the fabric smooth. In another moment she will dip her fingers once again

into the bowl and sprinkle water on the drying shirt. It is an intimate moment, one in which the young woman, completely absorbed in her work, is unaware she is not alone. Perhaps it is Degas himself who stands there, having arrived a little early to pick up his shirts, which are lying starched and finished at the left, while she hurries to finish the last one.

Degas was to live into his 80s, but around the time of this painting, he was profoundly depressed. Shortly after his 50th birthday, Degas wrote to a friend: "One closes, like a door, and not only upon friends…I was so full of projects; here I am blocked, powerless…I've lost the thread. I always thought I had time; what I didn't do…I never gave up hope of starting one fine day. I hoarded all my plans in a cupboard of which I always carried the key with me, and I've lost that key. I shall keep myself occupied…and that will be all."

Yet much of Degas' best known work was to come—his brilliantly colored pastels, the exquisite drawings, and the delicate sculptures of his ballet dancers.

Edgar Degas (1834-1917), *Woman Ironing*, begun c 1876, completed c 1887, French. Oil on canvas. 81.3 × 66 cm. Courtesy of the National Gallery of Art, Washington, DC; collection of Mr and Mrs Paul Mellon, 1972. © 1995 The Board of Trustees of the National Gallery of Art.

JAMA

THE JOURNAL of the American Medical Association

January 16, 1981

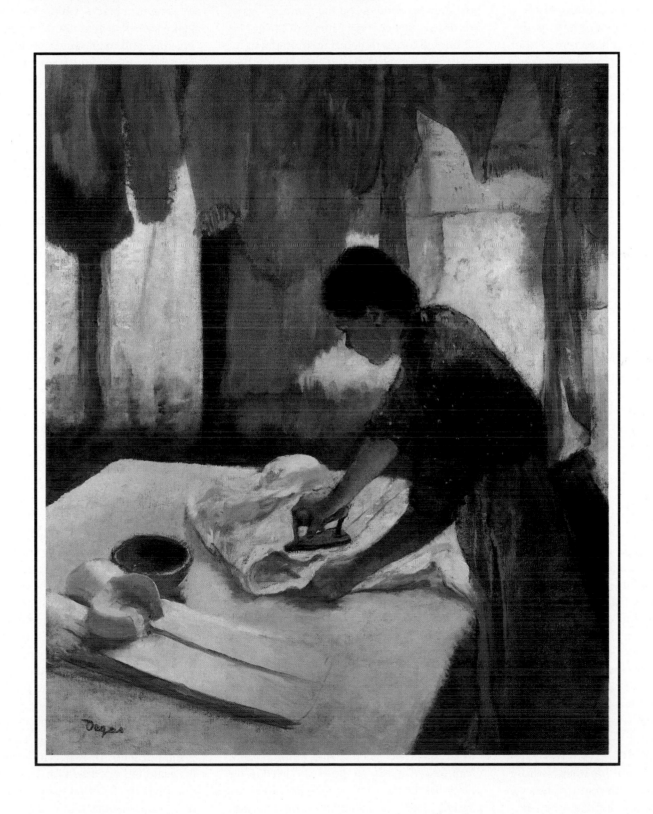

EASTMAN JOHNSON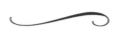

The Brown Family

In the beginning, a new country has no time for art, and no need of it. Its gods and its heroes are physically present, and its deeds are being lived. It is only later, when a people has a need to recall its heroes and its deeds, that pictures are painted and put in public places. Thus, there grows a class of paintings that are usually formal portraits of founding fathers, generals, and statesmen, as well as another class of paintings, history paintings, which depict battles, the signing of treaties, or other decisive events in the formation of the people. Still later, the people whose ancestors once spent all of their time clearing the frontier have the leisure to extol the beauties of the land for itself, and the huge landscape paintings are born. Finally, in a kind of need to establish a common identity, the people will wish to see themselves in all their varied and homely activities; the result is genre painting, small, anonymous, "typical" scenes of everyday life.

In mid-19th century America, certain families, usually affluent, wished to record themselves and the marks of their achievement and posed informally in their ordinary surroundings, usually their homes; the result is what is called a "conversation piece"; it is a kind of genre painting, except that instead of being an anonymous composite scene that is meant to generalize on an aspect of life, the surroundings are specific and the people have names, ancestors, and descendants. The conversation piece itself is the offspring of the small Dutch genre paintings of the 17th century and the English "estate portraits," the less formal portraits that show the "sitter" astride a favorite horse or standing in front of the manor home. In 20th-century terms, the conversation piece may be considered to be to the 19th-century parvenu what the annual Christmas letter is to today's middle-America.

Eastman Johnson (1824-1906) (early he dropped his first name of Jonathan), whose life spans most of the 19th century and even enters the 20th, and who lived as easily in the drawing room as on the frontier, recorded 19th-century American life in almost all forms of painting, from portrait to genre to conversation pieces. He was born in Lovell, Maine, one of three sons and five daughters of Philip and Mary Johnson. His father was secretary of state for Maine, later joining the Treasury Department in Washington, DC. Early on Johnson displayed remarkable ability at crayon portraits, and by the time he was 21 years old, he had set up a studio in one of the committee rooms of the US Senate building and was doing portraits of such people as John Quincy

> *...to make legitimate, at least this once, the universal human urge to peek into other people's living rooms.*

Adams, Daniel Webster, Dolley Madison, and the wife of Alexander Hamilton. The following year he was in Boston, where he did portraits of Longfellow, Emerson, and Hawthorne, among others. Despite his success, however, he felt the need for European study, and in 1849 he began a six-year course of work, the first two years in Düsseldorf, and the last four in The Hague, where he "discovered" Rembrandt and genre. In The Hague he was called the "American Rembrandt" and was even offered the position of court painter, but he returned instead to the United States, in 1855. From then on, with his ability at composition and his natural sense of draftsmanship, his fidelity to faces, and his feel for what was the "American scene," at least to those who lived in the latter half of the 19th century, his career rose steadily. He became known for his paintings of American blacks, Chippewa Indians, and genre scenes such as cranberry picking, corn husking, and maple sugaring, and he had portrait commissions from many of the industrial and political leaders of the time, among them George M. Pullman, William Vanderbilt, John D. Rockefeller, Grover Cleveland, and Benjamin Harrison.

In 1869, which was also the year of his marriage, Johnson was asked to do a "genre-portrait" or conversation piece for the James Brown family of New York City. It was to show him, his wife, and their grandson seated informally in the parlor of their home on University Place. In a sense the three people were intended to be only incidental to the painting, for the real subject was to be the room and its furnishings, which had been designed in 1846 by the prestigious Leon Marcotte in the Renaissance revival style. Now, the family was planning to move uptown to Park Place and the room soon would be dismantled.

The Brown Family is a somewhat altered version of the painting Johnson did for James Brown. In the original version, Johnson shows the room exactly as it must have looked, from richly carpeted floor to inlaid ceiling, with massive chandelier and a life-sized Renaissance statue. The result overwhelms the people, making them look quite out of place. In this second version, which Johnson may have done for himself, he simplifies by omitting the overpowering ceiling and upper third of the walls, the heavy chandelier, which hung at the left, and the statue, which rose, somewhat incongruously, behind the newspaper. This second version is much less forbidding and more intimate. Grandfather James sits enjoying a quiet moment, perhaps just after breakfast, with the financial pages. Eliza, his second wife, sits quietly by, knitting. The grandson, William Adams Brown, is insistent in getting his grandfather's attention. It is, however, the grandfather's face that is so arresting—at once amused, questioning, stern, indulgent—

Continued on p. 206

JAMA

THE JOURNAL of the American Medical Association

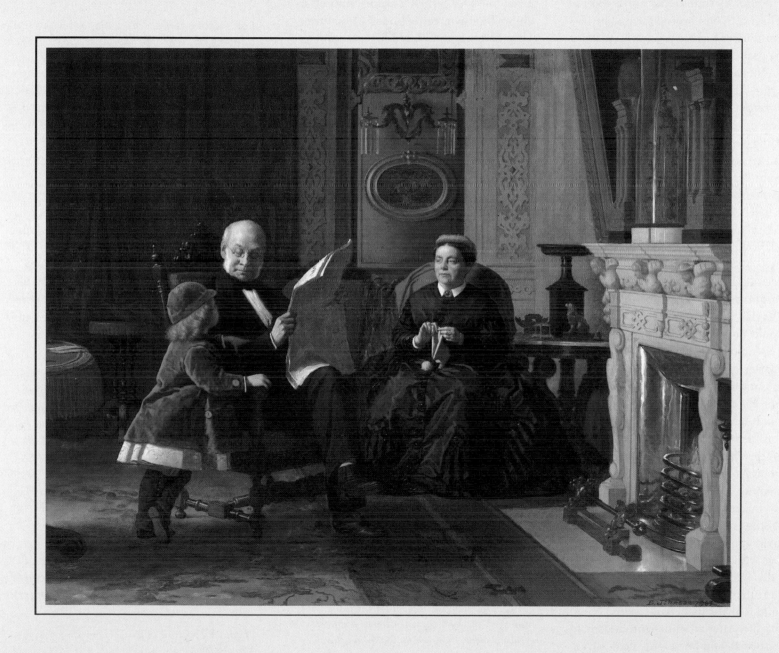

VINCENT VAN GOGH

Portrait of Dr Gachet

On May 21, 1890, the 37-year-old Vincent van Gogh (1853-1890) arrived in Auvers, a small village on the Oise River, about an hour by train to the northwest of Paris. His health had been poor, and he had had a number of bizarre psychotic episodes over the past one and a half years while living in the South of France. His moving to Auvers-sur-Oise was meant to accomplish several things: to remove him from the "madness of the South;" to put him geographically closer to his brother Theo, who lived in Paris, and on whom Vincent had had an absolute financial and emotional dependence for most of his adult life (even though Theo was four years younger); and to keep him under medical supervision, without, however, keeping him in an asylum. This medical care was to be provided by a 62-year-old homeopathic physician, Dr Paul-Ferdinand Gachet, who lived, largely retired at that time, in the village.

A would-be painter himself, Gachet had been a friend of many in the Paris art world for a quarter of a century, especially Pissarro, Cézanne, and Renoir, and had attended Manet on his deathbed several years earlier. All in all, it seemed a providential solution to the problem of Vincent: he could work freely in the village, he had family less than an hour away, and he had a physician keenly interested not only in nervous conditions such as Vincent had (Gachet had written his doctoral thesis on melancholy), but also one who could appreciate and discuss Vincent's paintings with him.

But this interlude was to differ little from all of the other hopeful beginnings, fresh starts, and rebirths that characterized Vincent's life. After an initial enthusiasm, his feelings soured, and he became possessive and quarrelsome and was overwhelmed by the conflict of his insatiable need for Theo's support and his awareness of Theo's own obligations to his wife and infant son. A crisis was reached when Vincent threatened to harm Gachet, but subsequently shot himself,

fatally. (A similar pattern had occurred some 18 months earlier in the South when van Gogh threatened his friend Gauguin with a razor, but later turned it against himself in the well-known "ear episode." At that time Theo had just announced his intention to marry soon, thus threatening a change in the financial and emotional relationship between the two brothers.)

For the moment, however, Vincent was happy and full of plans. Shortly after his arrival in Auvers, he wrote to Theo and his wife: "I have seen Dr Gachet, who gives me the impression of being rather eccentric, but

> *"Sad and yet gentle, but clear and intelligent— this is how one ought to paint many portraits."*

his experience as a doctor must keep him balanced enough to combat the nervous trouble from which he certainly seems to me to be suffering at least as seriously as I." A few days later he wrote, again to Theo and Jo:

Today I saw Dr Gachet again…He seems very sensible, but he is as discouraged about his job as a doctor as I am about my painting. Then I told him that I would gladly swap jobs with him. He said to me besides that if the melancholy or any-thing else became too much for me to bear, he could easily do something to lessen its intensity, and that I must not feel awkward about being frank with him. Well, the moment when I need him may certainly come, however, up to now all is well.

Early in June he wrote to Theo that Gachet "certainly seems to me as ill and dis-traught as you or me, and he is older and lost his wife several years ago, but he is very much the doctor, and his profession and

faith still sustain him." In the same letter Vincent describes a portrait Gachet had asked him to do:

I am working at his portrait, the head with a white cap, very fair, very light, the hands also a light flesh tint, a blue frock coat and cobalt blue background, leaning on a red table on which are a yellow book and a foxglove plant with purple flowers. It has the same sentiment as the self-portrait I did when I left for this place. M Gachet is absolutely fanatical about this portrait, and wants me to do one for him, if I can, exactly like it.

Also in the first half of June, Vincent wrote to his sister Wil: "I have found a true friend in Dr Gachet, something like another brother, so much do we resemble each other physically and also mentally. He is a very nervous man himself and very queer in his behavior." In this letter van Gogh also goes into considerably more detail about the por-trait he mentioned to Theo:

So the portrait of Dr Gachet shows you a face the color of an overheated brick, and scorched by the sun, with reddish hair and a white cap, surrounded by a rustic scenery with a background of blue hills; his clothes are ultramarine—this brings out the face and makes it paler, notwithstanding the fact that it is brick-colored. His hands, the hands of an obstetrician, are paler than the face. Before him, lying on a red garden table, are yellow novels and a foxglove flower of a somber purple hue.

A few days later, around the middle of June, he wrote to his mother and appended a few more lines to Wil about Gachet's portrait:

I painted a portrait of Dr Gachet with an expres-sion of melancholy, which would seem to look like a grimace to many who saw the canvas. And yet it is necessary to paint it like this, for otherwise one could not get an idea of the extent to which, in comparison with the calmness of the old portraits, there is expression in our modern heads, and passion—like a waiting for things as well as a

Continued on p. 207

JAMA

February 20, 1981

THE JOURNAL of the American Medical Association

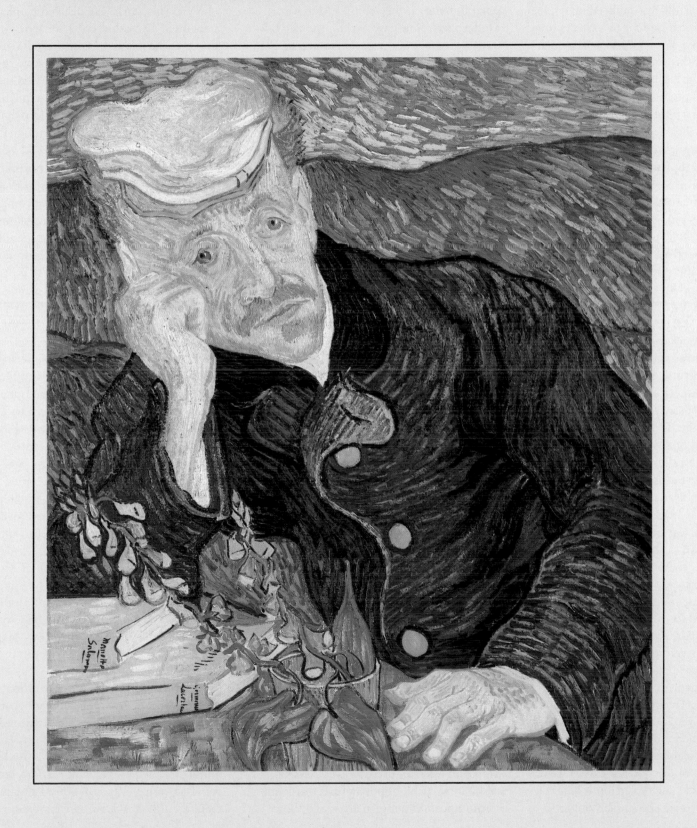

ARSHILE GORKY

The Artist and His Mother

In 1912, 7-year-old Vosdanik Adoian accompanied his mother to Van city on the shores of Lake Van in Turkish Armenia. The purpose of this short excursion from their home in the Aikesdan suburb of Van was to have a photograph made. It was not to be an ordinary photograph; it was to go to Vosdanik's father, Sedrag, who had four years earlier emigrated to America (Rhode Island) to avoid the Turkish army draft and thus eliminate any possibility of having to fight fellow Armenians. Left behind in Van were his 28-year-old wife, Shushanik, the 3-year-old Vosdanik, and three daughters, Akabi, Satenik, and Vartoosh.

Three years after the photograph was made, 10-year-old Vosdanik, his sisters, and his mother were forced to flee Aikesdan on a "death march" that eventually took them to Yerevan in Caucasian Armenia. In 1916, in the midst of war and starvation, the two older girls, Akabi and Satenik, left to join their father in America, while both Vosdanik and his youngest sister remained behind with their mother. By 1918, with the mother seriously ill, and both children working and providing the best they could, their only shelter had nevertheless been reduced to a roofless room in a small village near Yerevan. Finally, in March 1919, when Vosdanik was 14 years old and Vartoosh 13, their mother died of starvation in the boy's arms. She was dictating a letter to her husband. Six months later the children went to Constantinople, thence to Athens, and finally, in February 1920, they sailed for America on the *USS Columbus*, and Vosdanik finally saw his father for the first time in 12 years. The photograph meanwhile had not been forgotten, nor was the tragedy of the years following the photograph. The boy became the painter Arshile Gorky (1905-1948), and the photograph became the model for his most famous figure portrait, *The Artist and His Mother*.

Two versions of the portrait exist. Of the two, the National Gallery version is believed to be the earlier one. The similar, but later, portrait hangs at the Whitney Museum of Modern Art. Gorky worked on the two portraits for nearly ten years, beginning in 1926 and not finishing until 1935 (the same year that he was briefly married), or even later. The Whitney portrait differs in that Gorky has severed the Siamese twin-like connection at the elbows by painting a gray line between the two arms; also, instead of paralleling each other in a static pose as they do in the National Gallery version and in the photograph, the boy's feet in their Armenian slippers are almost at right angles to each other, the right one suggesting he is about to walk

> *"Eyes…are the soul of portraiture, the prime communication between artist and those who view his work."*

away. But even in the first version, Gorky has already isolated the mother and son in their separate worlds, their orbits unlikely to cross. The dead mother is emphasized by the pallor of her face, the pastel of her clothes, the hands that do nothing. In contrast, the living boy holds flowers, his face is deeply flesh-toned, and the emphatic hairline, shaped like a palette, suggests that he works as a painter. (The same shape, a favorite of his, is repeated in his slippers.) But whether in different worlds or not, the two figures—the absent mother and the remembered 7-year-old, already so charged with tragedy—look out at us, into us, through us, with a common eye. The boy-turned-man has condensed his life into a single gaze that holds us like an electric current. "Eyes," Gorky said, "are the soul of portraiture, the prime communication between artist and those

who view his work." He disliked being told he painted "Picasso eyes." They were Armenian eyes, he insisted. "Our eyes," he said. "The eyes of the Armenian speak before the lips move and long after they ceased to."

On another occasion Gorky wrote of his mother's apron: "My mother told me many stories while I pressed my face into her long apron with my eyes closed. She had a long white apron like the one in her portrait, and another embroidered one. Her stories and the embroidery on her apron got confused in my mind with my eyes closed. All my life her stories and her embroidery keep unravelling pictures in my memory." Indeed, the world always remained for Gorky, especially as he became more abstract and expressionist, a child's garden of shapes, and it was these remembered childhood shapes that formed so much of his work of later life.

Likewise, the facts of Gorky's life are as elusive and as fluid as the shapes and lines of his drawings. They drift in and out and, like the shapes, become whatever is needed. Deeply spiritual, even mystical, and Eastern, he did not consider facts important—it was meaning that was essential. A few facts can be pinned down, however. He adopted the name of Arshile Gorky in 1925, when he was 20, the Arshile being an Armenian royal name and Gorky being Russian for "bitterness." (He was no relation to the Russian playwright Maxim Gorky, although Arshile apparently did little if anything to correct the widely publicized misconception that they were first cousins; even Arshile's obituary noted the kinship. Curiously, Maxim's surname was also a pseudonym.) In the depths of the Depression, in 1933, Gorky joined the Civil Works Administration's Public Works of Art Project, later becoming part of the new Works Progress Administration's (WPA) Federal Art Project. It was during this period that he did his modern murals for the new Newark Airport, ten panels covering a total of 466.34 square meters, entitled *Aviation: Evolution of Forms*

Continued on p. 207

JAMA

The Journal of the American Medical Association

May 8, 1981

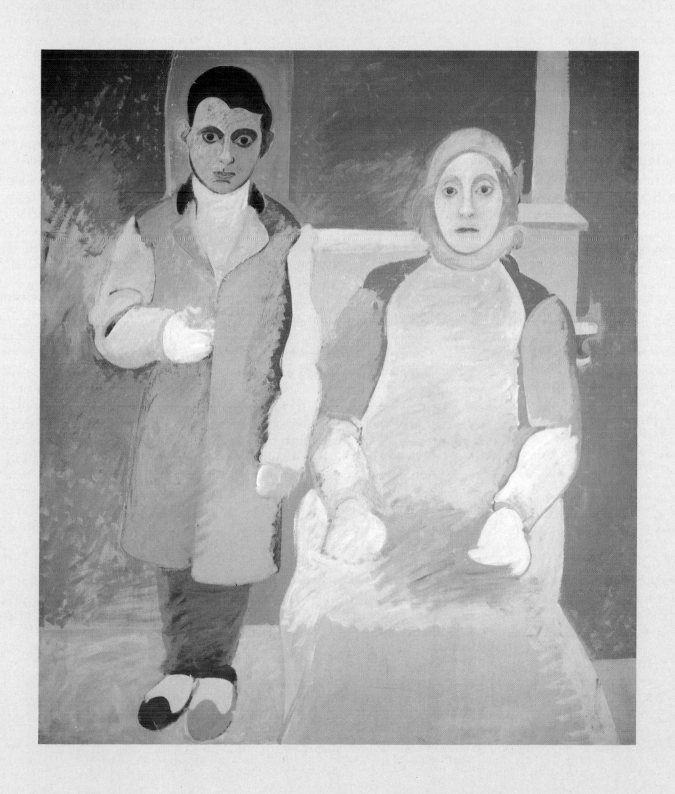

FRANCIS WILLIAM EDMONDS

First Aid

It was the time of Ichabod Crane, Jacksonian democracy, the "common man," and the making (and losing) of fortunes. It was the time of Emerson and Irving and the dwindling days of Aaron Burr. It was the second quarter of the 19th century and a brand new nation was feeling its oats. Banks rose, flourished, and failed. The population was doubling. The future was in land.

Meanwhile, in 1841, one of its native sons, 34-year-old Francis William Edmonds (1806-1863), amateur painter and professional banker, was in England winding down an eight-month journey he had taken through the south of Europe to look at paintings and to recover his health following some banking reverses and the death of his wife a year earlier. Whether or not the trip helped can perhaps be gathered from one of the closing entries in his travel journal:

If I restrain my ambition and not be too anxious to do too much: be patient; take things easily; allow nothing to fret me; submit to the changes and chances of fortune with perfect good nature; mingle freely with society; avoid being too much alone; use every convenient opportunity by reading books of travel to refreshen my impression of the countries thro' which I have passed; paint but little and rather for pleasure than reputation; finally think slowly, work slowly, eat slowly and walk slowly, I shall get a good appetite, sleep soundly, digest well, and live happily.

But his wishes and resolutions belied his circumstances, for only a few days earlier he had had another attack of the illness for which his physicians could find no cure and

"Oh, for the ministering hand of some kind female!"

he had recorded in his journal: "How dreary it is to be unwell in a foreign land among strangers! Oh, for the ministering hand of some kind female! But this is denied me." Not for long, however. Within six months after returning home Edmonds was to be married for the second time. And his marriage was but a prelude to a decade of artistic and financial success.

First Aid belongs to this decade of Edmonds' work and is an example of genre painting, which reached its heyday in this period of America's youth. It is unabashedly sentimental (is this perhaps the "ministering female" Edmonds had so longed for in England?), it points a moral, and it celebrates the virtues of rural common folk. On the other hand, as noted in an exhibit where this painting was recently shown, this is not the typical genre painting. Subject matter was equally as, if not more, important to 19th-century critics than was the quality of the painting; any scene suggesting distress or illness was unlikely to be thought well of. Indeed, Professor Gerdts suggests that even the title, *First Aid*, is more modern than the work itself. Perhaps because Edmonds was an amateur (in its original root sense, *to love*) painter and derived his livelihood from considerable success as a banker, he did not feel constrained to feed the popular taste.

On the other hand, he did please the critics enough to be made a member of the National Academy of Design.

First Aid has the look of a 17th-century Dutch courtyard scene transplanted to America, perhaps even to Edmonds' native town, Hudson, New York. It is known that during his visits to the European museums Edmonds had a strong preference for the Dutch painters, especially Teniers, Ostade, and Metsu. The line, with its unmistakable perpendiculars and definite angles, has the cleanness and certitude of the Dutch line. The color is limpid and balanced with touches of what has come to be known as "Edmonds' red" in the breast of the bird and in the upper sky. Likewise, shapes are balanced by similars or opposites, while the group of figures gathered in the center is posed in the classical pyramid shape. The story tells itself.

In 1855, misfortune came once again to Edmonds; he was charged, in a newspaper account, with embezzlement of the Mechanics Bank. However, the fact that he lost his job as a cashier but remained as a director attests more to the loose and speculative banking practices of the 1850s than to the gravity of a similar charge made today. Edmonds died suddenly and unexpectedly several years later of heart failure. He was 56.

Francis William Edmonds (1806-1863), *First Aid*, c 1840-1845, American. Oil on canvas. 43.2 × 35.6 cm. Courtesy of Henry Melville Fuller, Marlborough, New Hampshire.

JAMA

THE JOURNAL of the American Medical Association

June 26, 1981

WILLIAM MCGREGOR PAXTON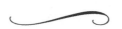

The Girl at the Telephone

By 1935, when he was 65 years old, William McGregor Paxton (1869-1941) had won the Corcoran Popular Prize for the fourth time. Justifiably, he was called "America's most popular painter." Yet until recently he has been eclipsed, not only by his friends and fellow Boston Impressionists DeCamp, Tarbell, and Benson, but by painters in the more "modern" tradition. Recently, however, this lapse has begun to be corrected, thanks to an exhibit organized by the Indianapolis Museum of Art, which has also been seen in El Paso, Omaha, and Springfield (Massachusetts).

Paxton was born in Baltimore, where his father, a caterer, had gone looking for better working opportunities. Before the boy was a year old, however, the family had returned to Newton, Massachusetts, and it was there that Paxton was to grow up, attend school, marry, and eventually die. His early art studies were at the Cowles School of Art in Boston where he worked, under scholarship, with the famed Bunker. Two years later, barely 20, he sailed for Paris and studied at the École des Beaux-Arts and the Académie Julian with Bunker's own teacher, the academician Gérôme. One can imagine the young American's feelings when the great master singled him out for favorable mention shortly after his arrival at the atelier. And one can share equally in what must have been puzzlement and dismay when, after four years of study, Gérôme told him that he showed none of the promise he had had on arrival from Boston. Still, Paxton's Paris studies had netted him not only a sure sense of color and contour, but most of all, a secure sense of draftsmanship, qualities he was to continue to develop and refine with continued study and practice.

Back in Boston, Paxton returned to the Cowles Art School where he met a young student from Rhode Island, Elizabeth Okie. They were married in 1899, when, nearly 30, Paxton was achieving some financial success. Elizabeth was 22, an artist in her own right, and very beautiful. In fact, she served often as her husband's model; more than 40 years of Paxton's work document her maturing beauty.

Between his marriage in 1899 and his death in 1941 Paxton continued to paint in Boston, his life being punctuated only by periodic trips to Europe, where he was most influenced by the paintings of Velázquez and Vermeer, and by summers in Provincetown, Rockport, or other nearby artists' colonies. Meanwhile, through an accumulation of exhibits and prizes and one-man shows, his reputation rose steadily. He was easily the most popular painter in America. Disaster

> *...the peaceful coexistence of the loveliest in art with the newest in science.*

touched him once, in 1904, when a studio fire destroyed most of his work, sparing only what was currently in an exhibit at St Botolph's Club in Boston. Most devastating was the loss of all of his early studies.

The Girl at the Telephone is one of the first works to be completed after the studio fire and shows Paxton as he was to be in his maturity. His subject is the Vermeer-like interior he was so fond of, the model is his wife, and the background is a mélange of old and beautiful objects, each essential to the design of the work. The colors, understated as they are, are warmed by the background and accented, but delicately, by his favorite lavender. Except for the insistent presence of the telephone, which intrudes on the eye like the jangle of its bell on the ear, we could be in an 18th-century parlor, with the mistress of the house addressing invitations to a *fête galante*. Instead, we have the 18th and 20th centuries contraposed: the mistress of the house sits on a Sheraton chair at her Empire desk beneath a Lancret painting, *Lacamargo,**

using the newly invented telephone to issue invitations to her own party. The painting is a paean to the peaceful coexistence of the loveliest in art with the newest in science.

Paxton also demonstrates his superb draftsmanship, his sense of structure, and his love of the curved line. For example, the lower right corner of the Lancret painting meets the corner of the Sheraton chair, and this point divides the painting vertically into fifths, while horizontally it approximates the ratio of the Golden Mean. From here the line leads directly to the model's face. In like manner, the subtle curves of the Sheraton chair are balanced by the curves of the model's arms, the lines again eventually coming to rest in her face. The left third of the painting is balanced by the strong verticals of the desk, of the dancing figure, and, of course, the still incongruous telephone.** Typical of Paxton's other work, the model's eyes are averted; any questions we may have for her must remain unanswered.

Paxton's popularity was to continue for many more years, although by the time of his sudden death in 1941 he had become largely ignored. His *New York Times* obituary notice called him "iconoclast" and "old fashioned" and remembered him chiefly for portraits he had made of Calvin Coolidge and Grover Cleveland. Paxton's own philosophy was summed up in his advice that one should always give the public what it wants, but make it better.

Lacamargo was Marie Anne de Cupis de Camargo, an 18th-century French dancer often painted by Lancret. She is noted chiefly for raising the dance skirt a few inches off the ground and introducing the heeless shoe, making possible the elevated dance steps, as shown in the painting.

**At the time of this painting the telephone was less than 30 years old. In addition to the desk set shown it was available in one other model: the wall set with hand crank. Calls were placed through a central operator and private lines were available. According to a Bell Telephone annual report issued in Boston

Continued on p. 208

JAMA

July 10, 1981

THE JOURNAL of the American Medical Association

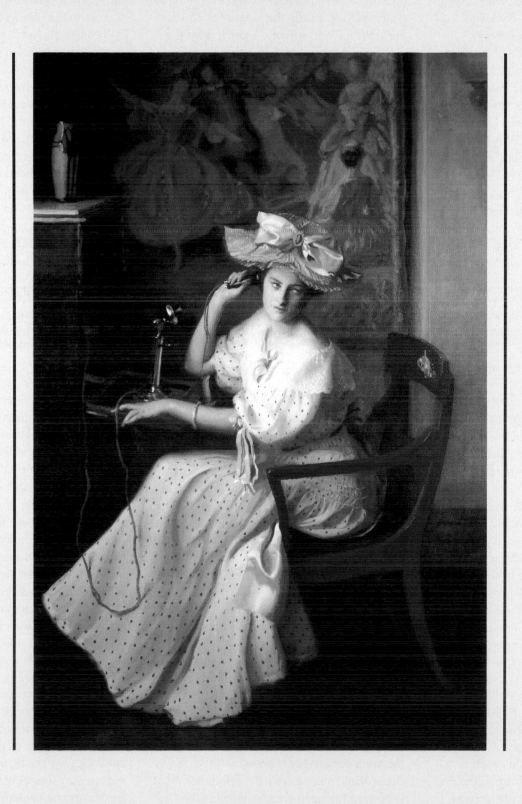

DAVID TENIERS THE YOUNGER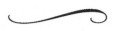

Tavern Scene

Rubens may have been the Flemish king of the Baroque, and Van Dyck was surely its prince, but tiny 17th-century Flanders also produced a whole aristocracy of other painters whose names remain familiar today: Jacob Jordaens, Paul and Cornelis de Vos, Jan Fyt, Frans Snyders, Jan (Velvet) Bruegel the Elder, Adriaen Brouwer, and David Teniers the Younger (1610-1690). Like a member of the aristocracy, Teniers the Younger, though often considered a minor painter, had an artistic lineage that, through marriage, stretched back to the High Renaissance. Great-grandmother Mayken Verhulst, herself a miniaturist of note, started it all by having a daughter who married the painter Pieter Bruegel the Elder. They had a son, painter Jan (Velvet) Bruegel the Elder, who in turn had two children, Jan Bruegel the Younger, again a painter, and daughter Anna, who became a ward of Rubens. Meanwhile, on the Teniers side, Mannerist painter grandfather Juliaen the Elder had a son, painter David Teniers the Elder, who fathered three painter sons, Abraham, Juliaen the Younger, and David the Younger. David the Younger married the ward of Rubens, Anna Bruegel, and they extended the lineage with painter son David Teniers III. But it is David the Younger and his genre paintings of peasant life with which we are here concerned.

Tavern Scene, painted in 1658, when Teniers was nearing 50, is one of some 2000 paintings he did during his 80 years, most of them genre paintings and in their day highly sought after. One suspects Teniers could not turn them out fast enough to satisfy the new art-buying middle class. (Like his father before him, David the Younger was, in fact, also an art dealer, and as a result very well-to-do.)

The scene is perhaps one of a bawdy group of peasants celebrating a belated Twelfth Night, or perhaps it is simply a normal evening out for a Netherlandish peasant. What immediately compels the eye, however, is the young man at the left who proudly shows his hand—two aces, a king, a club card, and a fifth, the identity of which the artist has adroitly kept hidden from the viewer. The young gentleman has anything but a poker face, while the face of the older man remains as inscrutable as his cards, which we are not permitted to see. One wonders whether the gleeful expressions of the kibitzers are honest indications of a good hand for the old man or whether they are only contrivances intended to outwit the confident youngster—already probably witless from the contents of the tankard that he so conspicuously displays (does he hold

> *...the only wisdom and truth to be found in the room that night are the owl and the candle...*

his liquor as easily?) and half drugged from the strong tobacco of the time. Judging from his clothes, perhaps he is a traveler from the city, stopping by the tavern for a night's lodging, unaware that he is the fall guy being set up by a group of wily country folk. In a satiric broadside, Teniers tells us that the only wisdom and truth to be found in the room that night are the owl and the candle almost directly above the young man's head, if only he would care to look up.

Teniers' composition is skillful and typically Baroque. Two groups of figures, one warming themselves at the fire in the right background and the other playing cards in the left foreground, form a strong diagonal that is bridged by a besotted patron sleeping on a bench in the midground. Mystery and infinity are added by the young woman at the open door. What is her errand? To deliver more drink, more tobacco? To procure? What is beyond the open door? A kitchen, the family living quarters, a snowy night? Accents to the diagonal are added not only by the strongly horizontal bench with its sleeping man but also by the equally strong vertical roof supports, which also divide the painting roughly into thirds. Diagonals, in a minor key, are added by the wood stacked in the right foreground, by the "V" support of the roof, and by the foreshortened table and benches in the left foreground, matched in turn by the foreshortened open door in the rear. Diversity of shape is accomplished by the various objects on the shelf on the back wall, the shelf and its support themselves nicely echoing the bench and roof supports. In the right foreground is the round dish, matched by the shape of the curled-up dog—perhaps the only living creature in the room impervious to tomorrow's woes. The barrel on which the dish sits is counterpoint in a major key to the almost unnoticed niche in the rear wall.

Teniers likewise uses the light in diagonal fashion, with the figures in the right rear shadowy and the light gradually increasing downward and leftward until it focuses our attention on the brilliantly lit group of card-players. The light that falls on the sleeping man is intermediate between the two groups, again providing a bridge, while his red hat leads our eye in an oblique line to the red hat of the jolly kibitzer, and finally to the vivid red of the hat belonging to the vainglorious young man who will shortly, we are sure, collect his comeuppance from the crafty old man who sits opposite him.

Teniers the Younger is often criticized in his genre scenes for being too obvious, too trite, and not fully faithful to the life of the Flanders peasant. Moreover, he is often judgmental, as the owl and the candle remind us. What is not disputed, however, and what makes him unique among his Flemish counterparts, is his use of color, at once brilliant, subtle, and speaking in the most pleasing harmonies. Teniers was especially noted for his greens, evident in its various hues

Continued on p. 208

JAMA

THE JOURNAL of the American Medical Association

January 15, 1982

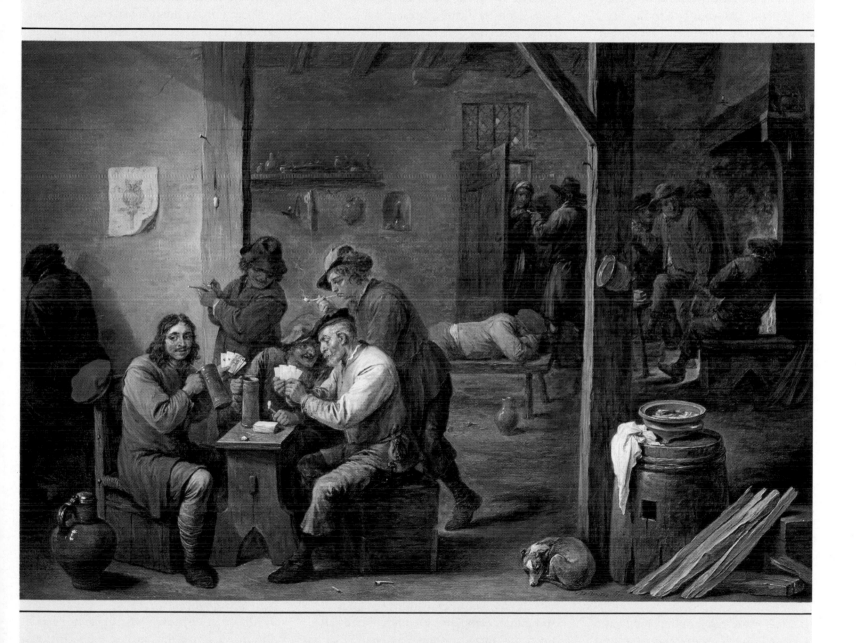

GERARD TER BORCH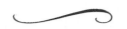

The Suitor's Visit

The Dutch War of Independence lasted for 80 years, beginning shortly after Philip II received the Spanish inheritance from his father, Charles V, and ending only in 1648 with the ratification of the Treaty of Münster. During this time, at the Union of Utrecht in 1579, The Netherlands, which were a Spanish possession, became divided into northern and southern provinces. The south remained loyal to Spain and became known as the Spanish Netherlands, while the seven northern provinces broke away, later formed a constitution under the chairmanship of the province of Holland, and became known as the United Provinces and its people, the Dutch. Today we know the northern and southern provinces as Holland and Belgium. Profound religious differences also distinguished the north and south, with the Spanish Netherlands remaining Catholic while the United Provinces were Lutheran, Anabaptist, and, later, Calvinist. These circumstances also created profound differences in the art of the two countries. In the north, religious painting and sculpture largely disappeared, while in the south they flourished.

Meanwhile, in spite of the lengthy war for independence, the United Provinces and the Dutch people prospered. Amsterdam became the center of world trade, the nobility, which had had ties to Spain, declined, and a wealthy middle class came into prominence. Art, too, prospered, in spite of the iconoclasm, but for reasons quite different from those existing to the south. Whereas royal patronage had customarily secured an artist's livelihood, the Dutch Independence now made this impossible. At the same time, the increasingly large and rich middle class was eager to display its wealth. Thus was created in the Dutch cities an art market, much like the tulip market and the foreign-import market, where the laws of supply and demand determined not only price, but even the general subject matter of the paintings. Thus were also created several generations of artists who catered to this taste and who made the 17th

century the golden century of Dutch painting. Among the most popular of the paintings were scenes of everyday life, or what we today call genre, and small portraits. Homely virtues, vices, and the many Dutch proverbs were frequent subjects. Often there were hidden jokes and even double entendres—not surprising when one considers that each artist specialized in a narrow range of subjects that he painted over and over again, so that he would occasionally like to surprise the viewer with something hidden.

> *Ter Borch, like the expert teller of a joke, has said everything, but explained nothing.*

Into this cultural milieu was born Gerard Ter Borch (1617-1681), whose life spans nearly the whole of the golden period of Dutch painting. His first drawing, showing a horse and rider moving away from the viewer, was done when he was 8 years old and indicates that he was something of a prodigy. At age 17, he left his native Zwolle and was in Haarlem. His earliest paintings, also of horses and of barracks scenes, date from this period. The following year he was in London. By the time he was 33, he had also visited Rome and Spain, where he saw the works, not only of the Italian masters, but also of Velázquez, with whom he is sometimes compared. He undoubtedly also knew the works of Rubens and Van Dyck, as well as those of his compatriots, Rembrandt and Hals. In 1648 he was in Westphalia, where he painted his most famous work, *The Ratification of the Treaty of Münster*, commemorating the beginning of the Dutch peace. Two years later, he settled permanently

in Holland in the small town of Deventer, where he remained, isolated from the Dutch art centers, and painted his small genre scenes, until his death some 30 years later.

Typical of Ter Borch's genre scenes, especially in his realistic treatment of fabrics and textures, is *The Suitor's Visit*, done about 1658 in Deventer. Small and jewel-like in its glossy, enamel-like finish, the painting is as elegant as an Elizabethan sonnet. A sumptuously dressed woman, in salmon-colored velvet bodice and white satin skirt bordered with gold, stands quietly to greet a more somberly, but equally luxuriously dressed aristocratic gentleman. Behind, on a table covered with an intricately patterned Turkish carpet, she has left her viol. The gentleman bows with a flourish of his wide-brimmed felt hat. The lady's *kookikertje*, or little spaniel lapdog, waits, somewhat quizzically, between them. A young girl remains sitting demurely at the table playing the bass lute, or theorbo, her eyes modestly on her music book, while in the background a second man stands inconspicuously, but nevertheless carefully overseeing the entire scene. The painting is an anecdote waiting to be told.

The conventional story is that of a wealthy upper middle-class Dutch family welcoming the daughter's suitor. The mother stands to greet him, while the daughter shows her skill with the lute and the father quietly appraises him. On the other hand, Ter Borch was also known for his *bordeeltjen*, or bordello scenes. In fact, one of his better known paintings, interpreted as a tender family scene by no less than Goethe and long titled *The Parental Admonition*, was reinterpreted in 1959 to be such a *bordeeltjen*.

Although Ter Borch has put certain signs into this painting that suggest the intentions behind the suitor's visit (the lute and the hands of the lady and gentleman have especial significance), he has been so delicate as to leave us in doubt as to what he intended. The scene leaves itself open to endless guessing. Is it a brothel scene, a family scene,

 Continued on p. 208

JAMA

February 12, 1982

THE JOURNAL of the American Medical Association

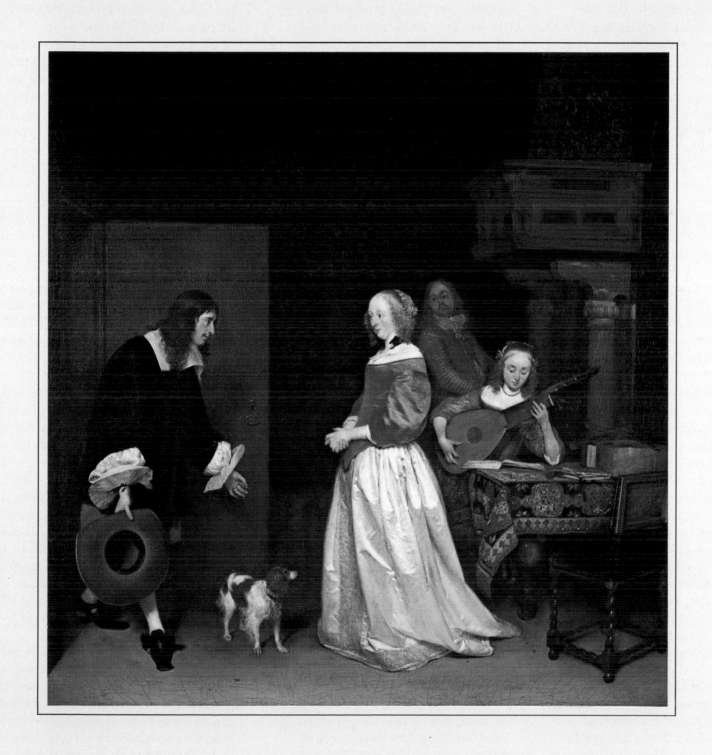

JOHN SLOAN ⌒

The Lafayette

On February 3, 1908, a group of artists, most of them journalists from Philadelphia, held an exhibit at the Macbeth Gallery in New York City; it marked the first major movement in 20th-century American art. Organized as a revolt against the prevailing turn-of-the-century American style that emphasized prettiness and technique, the 1908 exhibit was decisive in that it led to a no-jury show in 1910, to the Armory Show in 1913, and finally, in 1917, to the establishment of the Society of Independent Artists.

The group seemed to have as many names as Beelzebub. Because their paintings departed from the conventional light palette, pretty subject, and airy style favored by the National Academy of Design, the group was called variously the "Black Revolutionaries," the "Apostles of Ugliness," the "Black Gang," and "Outlaws." But it remained for a reporter for the *Evening Sun* to give the group their definitive name, the name by which they are known today, "The Eight," after the number of members in the group. (The other name by which the group is known today, "The Ashcan School," so called because some of the paintings by members of the group pictured garbage cans, did not become popular until a quarter of a century later, during the Great Depression, and included many other painters as well.) Led by the somewhat older Robert Henri, their mentor and teacher, the other seven members of the group were William Glackens, George Luks, Everett Shinn, Ernest Lawson, Maurice Prendergast, Arthur B. Davies, and the painter whose work most shocked the viewers, John Sloan (1871-1951).

Sloan was born in Lock Haven, Pennsylvania; at age 6 he moved to Philadelphia, where he went to school, grew up, and worked until his mid-30s. Two of his high school friends were Glackens and Albert C. Barnes, later the Argyrol entrepreneur and art benefactor. In his teens, Sloan taught himself to etch from a book, took drawing classes, and, when he was 21 years old, went to work in the art department of the *Philadelphia Inquirer*. He also began to study art seriously, with Thomas Anshutz, and met Henri, seven years his senior, who was to encourage him and with whom he was to lead the 1908 "revolution." In 1895, Sloan moved over to the *Philadelphia Press* and finally, urged by Henri, who had already been there for some time, moved to New York. He continued to submit work to the *Philadelphia Press*, however, to support himself. In 1912 Sloan began a two-year stint as art director to *The Masses* and also contributed to *Harper's*, *Collier's*, *Scribner's*, and

> *He called New York his "cosmopolitan palette where the spectrum changed in every side street."*

Everybody's. During all this time, although he continued to paint, exhibit, and win prizes (he had seven paintings in the Armory Show), Sloan did not sell a single work. His first sale was made at the age of 42 (to his high school friend, Barnes), and he did not sell to a museum until he was 49 years old. In fact, he never became self-supporting from the sale of his works until he was in his 70s.

Meanwhile, however, Sloan had acquired the eavesdropping eye characteristic of the good journalist and he continued to observe and to paint the vagaries of New York City life—the small, intimate dramas he saw each day as he wandered the streets, rested on a park bench, or watched from the window of his apartment. He called New York his "cosmopolitan palette where the spectrum changed in every side street." Hastily he would make his notes on a sketch pad and

only later would he make the painting, from memory. So familiar did these New York scenes become to viewers that they were called, generically, "Sloans."

The Lafayette is one such scene of New York life in the late 1920s. Although this building has now been missing from the city for more than 30 years, having been replaced by a multistoried apartment building, in its day it was a symbol of "old world elegance and hospitality" and "one of only two good old hotels left in New York." Built in 1902, at the southeast corner of University Place and Ninth Street, the 65-room brick Hotel Lafayette had a basement, a lobby level, and three upper floors for guests. Its restaurant was noted for its food and fine wines, and was a meeting place for literary and other celebrities. At about the time Sloan painted *The Lafayette*, its builder-owner, Frenchman Raymond B. Orteig, posted a $25,000 prize for the first nonstop airplane flight between New York and Paris, a prize earned by Charles A. Lindbergh on May 20 and 21, 1927.

Looking back on this painting some years later, Sloan was satisfied with it and had this to say: "This old hostelry on University Place has always been famous for the fine quality of its cuisine. It has also been a favorite resort of literary and artistic personages. To the passerby not looking for modern glitter, it has always had a look of cheer and comfort, particularly on such a wet evening as this. I will admit that in painting its exterior I chose the aspect most familiar to me. The picture seems to me to be a successful example of chiaroscuro [arrangement of light and dark parts]. Color and form are separate and simultaneous."

Shortly after he painted *The Lafayette*, Sloan had his first big sale: 32 paintings were sold for $41,000 in 1928. Already in his late 50s, Sloan was nevertheless still not able to make a living from his painting. In his autobiography, written some ten years later, he said: "Though a living cannot be made at art, art makes living worth while. It makes

Continued on p. 208

JAMA

THE JOURNAL of the American Medical Association

April 2, 1982

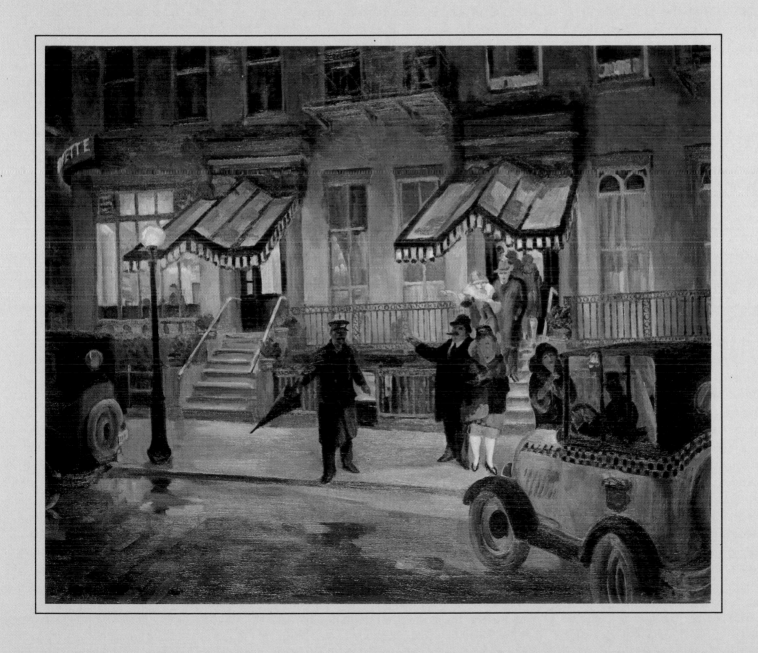

BERTHE MORISOT

The Artist's Sister at a Window

In the Paris of the 1850s, women were not yet admitted to the École des Beaux-Arts, nor were they allowed to compete for the Prix de Rome. Above all, they were not allowed to study from the nude. Indeed, in an article published in the *Gazette des beaux-arts* in 1860, Leon Lagrange consigned women artists to the sphere of pastels, portraits, miniatures, porcelains, and flower painting. "Who else but women would have the careful patience to hand-color botanical plates, pious images, and prints of all kinds?" he asks. And, "To women, above all, falls the practice of the graphic arts, those painstaking arts which correspond so well to the role of abnegation and devotion which the honest woman happily fills here on earth, and which is her religion."

Thus, when young Berthe Morisot (1841-1895) and her two older sisters, Yves and Edma, wished to paint, they were sent for private lessons to the studio of A. M. Chocarne. Of the three, Yves was to abandon her painting only a few years later, apparently not wishing to pursue a career. Edma and Berthe, on the other hand, carried on studies with Corot, and in the Salon of 1868 both young women, still in their 20s, had paintings that came to the favorable attention of Zola. A year later, however, Edma, whose painting Corot preferred to that of Berthe, was married to a young naval officer from Cherbourg and relinquished her career. But Berthe continued, becoming interested in painting from nature, and also in the effects of light.

With this turn of mind, and with the friendship of Édouard Manet, for whom she posed on occasion, it was only natural that Berthe should become part of the most innovative group of painters in Paris at that time, later to be called Impressionists. She showed works in all eight of the Impressionist exhibits, from 1874 to 1886, save one, that of 1879. Only Pissarro exceeded that number, exhibiting in all; Degas and Rouart also missed only one. At the Impressionist auction of 1875, Morisot's work brought better prices than that of Monet, Renoir, or Sisley.

The year 1874 was a landmark year for Berthe Morisot in more than one respect. Not only did she contribute nine works to the first group show of the Impressionists, but she also agreed never again to send anything to the official Salon, where she had been exhibiting for the past ten years. In 1874 Berthe also married Eugène Manet, brother of Édouard. She was 33. In 1879, the only year that she failed to send any paintings to the Impressionist exhibit, the couple's

> "Affection is a very fine thing, on condition that there is something besides with which to fill one's days."

only child, a daughter, Julie, was born. Berthe was by then 38 years old. For the next 16 years she was to be an active painter, continually developing and refining her art, organizing exhibits with her husband, and always remaining close to her family. Her home became a kind of salon, where artistic and literary persons gathered regularly to exchange ideas. Among them were Mallarmé, Baudelaire, Zola, Chabrier, Rossini (who considered her an accomplished pianist), Degas, Monet, and Renoir. Berthe took care to preserve their conversations in her journal. Then, in 1895, while caring for 16-year-old Julie, who was ill, Berthe herself fell ill and died. She was 54 years old.

The Artist's Sister at a Window was painted at Lorient in the summer of 1869, when the 28-year-old Berthe traveled from Paris to visit her sister Edma, who was newly married

to the naval officer, Adolphe Pontillon, and living at the marine base on the Bay of Biscay. The marriage, early that year, was the occasion of the first time the two sisters, who had also been constant painting companions, were separated. Both, apparently, had become depressed over the separation, and their letters to each other throughout the spring are filled with references to sadness, episodes of crying, melancholy, loss of friends, loneliness, and boredom. "Life here is always the same," wrote Edma after only a few weeks of marriage. "The fireside, and the rain pouring down." A short time before she must have written to Berthe mourning the loss of her painting, for in a reply Berthe, herself still single, remonstrates with her, saying, "Yes I find you are childish: this painting, this work that you mourn for, is the cause of many griefs and many troubles. You know it as well as I do, and yet, child that you are, you are already lamenting that which was depressing you only a little while ago…that lot you have chosen is not the worst one… Do not revile your fate…a woman has an immense need of affection." A month later, at the end of April, after Edma had been to Paris for a short visit, Berthe continued in a slightly different vein. "No matter how much affection a woman has for her husband, it is not easy for her to break with a life of work. Affection is a very fine thing, on condition that there is something besides with which to fill one's days." Then, acknowledging Edma's premonition that she might be pregnant, Berthe concludes, "This something I see for you is motherhood. Do not grieve about painting. I do not think it is worth a single regret."

In May, it was Berthe's courage that began to fail her. "I have done absolutely nothing since you left, and this is beginning to distress me. My painting never seemed to me as bad as it has in recent days. I sit on my sofa, and the sight of all these daubs nauseates me… Yesterday I arranged a bouquet of poppies and snowballs, and could not find the

Continued on p. 208

JAMA

THE JOURNAL of the American Medical Association

August 13, 1982

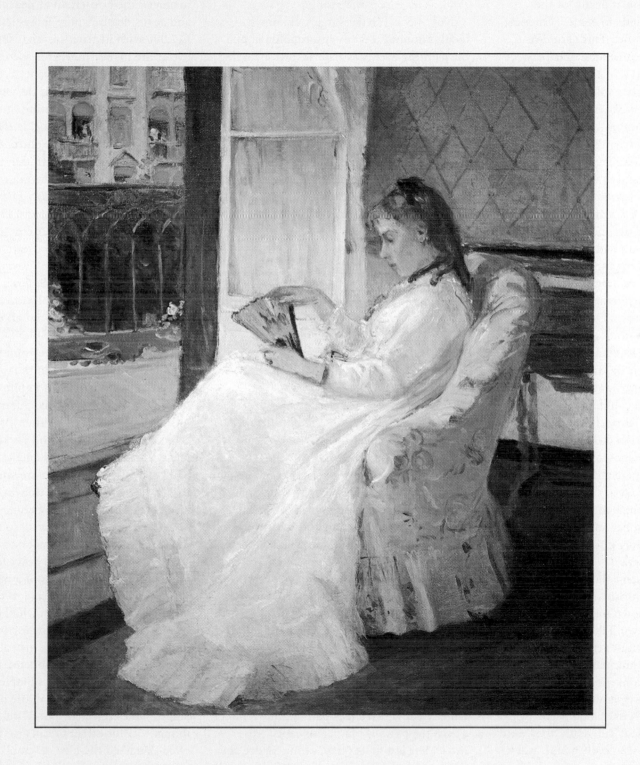

EDWARD HAYTLEY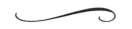

The Brockman Family and Friends at Beachborough Manor

"In the 18th century it is as if all Europe were waiting breathlessly for the tremendous revolutions to come," writes art historian Helen Gardner. This period of calm before the storm was the time between the death of Louis XIV, in 1715, and the American and French revolutions of the last quarter of the century. There were disagreements among the nations, to be sure, but they were more in the nature of family squabbles over the colonial territories in the New World. In England, it was the reign of George II and also a period of relative peace and prosperity. The aristocracy had entered its period of gradual decline, but the middle classes were rising, and with them, the cultural accoutrements of graceful living were in greater demand. Fielding and Smollett were the lights of the literary world, not to mention Samuel Johnson, soon to be followed by Boswell. Periodicals came into being, and newspapers could alter the course of events. In music, it was the German, Handel, who everyone went to hear. But in painting, England could again boast of native sons, notably Hogarth, who painted satires and conversation pieces, and Reynolds and Gainsborough, who painted portraits. Among the gentry there arose a demand for great manor houses set in vast parks. "The country houses of England in the 18th century, both in number and quality of design, are outstanding in European architecture," says Gardner.

Into this milieu came the English painter Edward Haytley (flourished, 1740-1761), who is almost unknown today. Little is known of his life beyond the dictionary entries, and they are not very satisfying. He was a painter of graceful portraits and landscapes, and of conversation pieces, those special kinds of genre paintings that were actually family portraits in a domestic setting. Or, to phrase it differently, they were portraits of the house, usually grand, and its inhabitants, also grand. Such a piece is *The Brockman Family and Friends at Beachbor-ough Manor* painted by Haytley in 1743-1746, as his career was rising.

Not only is Haytley largely unknown today, but until recently information about the painting itself was also lacking, including even the identity of the artist. Recently, however, Dr Emma Devapriam, curator of European art before 1800 for the National Gallery of Victoria, Melbourne, which owns the painting, recounted the interesting story of how the painting came to be identified. Referring to letters, journals, and cash books dating from 1644, Dr Devapriam not only conclusively identifies the painter as Haytley,

> *...the clean, well-ordered, tranquil life of an 18th-century Lord of the Manor.*

but she also identifies the various members of the Brockman family and their friends who are in the painting.

According to Dr Devapriam, Beachborough House had been the seat of the Brockman family since the days of Queen Elizabeth I. In 1743, which is the time of the painting, Beachborough Manor, located in a 300-acre park between Folkestone and Hythe in Kent, belonged to Squire James Brockman, who was born in 1696 and died in 1767. Squire James was 46 years old at the time of the painting. He had never married, but as the only surviving son, he inherited the manor and was head of the family. He is shown in the foreground in the brown coat and carries a large stick. Turning to face us from her easel at which she is painting the temple across the pond is Mary, also called Miss Molly. She is a first cousin of the Squire and lived at the Manor, although her father's (the Squire's uncle's) manor house was only

one and a half miles away. Mary apparently managed the household at Beachborough, and at his death, Squire James left her £12.000 with instructions that she was to live at the manor house for as long as she wished with as many servants as she wished. To Mary's left is Mrs Henckle, while behind her, at the left of the painting, strolling and reading a book, is Mr Henckle. The Henckles were evidently Squire James' close friends of long standing. In the right foreground of the painting, the figure in the blue riding habit is probably Elizabeth, also called Miss Betty or Betsy, and sister to Mary. She is shortly to be married to a parson, and her allowance from her cousin James is to be stopped. (However, she also received a bequest at the Squire's death, when she was a widow.) Next to her is the 8-year-old Miss Henckle, daughter of the previously mentioned couple. The other two figures in the painting, the young woman who has pulled a fish from the water, and the parson who is about to remove it from her hook, are possibly Miss Susannah Highmore, daughter of the painter Joseph Highmore, and the Rev Edmund Parker, a frequent visitor (and also a beneficiary of the Squire's will). Miss Highmore and Parson Parker are also linked in a drawing by Haytley immortalizing a small tragicomedy that occurred during another visit to the manor house. While fishing in the pond one day, Miss Highmore "tumbled down a steep bank into it," in the words of a neighbor. The Reverend Mr Parker had to pull her out by the leg. It is not known whether their relationship progressed any further. Insight into the Squire's character may also be gained from the correspondence of the time. Casting about for a suitable name for the body of water shown in the painting, Squire James rejected "pond" and also thought it "too small to call a serpentine river." He liked the idea of "pool" and a neighbor proposed calling it a "temple pool" or a "sacred pool."

Continued on p. 209

JAMA

THE JOURNAL of the American Medical Association

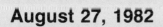

August 27, 1982

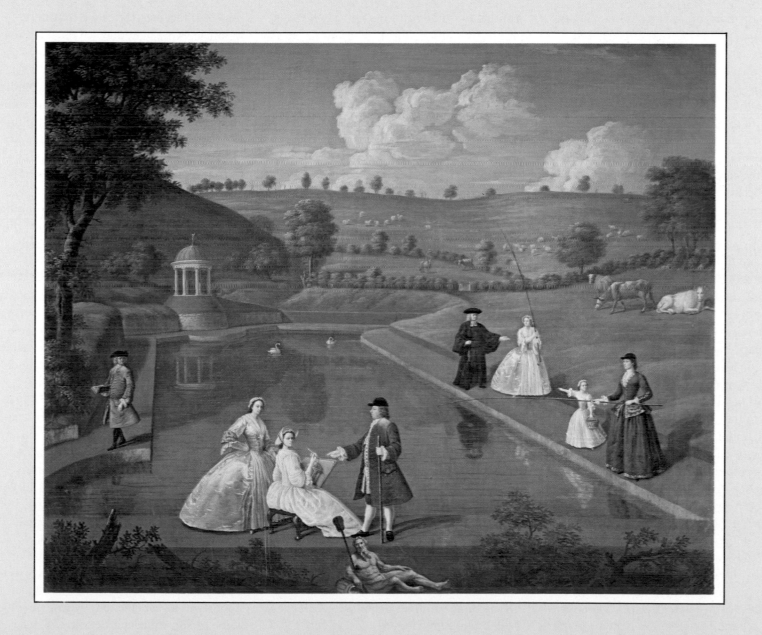

PIERRE AUGUSTE RENOIR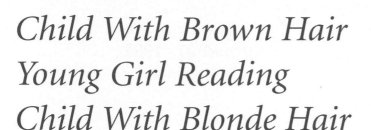

Child With Brown Hair
Young Girl Reading
Child With Blonde Hair

In his memoirs of his father, Pierre Auguste Renoir (1841-1919), film director Jean Renoir recalls his father's philosophy of life: "One is merely a cork," the painter said. "You must let yourself go along in life like a cork in the current of a stream…You go along with the current…You swing the tiller over to the right or left from time to time, but always in the direction of the current." And so the elder Renoir lived: Apprenticed to a porcelain painter as a teenager, copying at the Louvre, studying at the studio of Gleyre, painting in the forest of Fontainbleau with Monet, Sisley, and Bazille, sharing studios and living quarters with Monet and Bazille, exhibiting at the Salon, fighting in the war of 1870, and, finally, in 1874, exhibiting with his friends in the first of the four Impressionist group shows in which he was to take part. But then, as he was approaching his 40th birthday, Renoir entered a period of crisis. He stayed with the current, but he had to put his hand to the tiller. He traveled to Algiers, to Italy, where he saw the work of Raphael, to the Midi, and back to Algiers. He also refused to exhibit any longer with the Impressionists.

In the spring of 1881, however, he was still hopeful as he wrote to his dealer, Durand-Ruel, from Algiers, "I think I'm quite fit again now. I'm going to be able to work hard and make up for lost time." But by autumn he was writing to Durand-Ruel, "I am still bogged down in experiments…I'm not satisfied, so I clean things off, again and again…I am like a child at school. The new page is always going to be neatly written, and then pouf!…a blot. I'm still making blots…and I am 40 years old." Once he had seen Raphael's works, he concluded that he knew neither how to paint nor how to draw. He developed a dislike for Impressionism. He turned from plein air

painting to studio painting. He had entered a long, fallow period, during which he did relatively little painting.

Between 1885 and 1895, the decade surrounding his 50th birthday, he traveled much, to the south of France, to Italy, Spain, Brittany, London, and Holland. He was a close friend and frequent guest of Berthe Morisot Manet at her Thursday evening

> *…he has nevertheless captured the innocence and abandon of childhood.*

dinners, along with Mallarmé and Degas. Renoir had married in 1882, and in 1885 his son Pierre was born. In 1894 his second child, Jean, was born. In 1888, the first signs of the rheumatoid arthritis that was to progressively cripple him during the remaining years of his life appeared. Most important was his realization that, for him, Impressionism was dead. He had, in his own words, "wrung it dry." One might be understandably tempted to believe that these were the years of normal decline for any man, but Renoir was not any man. He was Renoir. For him they were years of searching and of sowing in the newly tilled earth.

To this critical period of Renoir's life belong three paintings of children: *Child With Brown Hair* (top left); *Young Girl Reading* (right); and *Child With Blonde Hair* (bottom left). Little more than sketches, and the largest hardly larger than a filing card (they are shown here only slightly reduced), they were all painted between 1887 and 1895, when Renoir was in his mid-40s to his

mid-50s. Together, they are a charming montage. Separately, they tell us something of Renoir's journey through the years.

The painting of the brunette (top left), with its cool, spare, lean line, shows Renoir as he was learning to draw again. The young girl's piquant expression has all the freshness of a peppermint stick. She is hesitant and tentative, as was Renoir at this time. The lines are clean, like the paintings he once did on porcelain. She mirrors reserve and restraint, just as did Renoir, who was holding back from the luscious and exuberant color we associate with him. With *Young Girl Reading* (right), by contrast, which was painted the following year, Renoir has returned to his profusion of color as to a September garden or an Arabian bazaar. Despite the exuberance, however, the color is controlled by his newly found line, delicate and subtle, as in the rounding of the shoulder and the tilt of the chin. The girl's total absorption in her book is matched by her unconscious and becoming air of grace and modesty. The blonde child (bottom left), which was done in 1895 as Renoir neared the end of his crisis, hints at the mature Renoir of the last 25 years of his life. Little more than a hasty sketch of a sleeping child, caught on the wing, he has nevertheless captured the innocence and abandon of childhood. The face is relaxed and full of color, like a sturdy 3-year-old who has suddenly dropped after strenuous play. Most important, he uses the reds by which we have come to know the later Renoir, which he wished to be "sonorous, to sound, like a bell."

Beginning as early as 1864, Renoir was to paint children hundreds of times. How does one explain his special affinity for children? Perhaps it was the challenge of color in their complexions, the delicacy of their skin,

Continued on p. 209

JAMA

September 10, 1982

THE JOURNAL of the American Medical Association

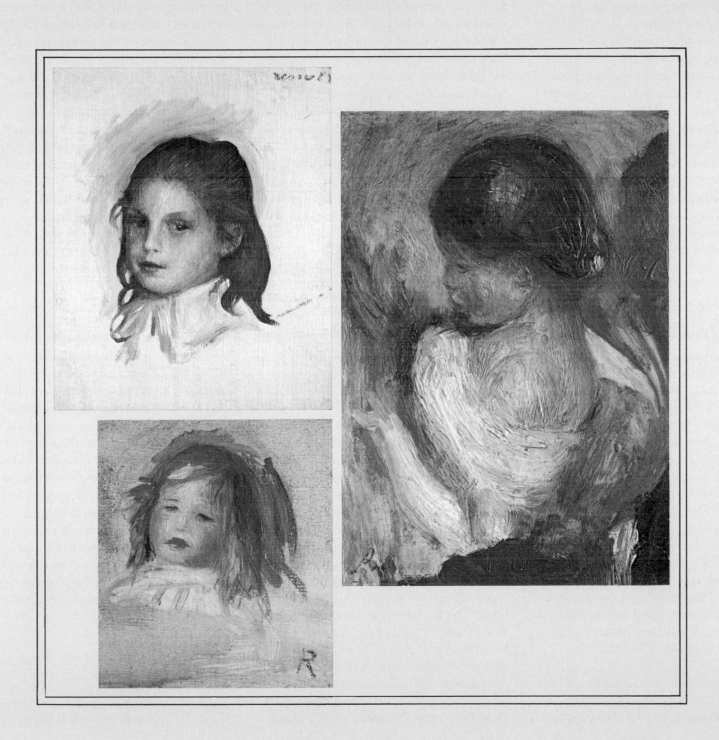

MAURICE DE VLAMINCK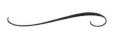

The Old Port of Marseille

In 1905, at the Salon d'Automne in Paris, a group of young painters exhibited works, the likes of which had never before been seen. Gone were the subtle color fusions of the now-familiar Impressionism. Instead, canvas after canvas was violent with color; large areas of green were juxtaposed against equally large fields of red; blues were pierced by pillars of orange, purples fought with yellows. All were vivid, brilliant, intense, unmixed colors, just as they came from the tubes. "Wild beasts," muttered a French journalist and the name stuck: *Fauves*. As a movement Fauvism did not last long; it was essentially over by 1908-1910. Among the young men so christened that day, however, was Maurice de Vlaminck (1876-1958). Born in Paris of Flemish descent, Vlaminck had a Flemish heart that loved van Gogh.

Everything Vlaminck did, he did with a flair and a passion. Married at the age of 18, he raced bicycles for a living, indulging, as he called it, his love of "open air, space, and liberty." He began painting to express what he felt about the French countryside seen from his bicycle. "I applied my colors with only one idea…to express what I felt." He took a job as a violinist in a gypsy orchestra on Montmartre so that his days would be free for him to roam the banks of the Seine and to paint. He painted for himself and for no one else. He was in love with nature. "It seemed to me that water, sky, clouds and trees understood the happiness they gave me." He wrote novels, and poetry, and anarchist articles. But it was for nature that he reserved his greatest passion. "One does not flirt with nature," he said. "One possesses her."

Vlaminck did not travel much beyond the Seine. He had the burgher's satisfaction with the place of his birth. In 1911, however, his dealer Vollard urged him to go to London to paint. The trip was not a success. The English mood was not to his liking. In 1913 his Fauve friend Derain urged him to join him in the Midi where he was painting, enchanted by the light. Vlaminck, who did not expect to be influenced by anything outside himself, reluctantly made the trip to Marseilles. He describes it in his autobiography, *Dangerous Corner*: "I was enchanted on my arrival at Marseilles. The old harbour was bathed in golden light; the pier, houses and anchored ships were impalpable…everything was seen through a silken gauze, as in a fairy tale, and

> *"…the light which touches up nothing, nor embellishes by artifice the appearance of people and things…"*

the rosy blue tints, touched with gold, made me think of some immaterial world…"

But in spite of the extraordinary light of the South, light that van Gogh claimed had driven him mad, Vlaminck still painted the dark, angry, brooding northern skies that were his Flemish heritage. "You come to Marseilles," said Derain, "and then wait till it gets dark [as in the North] before you start to paint." To Vlaminck it was all a part of truthfulness. The northern skies were in his blood. The southern skies were not. "Instinctively, I love the light of the north which leaves objects as they really are," he said, "the light which shines over Flanders and makes the waters of the canals so cold and still, which leaves verdure green and does not try to improve upon the whites, blues and reds

of forlorn barges; the light which touches up nothing, nor embellishes by artifice the appearance of people and things; the light which does not embrace earth, sky and water for its own sake." But he did paint nevertheless. *The Old Port of Marseille*, painted in 1913 when Vlaminck was in his late 30s, was one result of this trip.

It is perhaps dawn, such as Vlaminck first saw the old port. In the foreground, boats are piled higgledy-piggledy against each other as if beached by a storm. A bayonet of a bow juts off into space. A jumble of masts stretches upward. In the background, catching the first rosy rays of sun, are the houses of Marseilles, piled up Cézanne style, almost cubed. In between, reflecting the first light of day, is a deep and unforgiving water. Above, an angry sky holds on to night, threatening to withhold the day. Two small human figures, dwarfed, and almost an afterthought, trudge along the pier or fish off the side of a boat. The color, muted from his Fauve days, is nevertheless a cacophony of cerulean, golden umber, and greens, oranges, and yellows, outlined in black. The canvas is a slapdash of brushstrokes. Yet, the painting is anything but disordered. Over it there exists a strange harmony, a fought-for peace, like a passion that is spent or a night that has passed. Vlaminck is like that.

Nature was to be Vlaminck's temptress, his seductress, his mistress to the end of his life. His canvases are the record of how he struggled to possess her. For Vlaminck and his mistress it was a mutual seduction and an agreeable one.

Maurice de Vlaminck (1876-1958), *The Old Port of Marseille*, 1913, French. Canvas. 73 × 90.4 cm. Courtesy of the National Gallery of Art, Washington, DC; Chester Dale Collection, 1963. © 1995 The Board of Trustees of the National Gallery of Art.

JAMA

THE JOURNAL of the American Medical Association

October 8, 1982

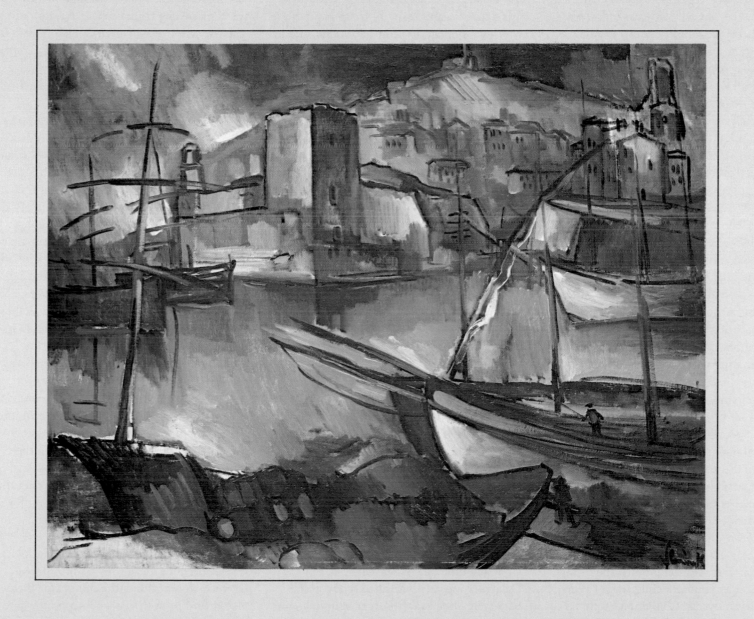

EUGÈNE DELACROIX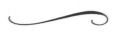

Vase of Flowers

Baudelaire called him the "most worthy representative of romanticism." Renoir called him "the greatest artist of the French school." Others named him heir to Rubens. His first entry to the Paris Salon, which is often credited with siring Impressionism, came when he was only 24 years old; it was not only accepted, but bought by the state for 1200 francs. He was Ferdinand Victor Eugène Delacroix (1798-1863).

Delacroix was the scion of a romantic age. Napoleon was emperor, and both of his older brothers fought in the Napoleonic wars. He greatly admired the poet Byron, who had rushed off to join the Greek war of independence and died at far-off Missolonghi, if not in battle, at least of war-related illness. He was a close friend of Chopin and was himself accomplished in music, as well as in writing. He was a devotee of Faust, Hamlet, and the novels of Sir Walter Scott. In his personal life he remained the perpetually available bachelor, forming frequent, and often long-lasting, liaisons, but never committing himself to the permanency of marriage. Even the illness that was to dog him for the last 30 years of his life with alternating periods of feverish activity and lethargy had the ring of the romantic: It was tuberculosis. But it was the circumstances of his birth that gave rise to the most romantic speculation about Delacroix, for his natural father was rumored to be none other than the noted French statesman Tallyrand. Moreover, there also appeared to be an elaborate attempt at a hazardous cover-up before his birth.

Eugène was the youngest of four children of Charles and Victoire Delacroix, aged 40 and 58 years, respectively, at the time of his birth. The next youngest child was 14 years old. For several years, Charles had suffered from a tumor of the testicles, most likely a sarcocele, which had deprived him of "all the advantages of virility." Now, however, a mere seven months before Eugène's birth, he elected to have the tumor removed. The operation, which was preceded by a luncheon

for his physicians at which a gracious Charles presided, lasted two and a half hours and had four intervals. At the last interval the patient said calmly, "My friends, that makes four acts of your operation, may the fifth not turn it into a tragedy." The operation was a success, and two months later Charles, with the pregnant Victoire at his side, and in the presence of witnesses, signed a document declaring his full recovery. The following month a government publication described "The operation for *sarcocèle* performed… upon Citizen Charles Delacroix. In April 1798, 13 days before the birth of Eugène,

> *"…a volcanic crater artistically concealed behind bouquets of flowers."*

the account was again published, with illustrations, in the government periodical *Le Moniteur Universel*. Nonetheless, speculation persisted, and even persists to the present day, regarding the identity of Eugène's father. While Charles went through elaborate and public declarations of his virility, it was the highly placed Tallyrand who took a special interest in Eugène's career, quietly opening doors that otherwise may not have been so readily opened. Moreover, Eugène bore an uncanny facial resemblance to Tallyrand and none whatsoever to his putative father.

By the time he was 30 years old, Eugène Delacroix was an established figure at the Salon. His themes were larger than life—war, revolution, and massacre—and were taken from history, mythology, literature, and religion. His paintings were not always well liked, but they were well known. Then, in 1832, at age 33, there occurred the most decisive event of his artistic life. Delacroix

was invited to accompany the Count de Mornay to Morocco. France had recently taken Algiers and it was deemed advisable to establish friendly relations with its next-door neighbor, the Sultan. Delacroix was to accompany the Count as a kind of "artist in residence." The trip lasted six months and the country overwhelmed Delacroix with its intense light, its often painfully vivid colors, its customs, its people, and its scenery. He was to paint these colors and customs for the rest of his life.

Vase of Flowers was painted in 1833, the year after Delacroix returned from Morocco. It was painted at the estate of his close friend, Frederic Villot, at Champrosay, near Fontainbleau, where Delacroix often sought rest, and where he himself eventually bought a cottage. The work originally belonged to Villot, a painter as well as a curator at the Louvre. Villot sold it in 1865 for 325 francs, and after passing through several sales the painting was confiscated by the Nazis from the Goldschmidt family. Eventually returned to them in 1958, it passed through other sales to its present owner in Scotland.

Why Delacroix did this relatively small easel painting at this time is a matter for reflection, for it is unlike the large, heroic themes and canvases he had done until then. It is in fact the first flower piece we know of. The other flower pieces, of which there are about half a dozen, date from his later years. However, certain facts concerning this period can perhaps explain the reason for the painting. In 1833, Adolphe Thiers, who had championed Delacroix as early as 1822, became Minister of Trade and Public Works. He secured for Delacroix the monumental commission of doing the murals for the Salon du Roi in the Palais Bourbon, where Louis-Philippe presided at legislative sessions. It was his first such commission and amounted to 35,000 francs. From this it is not difficult to imagine a tense and weary Delacroix, physically and mentally tired from his strenuous mural painting, with its

Continued on p. 209

JAMA

THE JOURNAL of the American Medical Association

October 22/29, 1982

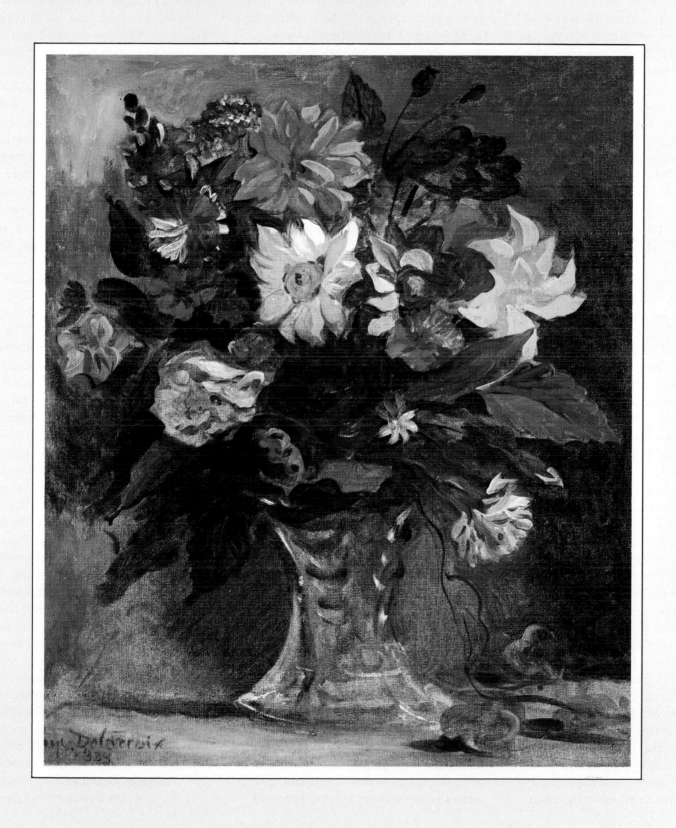

CAMILLE PISSARRO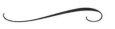

The Farm (La Ferme)

Impressionism reached its fullness in the 1870s, but the decade was less than kind to the man who has been called "the dean of the Impressionists," Camille Pissarro (1830-1903). Already in July of 1870 there was war, and the 40-year-old Pissarro, with two children and the pregnant Julie, not yet his wife, was forced to flee from France to England. He left everything behind, including furniture and some 1500 paintings, the fruit of his work since he had arrived in Paris from his native Danish West Indies in 1855. The couple's child, a daughter they named Adèlle-Emma, was born in the autumn but died two weeks later of an intestinal infection contracted from the wet nurse. While in England he heard that the Prussians had occupied his house in Louveciennes and had destroyed most of his canvases, the work of 15 years. When he returned, in 1871, he found his house pillaged and the canvases that had not been totally destroyed by the Prussians were being worn, painted side in, as aprons by the village women when they washed clothes.

Things temporarily brightened in 1872 when, for the first time in his life, the 42-year-old Pissarro became self-supporting, being no longer dependent on his mother, Rachel, to supplement his income. His good fortune increased when, at an auction the following year, his paintings sold at prices between 270 and 950 francs. At that time, an industrial worker earned 5 francs per day, an office worker 100 francs per month, rent was 150 to 200 francs per year, and food and fuel were 1000 francs per year for a family with two children. For the first month of 1874, Pissarro's dealer paid him more than 1800 francs. But the relative prosperity was short-lived. The country's financial crisis of 1873 caught up with the art market and his dealer made no more payments to him for the next five years. In the spring his oldest daughter, Minette, aged 9 years, contracted an upper respiratory tract infection and died.

Also in 1874 Pissarro faced the agonizing decision of whether to exhibit at the Salon, or whether to withdraw and exhibit with the then-unknown group of rebel painters who would become known as Impressionists. Despite the greater possibility of financial success through the Salon, he chose the latter because of his artistic beliefs. Their exhibition, the first for the Impressionists as a group, was not a success and the exhibitors were subjected to public ridicule. Nevertheless, once on a path Pissarro rarely swerved, and he eventually exhibited in all eight Impressionist shows, the only artist to remain so loyal. Self-doubt was a constant companion, however, and between 1876 and 1878 Pissarro averaged less than one completed painting a week. When he was able to sell them at all, he received 50 francs for a small (50.8 × 63.5 cm) canvas and 100 francs for the larger (63.5 × 76.2 cm) ones.

...a bourgeois who called himself a "proletarian without overalls."

The nadir of the decade came in 1878. Nearing age 50, Pissarro described himself as being in a "hell of inaction." His closest and most intimate friend, who had sustained him both financially and emotionally for many years, died suddenly at the age of 52. At auction, the prices of his paintings dropped to a low of 7 to 10 francs for a painting. His wife, Julie, pregnant at the age of 40, was bitter, lonely, and nagging at their penniless condition, not comprehending his single-minded devotion to painting. Pissarro wrote to his dealer: "It is no longer bearable. Everything I do ends in failure." On the other hand, he could also still write: "What I have suffered you can't imagine and what I am still suffering is terrible, very much more than when young, full of enthusiasm and fervor, convinced as I now am that I am lost and without a future. Nevertheless it seems to me that I would not hesitate, if I had to begin all over again, to follow the same path."

The Farm (La Ferme), also called *Woman With a Goat*, was painted at the end of the decade. Looking for new motifs, Pissarro had moved from Louveciennes, a suburb of Paris, in 1872, to Pontoise, an old Roman town with a population of several thousand about 3.2 kilometers from Paris, where it was picturesquely situated high on a bank of the Oise. Here he roamed its countryside for the rest of the decade in all weathers, in the worst heat, in the rain, in frightful cold, painting its landscape, its seasons, its people, its humble occupations, in short, its heart. *The Farm* is a broad, impersonal autumn landscape made intimate by a glimpse of a peasant woman performing one of her homely, daily chores, that of finding a spot for her goat to graze. The morning is crisp and clear. The sun has just risen, to the left. It shines full and brilliant on the left facade of the farmhouse, catching and flaming a few of the dying leaves on the large tree. The scene is timeless and rustic, nearly trite, but it is also one whose serenity and idealization belie its everyday harsh reality. Beneath the pastoral qualities Pissarro shows us a sense of isolation, even desolation, at the loneliness, the thinning leaves, at the departed summer, the imminent winter. The woman performs her task automatically, with little awareness of the glorious morning. The sun shines with false courage. A chill still clings to the landscape. One can only imagine the dankness and darkness of the interior of the almost windowless stucco farmhouse, an interior that is perhaps shared at night by the goat for the warmth it gives, in addition to its milk and cheese. The woman's peasant body is thickened by layers of clothing, her feet shod in heavy clogs, testimony to the penetrating dampness and cold, both inside and out. The skin of her hands is reddened and cracked by laundry soaps, by wet, and by cold. As Pissarro portrays her, her life is,

Continued on p. 209

JAMA

THE JOURNAL of the American Medical Association

November 12, 1982

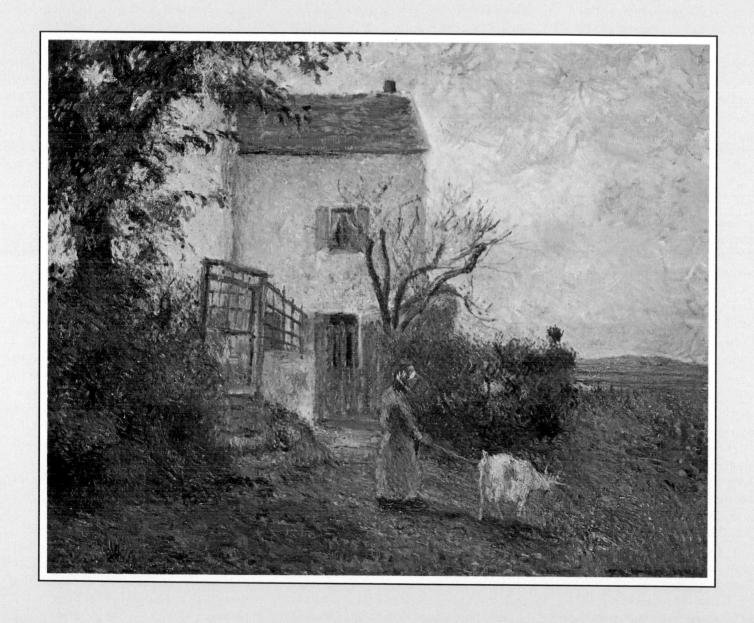

AMEDEO MODIGLIANI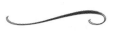

Gypsy Woman With Baby

In the Paris of World War I, where he worked the last 15 or so years of his life, he was known only to other artists and writers. His paintings sold for little, and he often gave away his drawings in the bars and cafés of Montparnasse. He painted on both sides of the canvas, to save money. Sculptures he carved in Italy are rumored to be at the bottom of the Reale Canal in Livorno, dumped there by himself when his friends laughed at their primitive shapes. His behavior was eccentric and shocking, even by Paris standards of the teens. He took hashish pills, which he bought for 25 centimes each (a modest meal cost 300 centimes), used cocaine and ether, and drank absinthe, gin, and brandy to excess. On several occasions he removed all his clothes in public. He was promiscuous and sexually abused his women. His favorite book, which he carried on his person and could quote from memory, was Lautréamont's *Les Chants de Maldoror*, a work of bizarre and sadistic imagery that was to influence the Surrealists greatly. He could also recite Dante by heart. In his youth he was a devotee of Nietzsche and believed that persons of moral superiority, such as he believed himself to be, lived by a separate ethic. His ego was fragile, he was insecure and timid, and he compensated by being aggressive. He was demanding and self-centered, his spirit anguished and tormented. Yet on his death at the age of 35, every artist and writer in Paris followed in his funeral cortege and he was buried in Père-Lachaise cemetery. Not surprisingly for a man who had become a myth almost before he was dead, the prices of his paintings skyrocketed almost immediately. Two days after his death, prices went up ten times. Ten years later paintings that had sold for 150 francs at the end of his life were selling for 500,000 francs, and persons who had received the giveaway drawings were seeking to authenticate them. The canal at Livorno was dredged, but the sculpture was not found.

For one who has become such a legend, it is impossible to sketch his life in any but the broadest strokes. Amedeo Modigliani (1884-1920) was born in Tuscany, in the Italian seaport town of Livorno (Leghorn), to a cultured, liberal, bilingual (Italian and French) Jewish family, the youngest of four children. On the maternal side the history of mental instability was strong. Modigliani, called "Dedo" by his family, was a sickly child, with numerous pulmonary illnesses. He did poorly in school, until, in 1898, at the age of 14, he began taking lessons in drawing, portraiture, landscape, and the nude in Livorno under

> *...as though she had come into possession of a secret, primal knowledge.*

Micheli, student of Fattori. He was best at the nude. In 1901, after a serious attack of pleurisy, his mother took him to Capri. From there Dedo went on his own to Rome, Naples, and Misurina. To a friend he expressed his adolescent hope: "I should like my life to be as an opulently abundant river flowing over the land with joy." The following year Modigliani left home for good, going to Florence to study under Fattori at the Scuola Libera di Nudo, but soon he went to Venice for similar studies. Here he lived in a heady, decadent atmosphere, and it was also here that he was first introduced to hashish pills. In January 1906, at the age of 22, Modigliani left for Paris where he was finally to paint seriously, almost always portraits of nudes, and where he was to spend the rest of his short life. He settled in the artist colony of Montmartre, where he was soon drinking absinthe with Utrillo and befriending Soutine.

In Paris Modigliani had grave difficulties with women; his reputation with them was unsavory. Nevertheless, in 1917, when he

was 33 and far gone with drink and drugs, he met the sheltered Jeanne Hébuterne, an art student, aged 19. She attached herself to him with fanatic devotion, but their relationship was more that of a wolf and a lamb, who, as Lautréamont says, "may not look at each other with gentleness." In November 1918, the couple's only child, a daughter, Giovanna, was born in Nice, where the couple had gone some months earlier for Modigliani's health. He returned alone to Paris the following May, but Jeanne, pregnant again, joined him a month later. It was only during this last summer of his life that Modigliani's paintings began to bring decent prices. Jeanne, on the other hand, could cope with neither housekeeping nor child care. The studio was dirty, the child was put out to a nurse, Modigliani ate in restaurants. He was frequently ill. Jeanne's drawings of him show him in bed, reading. His last photograph, taken in late 1919 or early 1920, shows him unkempt, tired, and worn, but still handsome, as he had always been. In January 1920 Modigliani was stricken with a kidney ailment. He was also coughing blood. He died ten days later of tuberculous meningitis, which his physician said had been smoldering, unrecognized, for some time. For Jeanne, now nine months pregnant and estranged from her parents, it was the ultimate loss. She did not wait for the baby to be born. Two days after Modigliani's death, at 4 o'clock in the morning, she threw herself from a fifth floor window of her parents' home.

Gypsy Woman With Baby, also called *Maternité*, or *La Bohémienne*, was painted during the last year of Modigliani's life. It is not known who the model is, nor whether the work was painted in Nice or in Paris. However, Modigliani had an infant daughter at the time, toward whom he had the tenderest feelings, and it is possible that the pose reminded him of Jeanne and their baby.

The canvas is dominated by the sculptural figure of a woman, as cool and remote as an

Continued on p. 210

JAMA

December 3, 1982

THE JOURNAL of the American Medical Association

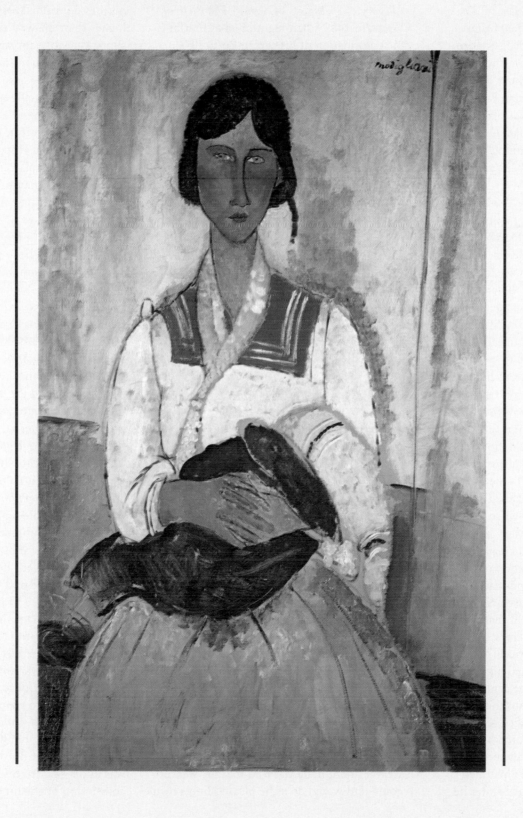

SANDRO BOTTICELLI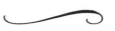

Madonna and Child

Called the "brightest star of the Florentine galaxy in the latter part of the [15th] century" and "one of the greatest painters Italy has ever produced," Sandro Botticelli (1444-1510) was nevertheless forgotten until just over 100 years ago, when he was rediscovered by Victorian England. No small part in his eclipse was played by the rise of the three stars of the Florentine High Renaissance at the beginning of the 16th century: Leonardo, Raphael, and Michelangelo.

Sandro Botticelli was born Alessandro di Mariano Filipepi, the son of a not very prosperous leather tanner in Florence. He was the youngest of eight children, four of whom survived. As a boy he was sickly, and although, according to the 16th-century biographer, Vasari, he was given good schooling, he was always discontented. He would learn what he wanted to learn, and he especially took no pleasure in "reading, writing, or accounts." In his teens he was apprenticed to the goldsmith Botticello, according to Vasari, who is, however, not always reliable. What is certain is that around 1464, when he was 20 years old, Botticelli entered the workshop of the Carmelite monk and painter Fra Filippo Lippi—the same Fra Filippo Lippi who had caused such a scandal in Florence eight years earlier when he eloped with the model for a Virgin Mary he was painting, the beautiful nun Lucrezia Buti, on the occasion of her veneration of the Girdle of Our Lady. (The pupil-teacher-pupil cycle was to complete itself eight years later, in 1472, when the fruit of that union, the future painter, Filippino Lippi, age 15, entered the workshop of Botticelli.)

From 1470, when he opened his own workshop, until the end of the century, Botticelli's career roughly spans the years of the rule of Lorenzo "il Magnifico" de' Medici, who greatly admired and favored him. His development can be marked by three of his most famous and most often illustrated works: *Fortitude*, in 1470, shortly after he opened his workshop; *The Primavera*, or *Allegory of Spring*, in 1477; and *The Birth of Venus*, in 1485, often mentioned as marking the culmination of his career. Botticelli's career declines only after 1496, when the apocalyptic Dominican preacher, Savonarola, who had been denouncing the paganism and Platonism of the Medici Florence to increasingly large and enthusiastic crowds, came to power. Although there is no evidence that Botticelli was ever a *piagnoni*, the name given to the official followers of Savonarola, his work becomes moralistic and tortured. For the last ten years of his life Botticelli

> *The paradox of the painting is in the Child, who looks older and wiser than the mother.*

painted little, although in 1504 he was a member of the commission charged with choosing the setting in Florence for Michelangelo's *David*. In his last years Botticelli went about on crutches and died after long illness and decrepitude. He was 66 years old.

Botticelli had a complex, neurotic personality. During his life he made much money, according to Vasari, but he lived immoderately, squandered, and mismanaged it. He was given to whimsical and eccentric behavior. He never married, and on one occasion, when he dreamed he had married, he was so distraught that he had to walk the streets of Florence all night. He was also fond of jesting and of the practical joke. Vasari records that Botticelli lived next door to a weaver whose eight looms shook his house so badly that he could neither paint nor even stay at home. When Botticelli spoke to the weaver about it, he was told that the weaver could and would do as he pleased in his own house. Botticelli then balanced a huge stone on the roof of his own house, which was higher than the weaver's. When the walls shook the stone threatened to dislodge and crush his neighbor's house and looms. In terror the weaver asked him to remove the stone, but Botticelli replied that he could and would do as he pleased in his own home.

Early in his career, when he was in the workshop of Fra Filippo Lippi and for a short time thereafter, Botticelli painted many Madonnas. So marked was the influence of Lippi that until the relatively recent revival of study of Botticelli, some of the Madonnas now attributed to Botticelli were once thought to have been painted by Fra Filippo Lippi or by his son, Filippino Lippi, whom Botticelli had trained. The theme itself dates back to about the sixth century. Three major types of Madonnas were developed in Byzantine art, each intended to recall a theological teaching: the regal Madonna, enthroned; the standing Madonna, holding the Child on her left arm; and the interceding Madonna, praying. In addition, there were two additional, more maternal types: the nursing Madonna (*galaktotrophousa*) and the Madonna with the Child caressing her cheek while she contemplates his coming Passion and death (*glykophilousa*). Western art at the end of the Middle Ages adopted these same general types, but gradually came to favor more personal and intimate representations. The interest was in the emotional lives of the Virgin and Child and the purpose was to evoke sentiment and piety rather than to teach theology. During the Renaissance and continuing well into the Baroque period, the *glykophilousa*, the Virgin contemplating the Passion, and its variants was the most popular representation. Botticelli's *Madonna and Child* is one such example.

Madonna and Child, like many others on the same theme that he painted, belongs at the beginning of Botticelli's career, when he was in his early to mid-20s. According to the convention of the time, as would have been

Continued on p. 210

JAMA

December 17, 1982

THE JOURNAL of the American Medical Association

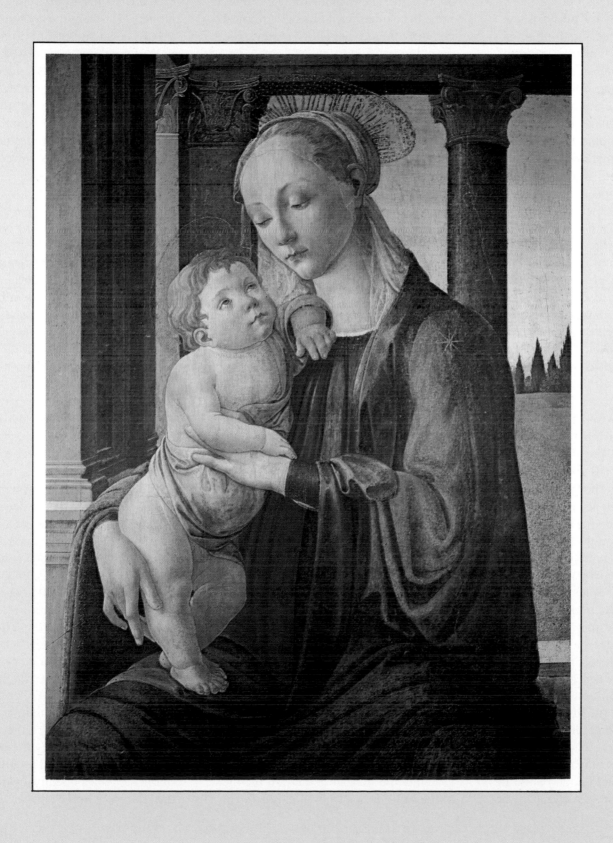

GABRIEL METSU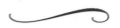

The Intruder

When the golden light of the 17th century shone on Holland, it saw that life was good indeed. Once subject to Spain, the Dutch were now newly independent, prosperous, a political and a colonial power, a rising sea power, a haven for the persecuted. Their pride was justified. But, deprived of religious images as a result of their Calvinist conversion, and little inclined to classical history or mythology, Dutch artists were denied many subjects traditionally interpreted by the painter. So they turned inward, to their own land, their sea and ships, their towns and streets, to themselves, even to their flowers, food, and stemware, and dead game and fowl. But while portraits, landscapes, and still lifes provided one kind of satisfaction and pride, the Dutch also wished to see themselves in context, engaged in their daily activities of home, business, and street. Thus arose the popularity of the so-called genre painting. Eventually, the genre painting, like an inquisitive camera, which at first had confined itself to activities in the courtyard or to merrymaking in the tavern, began to intrude into the more intimate life of the Dutch, poking into their brothels, even intruding into the privacy of their bedrooms. Moreover, the painters developed an extensive vocabulary of symbols, or iconography, so that what might look on the surface to be a simple, homely scene could be transformed by the addition of a few equally homely objects, such as a basin or an owl or a candle, into a painting that told, to the properly initiated, a quite different story. And the Dutch liked stories. So, also, did the Victorians two centuries later, but not, apparently, the same kind of stories. Thus, whereas the 17th-century Dutch were moralistic (many of their paintings, even a still life of flowers, for example, taught a lesson of life), the 19th-century Victorians were still puritanical, and while they could not expurgate a centuries-old painting, they could bowdlerize its title or other written descriptions. Even Goethe

did it. Thus, many a bold bordello scene came to be interpreted as a sweet musical evening at home with father, mother, daughter, and suitor (see Ter Borch, *The Suitor's Visit*). Still, part of the genius of the Dutch is to be ambiguous, and, thus, in many of the paintings one may see what one will see. Such are the paintings by Teniers (see Teniers, *Tavern Scene*) and Ter Borch. Such, also, is thought to be *The Intruder* by Gabriel Metsu (1629-1667). Even today, Metsu's painting remains largely in mystery. It is not so easily penetrated.

> *...an otherwise commonplace scene has been lifted into a singular harmony of color, line, and composition.*

On the surface, the events portrayed are simple enough. A young woman, partially in night attire, and her expression none too welcoming, rises hastily from her curtained bed, reaching to slip her foot into her slipper. A laughing cavalier, arrayed in rich black and gold, bursts through the door from an outer room and reaches to embrace her. A much-amused housekeeper, keys and purse dangling from her belt, only halfheartedly restrains him. Off to the left, in opulent velvet and ermine, her hair dressed and bejeweled, her face partially illumined by light from the unbarred window behind her, sits an equally amused older woman toying with a fine ivory comb. A sumptuous Turkish carpet covers the table to her left. On it, a baroque-framed mirror reflects her image. At her fingertips is a costly jewel box. At her feet, her little spaniel lapdog, or *kookikertje*, examines the scene quizzically. At the right of the painting, tossed over an intricately

carved chair, just as the young woman had probably left them the night before, are a red jeweled gown and ermine-trimmed jacket. In the foreground are a pewter ewer and a guttered candle set in its holder.

So much for the objects Metsu painted. It is when one comes to "read" the painting, at which the 17th-century bourgeoise patrons were highly skilled, that meanings shift and slide and slip away. The conventional interpretation is that a betrothal is represented. In Dutch society, a young man was required to make a public avowal of his fervor before the actual betrothal. This he is presumably doing by bursting into the bride-to-be's early morning boudoir in the presence of her mother and the housekeeper. According to Christian iconography, the mirror then represents purity; the pitcher and candle, virginity; the dog, fidelity. The bride is not wearing her shoes, an indication that the room is holy ground, the nuptial chamber.

Another, more recent interpretation, however, suggests that this may be a bordello scene, so popular at the time, or, as the Dutch called them, *bordeeltjen*, a specific term because the general term "genre" was not yet known. In this case, the iconography is read much differently. The mirror, because an image is reflected in it, becomes a symbol for vanity. Nor are the shoes a symbol for holy ground, for they are not truly empty; the young woman is slipping her foot into the left one. Finally, the configuration of the extinguished candle and long-necked pitcher have unmistakable anatomical reference to activity of the night before. The keys and purse at the housekeeper's belt indicate what kind of house she keeps.

This latter reading of *The Intruder* could probably be clinched if the position of the right hand of the woman in green could be explained. For example, if the seated woman could be shown to have once held a coin between her thumb and forefinger (and since erased by a onetime owner or dealer), then her place in the tableau would not be

Continued on p. 211

JAMA

February 11, 1983

THE JOURNAL of the American Medical Association

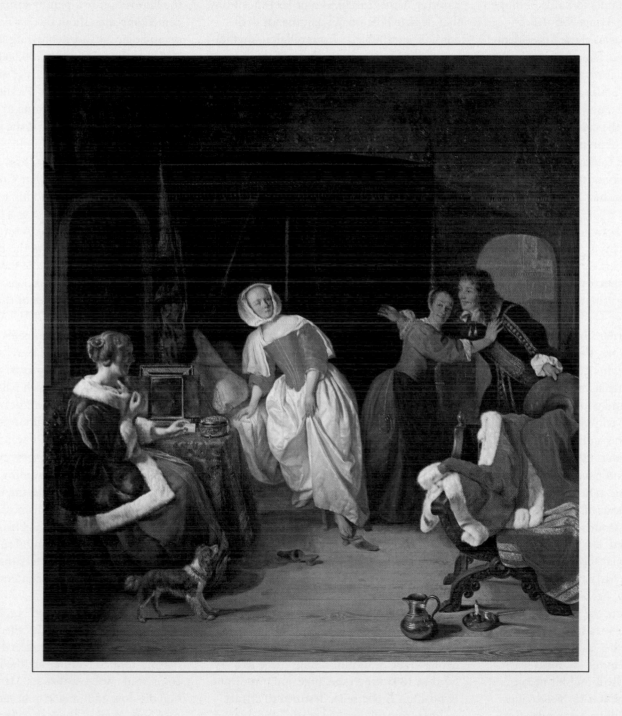

GUSTAVE COURBET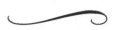

La Mère Grégoire

Europe, in 1848, was in a state of foment. Revolution and revolt were rampant. In Paris the workers rose up and Louis Philippe was forced to abdicate. Louis Napoleon, nephew of Bonaparte, was elected president of the Second Republic. There were, likewise, revolutions in Vienna, forcing Metternich to resign, and in Venice, Berlin, Milan, and Parma. In Switzerland a new constitution was adopted, making the country a federation. In Rome the papal premier was assassinated and Pius IX fled to Gaeta. Marx and Engels issued the *Communist Manifesto*, and John Stuart Mills published *The Principles of Political Economy*.

Living in Paris at this time was the 29-year-old (Jean Désiré) Gustave Courbet (1819-1877), arrived eight years earlier from the provinces in the conviction that he would revolutionize painting. The eldest in a family of four sisters, Courbet was born in the beautiful village of Ornans in the Franche-Comté region of the Jura, the son of Régis Courbet, a well-to-do vine grower, and Sylvie Oudot of Ornans, "a tenacious woman,… affectionate, simple, and good," on June 10, 1819. Educated in the conventional fashion of the provinces, he was a dilatory student, rebellious and boisterous, taking interest only in the drawing and painting lessons given by a local teacher. When, at the age of 21, Courbet left for Paris, his father expected him to study law, but Courbet was adamant in his intention to paint. His father responded with long-term financial support.

For Courbet, who was, as he foretold, to revolutionize painting, becoming the undisputed father of Realism, the year 1848 was likewise one of stirrings. Indeed, the seven-year period 1848 to 1855 is considered to be critical in his life and in his art, for it was during this time that he found his métier. Public taste at the time was formed by the Salons, the annual exhibits held under the auspices of officialdom that determined, often in a few seconds of deliberation on each candidate, which paintings should be

hung and which should be refused. The judges favored the traditional in French painting, large "machine-type" compositions that depicted the imaginary, the ideal, the heroic scene. Subjects from religion, mythology, and history covered the walls of the Salon each year. The Idealists, the Classicists, and the Romantics dominated. But Courbet, influenced perhaps by Daumier, wanted to paint tangible facts and seen reality, not ideas. When criticized for his choice, he retorted, "Show me an angel, and I'll paint one." And then, when he could carry the discussion no farther, he would close it with a

> *To paint the common man was dangerously Socialist.*

roar of his noisy and peculiar laughter, his huge frame shaking meanwhile. Nor did he wish to romanticize his facts. Hence he turned to the people and situations he saw every day—to the Ornans peasants awkwardly mourning his grandfather in a funeral cortege, to an old man and a young boy breaking stones for a road, to the preposterously fat wife of the proprietor of a brasserie he frequented. The Parisians didn't like his paintings. They were outraged. To paint the common man was dangerously Socialist. To paint him life-size, the size of gods and heroes, was blasphemous. To paint death was perhaps acceptable, but to paint it in its commonplace aspects, to omit its uplifting and enobling aspects, was heresy. Most important, to paint an ugly woman was to destroy art, which was art only when it depicted the beautiful. Things came to a head in 1855, when the huge and important Exposition Universelle, destined to attract visitors from all over the world, was opened in Paris. Courbet had two works rejected. It was about this time that he wrote to a friend: "Under the laughing mask you know, I hide

regrets, bitterness and a sadness that grips my heart like a vampire." He responded to the Exposition by opening his own unprecedented one-man show, the Pavilion of Realism, on an adjacent site, borrowing heavily to do so. He expected to gross 100,000 francs, but, like Shakespeare's Caesar, his "wisdom was consumed in confidence." Public turnout, even among those who came to ridicule, was sparse. Like a bad joke, the one-man show died.

It was about this time, 1855, that Courbet painted the portrait *La Mère Grégoire*. In 1848, Courbet had moved his studio to 32 rue Hautefeuille, where he was to remain for the greater part of his life. A few steps away, at 28 rue Hautefeuille, was the Brasserie Andler, presided over by the Bavarian proprietor, M Andler, and his Swiss wife, Mme Andler, the Mère Grégoire of the painting, who ruled over the cash desk and the ledger. Unlike the usual mirrored cafés of Paris, the brasserie was more like a German beer hall, a long room, dark and narrow, with long tables and benches at which patrons sat back to back. Sausages, hams, and cheeses hung from the ceiling. On the floor sat barrels of sauerkraut. A billiard table was at the rear. Here Courbet went almost every evening from 6 until 11 PM, consuming great quantities of food and beer, playing billiards, arguing his tenets of Realism, smoking, boasting, and laughing. "Realism may have been born in Courbet's mind in his studio… but the brasserie held it over the baptismal font," says Castagnary, a contemporary frequenter of the café.

As Courbet has painted her, Mme Andler, or Mère Grégoire as she is called, sits in her customary place at the cashier's desk. On the marble-topped counter are the ledger, a few coins, and a vase of flowers. Her ungainly body is dressed in black, relieved by the delicacy and detail of the lace collar and cuffs. The tiny flowers in the vase contrast with the outsize body and reinforce the delicacy of the collar and cuffs. In her left hand Mère

Continued on p. 211

JAMA

THE JOURNAL OF the American Medical Association

June 24, 1983

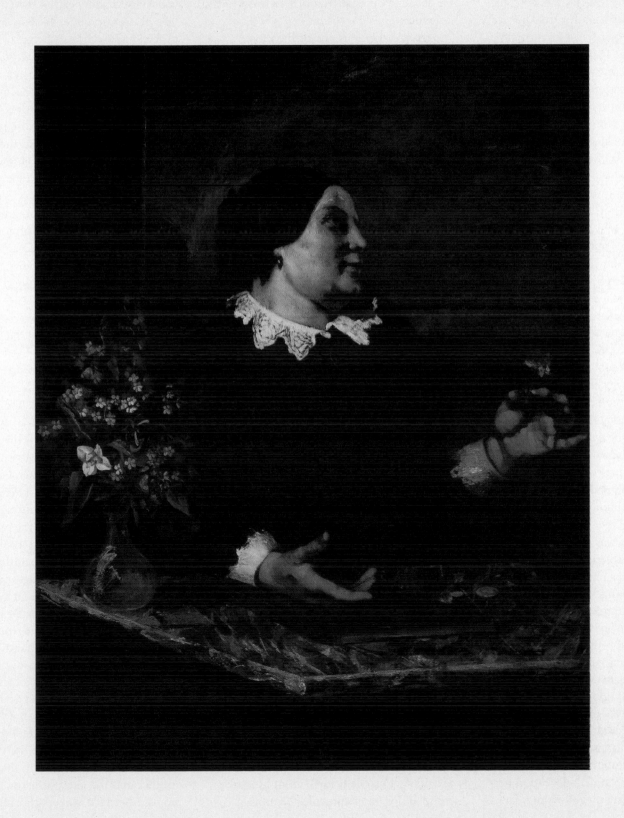

THOMAS EAKINS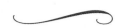

The Gross Clinic

In Europe, in Paris, Realism was born in 1848. Courbet was its father. In America, Realism was born a quarter of a century later, in Philadelphia. Thomas Eakins (1844-1916) was its father. In each case, it was a difficult child, shocking polite society, rejected by public and critics alike, and bringing their fathers much sorrow and hardship, but never once abandoned by them.

Eakins was born in Philadelphia on July 25, 1844, the first child of Benjamin Eakins, a writing master, and Caroline Cowperthwait Eakins. Three sisters, and a brother who died in infancy, followed. In high school Eakins showed special aptitude for mathematics, science, and drawing, and after graduation he worked with his father teaching penmanship. At the same time he attended the Pennsylvania Academy of Fine Arts, learning to draw the human figure. To advance and reinforce his knowledge, Eakins also enrolled at Jefferson Medical College, where he took anatomy and dissection classes under Drs Joseph and William H. Pancoast. In 1866, when he was 22, Eakins went to Paris where he entered the École des Beaux Arts to study with the traditionalist Gérôme. He returned four years later to the family home in Philadelphia, where he established and maintained his studio for the rest of his life.

The young Eakins was a strong, active man, vigorous and athletic, and his early Philadelphia paintings reflect his interests: scenes of rowing, fishing, sailing, and hunting. Especially did he like to paint the nearly nude body in motion, every muscle and joint portraying its appropriate action. In 1873 and 1874, he again attended Jefferson Medical College, taking Dr Joseph Pancoast's "General, Descriptive, and Surgical Anatomy," and Dr Samuel Gross' "Institutes and Practice of Surgery." A year later, when he was 31, Eakins began work on his first "big painting" in anticipation of exhibiting it at the forthcoming Nation's Centennial celebration to be held in Philadelphia the following year.

He chose to do a portrait of Dr Gross, today known as *The Gross Clinic*.

Professor Gross is one of the most eminent surgeons America has ever produced. His huge and profusely illustrated textbook (which Eakins probably read), *A System of Surgery*, was first published in 1859 and is called one of the greatest surgical texts ever written. In 1847, Gross was one of the founders of the American Medical Association. At a meeting of the Association in 1870, five years before Eakins painted *The Gross Clinic*, Gross was the first to suggest that the Association replace its

> *There is no fear in these hands, only confidence and control.*

unwieldy annual *Transactions* with a weekly medical journal—a suggestion that finally became a fait accompli on July 14, 1883, and which has continued ever since as *The Journal of the American Medical Association*, or simply, *JAMA*.

As Eakins depicts him, Professor Gross, then aged 70, stands within his milieu, the surgical amphitheater, performing and lecturing on the removal of a sequestrum from the femur of a young man. His brightly lighted head is the apex of a triangular composition of similarly lighted figures, while behind him, in deep shadow, the students rise in vertical and horizontal rows. Above him and off to the left, recording, sits the clinic clerk, Dr Franklin West. Below him, a woman, the patient's mother, required to be present because this is a charity operation, shields her eyes. Over at the right, the patient lies on a table on his right side, his left buttock and thigh exposed, his sock-covered feet visible below. About him are grouped five other surgeons, beginning

clockwise at the head of the table, Drs W. Joseph Hearn, James M. Barton, Daniel Apple, and Charles S. Briggs. The fifth surgeon is hidden behind Dr Gross, only his left hand, right shoulder, and right knee visible. Behind the surgeons, in the entryway, are two more shadowy figures, at the right Dr Samuel Gross, Professor Gross' son (who was to succeed his father in the chair of surgery at Jefferson), and Hughey O'Donnell, the janitor. All are portrait likenesses of the models. The composition is closed by an instrument table in the foreground. The colors of the painting are almost monochromatic, the only deviations being the pink cloth on the instrument table, the patient's gray-blue socks, and the blood on the scalpel and the surgeon's hands—shocking blood that the contemporary American realist Raphael Soyer notes is not like "the blood so harmoniously blended in Delacroix's battle scenes, [but] real blood, sticky, thick."

In an Eakins painting there are no trivia, only an ordering of detail, one to the other, and each an expression of an entire story. Consider, for example, just the hands of the principal figures. In the four surgeons clustered about the patient, each hand is painted according to its proper task: Hearn lifts momentarily the soft, lightweight chloroform cloth; Barton holds the probe, gently feeling inside the incision; Apple, with his left hand, hands up a tenaculum, meanwhile concentrating on the retractor in his right (the figure hidden behind Dr Gross holds the second retractor in his left hand, just visible at the far side of the wound); across the table Briggs has both hands firmly on the patient's leg, keeping it steady and extended; and in the background, West sits in a writing posture, his right hand responding to every word of Gross' case notes. But the highpoint of the drama is encapsulated in Eakins' juxtaposition of the hands of the two people most closely identified with the patient: the mother and the chief surgeon, hers, drawn up over her face, fingers clawing and taut,

Continued on p. 212

JAMA

THE JOURNAL of the American Medical Association

July 15, 1983

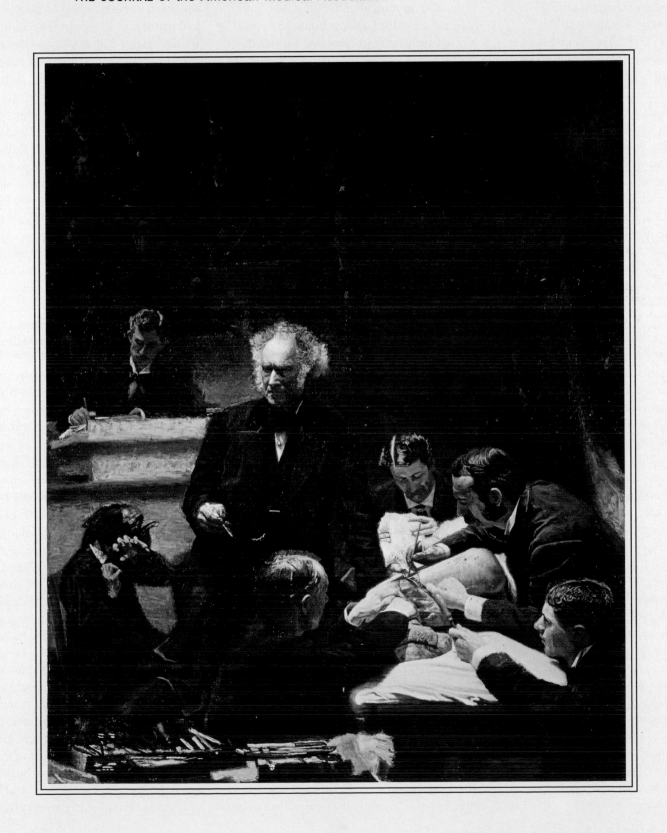

HENRI ROUSSEAU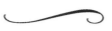

Tropical Forest With Monkeys

Until 1893, when he retired after 25 years as a petty bureaucrat in the customs house in Paris, Henri Rousseau (1844-1910) had been never more than an obscure little man, "a little small colourless frenchman,…like any number of frenchmen one saw everywhere," as Gertrude Stein described him. He lived alone, a widower who had lost all his family (except for a daughter, who lived with relatives), an innocent eccentric who wrote plays that were never produced, composed music that was never published, played the flute, the cornet, violin, and mandolin, and sang in a "sweet piping voice." To the neighborhood children he gave lessons in elocution, drawing, and music. For relaxation he took solitary walks to the Jardin des Plantes, where he spent hours observing the exotic plants and watching the animals. And he was a self-taught painter with an unshakable belief in his undiscovered genius.

Rousseau was born in the town of Laval, southeast of Paris, where his father had a hardware store. A mediocre student at best, he dropped out of school in his teens and joined the military. In 1868, upon the death of his father, he was released and settled in Paris, where he married Clémence Boitard, the daughter of a cabinetmaker, and began his career as a city customs clerk. But his ambition was to be a painter in the academic style of Ingres, who had just died, and to this end he drew and painted in his spare time. In 1884, when he was 40, Rousseau obtained permission to copy paintings at the Louvre; two years later he exhibited for the first time at the Salon des Indépendants, where, in contrast to the official Salon, virtually no painting was refused admission. The public laughed and the critics ridiculed, calling his work a "universal joke" and "stupefying," but for the next seven years (during which time Clémence died) Rousseau continued these annual exhibitions. Painful though they must have been, he never lost his serenity.

In 1893, at the age of 49, Rousseau resigned from the customs house to devote himself exclusively to painting. With virtually no training, and apparently still unaware of his lack of skill, he nevertheless retained complete confidence in his abilities. For the public he wrote that he was "on the verge of becoming one of our finest realistic painters" and that he possessed a "natural intuition" that "even my parents were unaware of." In a way he was prophetic, for only a year later Rousseau received his first favorable notice. It was only a single mention in the avant-garde press, but it heralded his discovery

…the garden, in its last delicious moment of indecision before yielding up its innocence.

by the young radical group of Paris painters and writers, among them Delaunay and Picasso. Affectionately nicknamed "Le Douanier" for his former customs work, he was appreciated, however, more for his humble social charm and naive eccentricities than for his work. In 1889, Rousseau married a second time, but the marriage ended four years later when his wife died. Finally, only five years before his own death, public recognition as a serious artist came at last to Rousseau in the form of an exhibition at the semi-official Salon d'Automne; his work was hung in the same room as that of the popular Fauves: Matisse, Derain, and de Vlaminck.

During these last years "Le Douanier" became the social lion of Montmartre. The famous "Banquet Douanier," given by Picasso in 1908 in his Bateau Lavoir studio, has been immortalized by Gertrude Stein in *The Autobiography of Alice B. Toklas*. It was intended as a "jokeful amusement" to honor

Rousseau and a painting of his that Picasso had just found in a grimy shop and bought for five francs. The studio was decorated and places were set for 30 guests at planks set across carpenter's trestles. The painting was decked with flags and a throne was set for Rousseau at the head of the table. When the food failed to arrive, however (Picasso having given the caterer the wrong day), the guests made it up with wine and the party soon degenerated into a noisy, riotous affair. The painter Marie Laurencin was one of the first to become drunk, and fell into a tray of jam tarts. Later, the poet Salmon became violent and had to be restrained. But throughout the long evening and into the morning, during the songs and the poetry readings, Rousseau sat happily on his throne, alternately dozing, with wax from the lantern above dripping on his bald head, or waking, playing the violin and singing songs. "Picasso," he exclaimed, his heart bursting with gratitude, "you and I are the greatest painters of our time." Fame and friends did not change Rousseau, however. He continued to live in the remote rue Perrel in a single room above a plasterer's shop. Here he painted, cooked, slept, and held his musical soirées on Saturdays.

The period was marred by only two events, both apparently the result of Rousseau's extreme credulity. In 1907, thinking he was doing a favor for an acquaintance, Rousseau become involved in bank fraud and was sent to prison. Later, touched by the childlike trust and obvious gullibility of this little bald man in his 60s—and swayed not a little by the strangeness of the painting he brought—the court released him on a suspended sentence. Not long after, Rousseau fell in love with Mme Léonie, the 54-year-old widowed daughter of one of his former coworkers at the customs house. In spite of her indifference, he pursued her with letters, gifts he could ill afford, and visited her at the department store where she worked. But if Léonie was cool, her father was adamant. No man who made such absurd paintings was suit-

Continued on p. 212

JAMA

THE JOURNAL of the American Medical Association

February 10, 1984

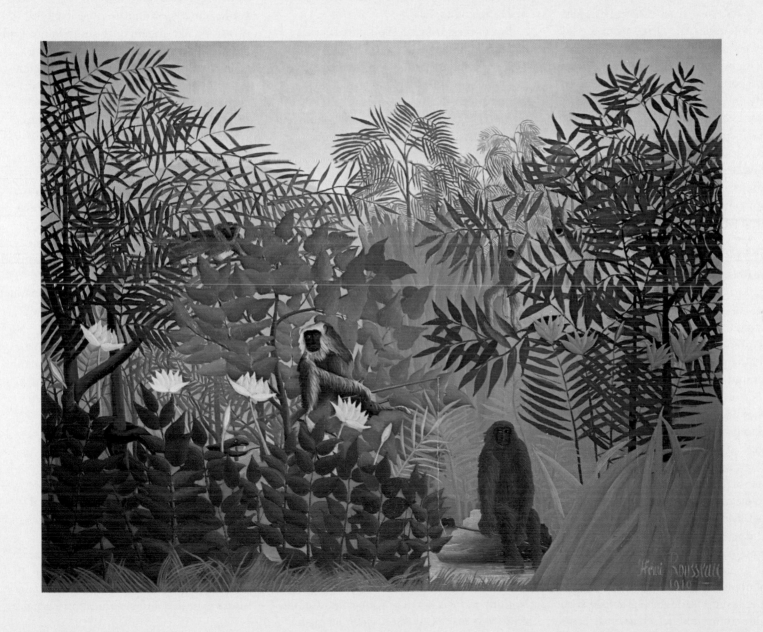

CLAUDE MONET

The Cradle—Camille With the Artist's Son Jean

The winter of 1867/1868 was one of a succession of many harsh times for Claude Monet (1840-1926), the bourgeois grocer's son, and the young daughter of a respectable family, Camille Doncieux, whom he had seduced three years earlier. Disinherited by both families, they lived from the sale of an occasional painting, prodigally when there was money, more often in sharp poverty after it was gone. Then Monet would live off the charity and forebearance of his friends, importuning them with wheedling, arrogant demands for sums in exchange for future paintings. Obsessed with his painting and bitter at his lack of recognition, Monet refused to marry Camille, and she, for whatever reasons she alone knew, stayed with him. December 1867 was typical in most respects: they were cold, they had no coal, and they had no money. But there was one difference: this winter they had a child, a son, Jean, born the previous August, and the child was sick. "I am without a penny," Monet wrote to his friend Bazille on New Year's Day, 1868, in one of his whining letters. "I have passed the whole of today nearly without a fire, and the baby is ill with a cold…For several days we have lacked the necessities, and even for so short a time it is not good to be without a fire with a baby and a wife."

Monet, an unorthodox, unknown, penniless painter of 25, had met Camille, a tall, darkly beautiful girl from a rigidly proper family, in 1864 when she was just shy of her 18th birthday. At the time, he was living with Bazille, who had dropped out of the École de Médecine to paint, in Bazille's studio. Monet was enchanted by Camille and, besides making her his model, formed a liaison with her. Camille committed herself at once. From that day forward, until her death 15 years later from uterine cancer, despite prolonged separations and even abandonments, she remained Monet's faithful model, mistress, and muse. Only much later did she become

his wife, and then only when she had promise of a small dowry. By then their son Jean was 3 years old and Camille's money was an escape, albeit a temporary one, from poverty and a renewed opportunity for Monet to paint, free of anxiety.

But in the spring of 1867, a fresh crisis had arisen in Monet's and Camille's lives. The 20-year-old Camille was pregnant, unwed, ill, and approaching term. The couple, living in Paris, was also again destitute, except for a small sum Monet had from the recent sale of two paintings. Monet placed Camille in the home of a medical

> *…it is Monet himself who is siphoning off the soul of Camille.*

practitioner of uncertain qualifications he had met through Bazille (most likely an ex-medical student acquaintance). Here she remained through the summer, while Monet went to Sainte-Adresse to live with his father's sister, where his father had promised him food and lodging, but not a penny to spend. In August, Camille was delivered of a healthy boy, but Monet, financially tethered in Sainte-Adresse, could not raise even the train fare for the trip to Paris to see Camille and his son until late September, when he turned up unexpectedly at Bazille's Paris studio. He had with him a "collection of magnificent canvases" he had managed to complete in Sainte-Adresse despite his desperate anxiety. Nothing more is heard of Monet and Camille until New Year's Day 1868, when he made his appeal to Bazille for money, this time for coal and other necessities for Camille and the sick Jean.

It was during this winter that Monet painted *The Cradle—Camille With the*

Artist's Son Jean. The composition is dominated by a central, bright triangle that is balanced on either side by the dark masses of Camille and the parental bed. The baby, borne up on its ribboned and rose-covered cradle, emerges from the labia-like folds of the drape like an emperor on his barge. Only a few millimeters of face and hands are visible, yet, with his glow of life, the infant dominates the entire painting. Bundled against the cold and rosy with fever, he is secure in his delicate world of pinks and pastel blues and yellows, except for one jarring accent of pure blue, which asserts itself on his bonnet. In contrast, Camille, though only 20 years old, has been transformed from the dark-haired, playful girl of earlier paintings to a drab, matronly domestic. Her body is thickened and her face is wan. It is as though, by some fiendish balance of spirits, the child can increase only as Camille decreases. More likely, it is Monet himself who is siphoning off the soul of Camille. Camille's shapeless body is a reminder of the difficult and precarious present; the bulky bed, a remembrance of a past liaison. It is in the cradle, which is connected to the bed by a diagonal fold of drape, that the future lies.

Monet has anticipated in color what T. S. Eliot would later paint in words: "Time present and time past/Are both present in time future,/And time future contained in time past…Time past and time future/Point to one end, which is always present." Thus it is only in the present, at its stillpoint, that time is transcended; it is in Camille, in the woman, the mother, that the breach between past and future is healed and becomes the eternal.

Claude Monet (1840-1926), *The Cradle—Camille With the Artist's Son Jean*, 1867, French. Oil on canvas. 116.2 × 88.8 cm. Courtesy of the National Gallery of Art, Washington, DC; collection of Mr and Mrs Paul Mellon, 1983. © 1995 The Board of Trustees of the National Gallery of Art.

JAMA

THE JOURNAL of the American Medical Association

May 11, 1984

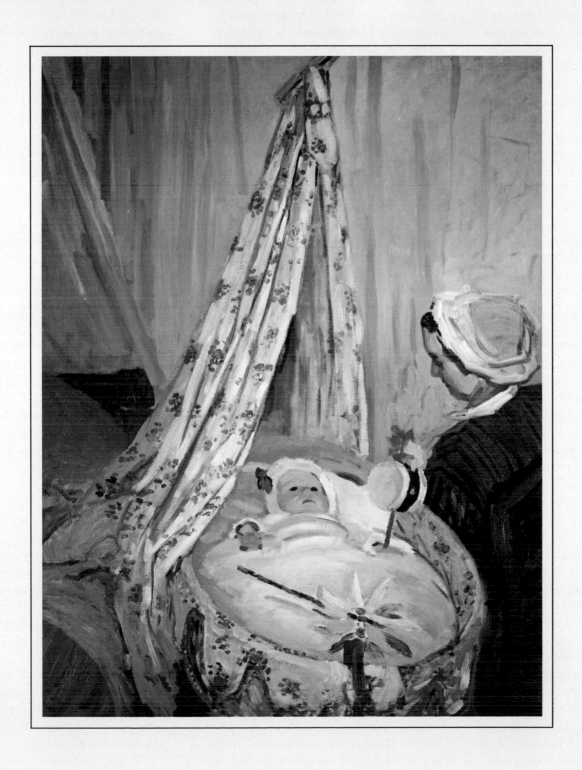

GEORGE WESLEY BELLOWS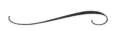

Dempsey and Firpo

George Wesley Bellows (1882-1925), sports hero of Columbus, Ohio, and Ohio State University, produced some 600 paintings in his relatively brief lifetime. Most were scenes of the life around him—tender portraits of women and children, New York tenements, vagrants, the jobless, riverscapes, snow scenes, urban renewal. Yet his reputation as a painter of prizefighting would suggest that it was his principal genre. In fact, he produced only six boxing paintings, three between 1907 and 1909, when prizefighting was legal only in self-styled "clubs" before small groups of "members," and three from 1923 to 1924, after boxing had been legalized as a general spectator sport in New York State. On the other hand, he did produce many boxing drawings and lithographs, which were widely reproduced.

Bellows was born in Columbus, Ohio, the only child of parents already well into middle age. His middle name was an invocation of the founder of Methodism, and testified to his mother's ambitions for this late-life child: She had hopes that he would become a bishop. Young Bellows, however, was interested in baseball and drawing and pursued both, adding basketball when he entered Ohio State. He was outstanding enough to be scouted by the Cincinnati Reds for shortstop, and for a time he played semi-pro baseball. At the age of 22, however, without taking a degree, he said good-bye to Columbus and enrolled in the art classes of Robert Henri in New York City. Success came quickly. In 1909, before his 27th birthday, he sold his first painting to a major museum, and also became the youngest associate member elected to the National Academy of Design. Four years later he became a full member. In 1923, the *New York Evening Journal* commissioned the now well-known Bellows to make a drawing of the upcoming prizefight between the heavyweight champion Jack Dempsey and the Argentine challenger Luis Angel Firpo.

For two months during the summer of 1923, the attention of the world had been riveted on the two principals: The relatively unknown, taciturn, and frugal Firpo, one-time butcher, brickmaker, and drugstore clerk from Argentina, had been boxing for only four years. In spite of the fact that he had never taken boxing lessons, had a reputation as a slugger with an inaccurate (though powerful) right, and had fought in only 26 matches (20 KOs), he was acknowledged as the heavyweight champion of South America and had drawn 80,000 spectators when he had fought Willard in the United States that summer. Dempsey, on the other hand, had been the world heavyweight champion the

> *"I don't know anything about boxing. I am just painting two men trying to kill each other."*

entire four years of Firpo's career, and while unpopular for a time because he did not defend his title often enough, was a veteran of 68 fights (46 KOs). The public was ready to readmit him into its kingdom of heroes or, if he failed, at least into its Valhalla. The press had all it needed. All summer its members vied with each other to create new hyperbole: The fight was to be a match between "fearless Firpo" and "man-killer Dempsey," between the "Wild Bull of Pampas" and "Grizzly Bear Jack"; it was to be the "battle of the Americas," the "Battle of the Century" (even though the century was not yet even at its quarter-mark), and the "greatest battle in the history of pugilism." The hype paid off. On the 14th of September, 1923, a Friday evening, 87,000 people—"bankers, brokers, lawyers, street cleaners, merchants," "three governors, two former governors, and two sons of a former president," "even women"— gathered under a starry sky at the Polo

Grounds in New York, having paid a total of $1,188,822.80 to see an "entertainment" that would be over in less than four minutes. Millions more heard it on the radio, or saw it in newsreels. Of this total, the federal government netted a modest $180,000, New York State $57,000, Dempsey a relatively untaxed $475,000, and Firpo an equally untaxed $100,000. Promoter Tex Rickard got a handsome $400,000. Movie rights were extra.

The action was as savage as it was brief. In the opening seconds Dempsey floored Firpo seven times, all but two with left hooks to the head, the other blows a right to the head and a left to the body. Moreover, after each knockdown Dempsey failed to go to a neutral corner, but stalked Firpo, hitting him again as soon as his gloves left the canvas. Referee Gallagher did not enforce the rule. Nevertheless, Firpo came back with his "relentlessly powerful right," hitting Dempsey nine straight times. The eighth, to the jaw, caused his head to drop and his knees to wobble; the ninth put him through the ropes into the laps of reporters, who obligingly pushed him back into the ring on the six-count (an action that even Dempsey later admitted was illegal). Firpo followed up with an additional 13 straight blows without Dempsey, his "brain dulled," returning a single punch. He was saved by the bell. Recovered for the second round, Dempsey knocked Firpo down twice in the first 57 seconds, the second time for the count. But it was anticlimactic; the celebrated moment, the moment everyone remembers (but ironically a moment few saw because of the poor seating arrangements at the Polo Grounds), was Dempsey through the ropes. It was also the moment Bellows, seated at ringside with the working press (it was into his lap he claims Dempsey fell), chose for his *New York Evening Journal* assignment and for his subsequent painting, *Dempsey and Firpo*.

Dempsey and Firpo, with its powerfully sculpted Greek-like figures arrested in mid-motion, has an eerie, silent, suspended

Continued on p. 212

JAMA

THE JOURNAL of the American Medical Association

May 25, 1984

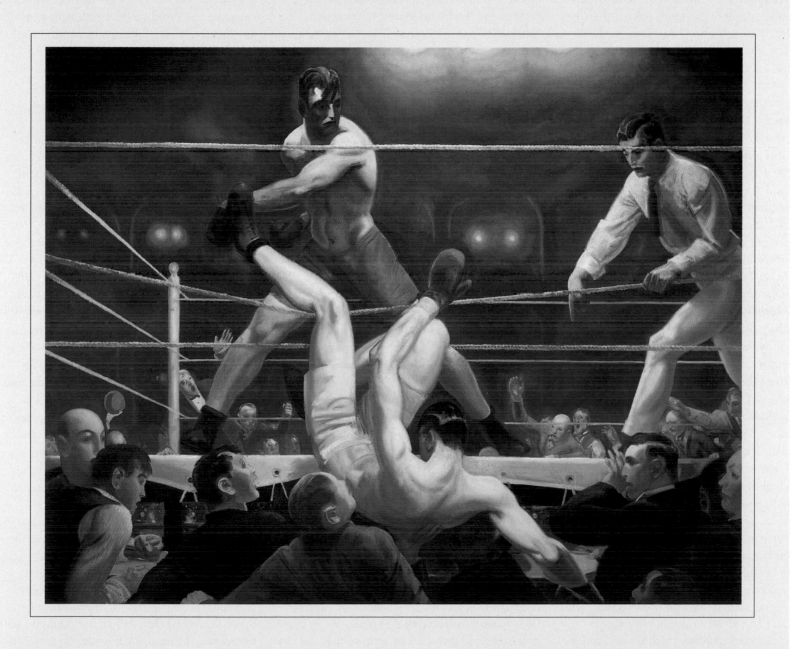

AMEDEO MODIGLIANI

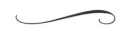

Madame Amédée (Woman With Cigarette)

Afirst encounter with a painting by Amedeo Modigliani (1884-1920), most of them portraits of his friends (and which were often done in exchange for a little wine that he drank as he worked), is apt to leave the viewer with an uneasy sense of their strange, almost grotesque, qualities. Only after a little familiarity does one come to discover their beauty. His portraits of young women are subtle harmonies of line and color that could be Botticelli in ragtime; his long and elegant necks recall Parmigianino's Virgins. His nudes, on the other hand, are bold and sensual harmonies of the cylinders, spheres, and cones Cézanne said one must look for in nature.

The sordid details of the short and tormented life of Modigliani have been recounted in numerous books and articles. His birth in a sense presaged his death. Only a few days before he was born, his parents, two sisters, and a brother, impoverished by the father's bankruptcy, had been forced to move into an apartment in a run-down section of the seaport town of Livorno (Leghorn). Under Italian law, officials confiscating a debtor's property could not seize the bed in which a woman had just given birth. Thus, the mother and newborn Amedeo ("beloved of God") lay in a bed that was piled high with the clutter of possessions the family had salvaged. Thirty-five years later, in Paris, in the early days of 1920, Modigliani lay nearly unconscious and dying in his squalid studio. The bed was littered with empty bottles and opened sardine tins dripping oil. His mistress, the 21-year-old Jeanne Hébuterne, near term with their second child, sat at his side uncomprehending, simply watching, unable to summon enough sense to get a doctor, or, indeed, anyone.

Modigliani left his parents' home when he was 18 years old to study art in Florence and Venice. There, besides Botticelli and Parmigianino, he was also introduced to hashish pills. He arrived in Paris in 1906, when he was 22, and soon was settled in Montmartre,

drinking absinthe with Utrillo. Over the next 14 years he would become a legend for his bizarre behavior and promiscuous sexual affairs and for his addiction to cocaine, absinthe, gin, and brandy. His two favorite authors were Dante and Lautréamont; he could quote from either with equal ease. Two years before his death, far gone with his excesses, he met Jeanne, the shy, sheltered, virgin art student, still in her teens. The following year, 1918, the couple, accompanied by several other artists and by Jeanne's mother, went to Nice, where they stayed for more than a year. In November of that year,

> *...she is the Madonna of middle age and she no longer has any illusions about her innocence.*

in Nice, the couple's only child, a daughter, Giovanna, was born. Less than 15 months later, Modigliani died of tuberculous meningitis. The depth of Jeanne's mute dependence on him became evident when, two days after his death, she threw herself from a fifth-floor window of her parents' home, killing herself and their unborn child.

Madame Amédée (Woman With Cigarette) is a departure from his familiar ladies with long necks. It was painted in 1918, the year of Modigliani's sojourn in Nice, but whether the painting was done in Nice or in Paris is unknown. Nor is anything known about the sitter beyond the safe assumption that she was a friend or acquaintance of Modigliani. Thus, whatever we are to know about Madame Amédée, we must learn from the painting. Madame Amédée is, on first acquaintance, a formidable woman, strong-willed, calm, imperious, confident. Feminine wiles are not her coin of the realm. Nor does

she need as her stock in trade the narrowed waist, the firm, high bosom, the trim ankle, the careless tress, exactly positioned. At one extreme, she could be the headmistress of an exclusive young ladies' seminary; at the other, the chief madame of a brothel. But whoever she is, it is certain she is someone we would not want to be owing the week's rent—nor even an overdue library book, for that matter.

On the other hand, closer acquaintance with Madame Amédée reveals more, permitting us to know her as perhaps Modigliani knew her. In contrast to the young, virginal Madonnas with the elongated necks, she is the Madonna of middle age and she no longer has any illusions about her innocence. Her eyes are sunken and world-weary; her gaze, cynical and calculating. Whatever she sees has its price, and Madame Amédée has seen it all. Her neck is clotted with chins, the lips rouged into a miserly Cupid's bow, and the cheeks are chubby. The sometime willowy body, which once could wear anything or nothing, hides its thickness in solid black and drapes the upper arms. The décolletage is hardly daring. And as if to further emphasize the cruel departure of her youth, Modigliani places her monumental body on a slender, fragile chair. Where once she could have sat with elegance and grace, she now sits incongruously, like a pyramid on a lily pad.

Modigliani has perhaps been unkind to Madame Amédée, but he did not stop with the obvious. Instead of the spheres and cylinders from which he built his female nudes, he has given us a virtuoso display of right angles and squares that has made her into a virago. The forearms, for example, are set perpendicular to each other, thereby conveying a sense of masculine strength. The V of the neckline of the dress is also a right angle, and its importance is stressed by placing its deepest part a little to the right of the center of the painting. The diagonals of the shoulders also form a 90-degree angle, its sides meeting at Madame Amédée's lips.

Continued on p. 213

JAMA

THE JOURNAL of the American Medical Association

July 6, 1984

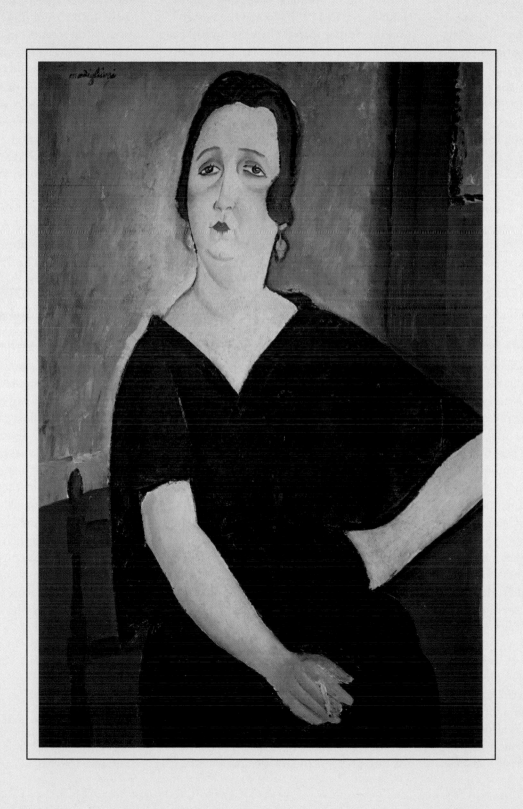

PIERRE-JACQUES VOLAIRE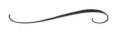

The Eruption of Mt Vesuvius

To the cultured person of the 18th century, the Grand Tour of the European continent was de rigueur, as indispensable to a mature view of the world as Homer and Livy to youth. Principal among the objectives, especially in the decade of the 1760s, was a sojourn in the city of Naples, to which one came after a day-and-a-half's journey by coach via Appia from Rome or by sea from Leghorn or Civitavecchia, sailing into the magnificent Bay of Naples in the shadow of Mount Vesuvius. Center of the Italian Enlightenment, Naples was the third most populous city in Europe, surpassed only by London and Paris. Under the newly installed Bourbon dynasty, it was a sophisticated center of opera, theater, and concerts, supported by the many balls and society gatherings of the nobility and middle-class intelligentsia of clergy, lawyers, and government administrators. Here came the poet, the writer, the artist, and the scientist to contemplate, to speculate, to dig a little at Herculaneum and newly discovered Pompeii, but most of all to hope for one of Vesuvius' spectacular shows. There arose, in fact, a "cult of Vesuvius," led in large part by Sir William Hamilton, the British ambassador to the kingdom of Naples from 1764 to 1800, who headed more than 200 expeditions to Vesuvius, including some 50 ascents to its crater. As if jealous of those who would pry the secrets of the past from the Roman citizens of 79 AD, Vesuvius responded like an angry god with a new series of eruptions. Between 1707 and 1794, there were no less than six spectacular outbursts, along with innumerable smaller ones.

Among those who came to Naples during this time was the French painter, Pierre-Jacques Volaire (1727-before 1802), who arrived in 1769. Son and grandson of painters, "le Chevalier Volaire," as he was also known, was born in the port city of Toulon on the Mediterranean coast, just south of Marseilles.

Few details of his life are available, but it is known that in 1754 he joined the French marine painter Joseph Vernet, who had been commissioned by Louis XV to paint all the ports of France. Together they traveled for eight years, Volaire assisting Vernet in some of the seascapes of his famous series. Volaire returned briefly to Toulon and, in 1763, settled in Rome, where he continued his marine paintings. At the end of the decade he visited Naples, where he began the numerous "vending machine" scenes of Vesuvius that became his specialty. During this time he climbed Vesuvius at least once,

> *...exploding like the Roman god of fire in a wild paroxysm against men who inquired too deeply into its secrets...*

in April 1774. Volaire died in Naples sometime around the end of the century. He has been characterized as an "energetic and prolific painter." He has also been called a romantic and theatrical painter who anticipated the moderns in his treatment of air, light, and space. He also foreshadows the fire and light of Turner and recalls the raining brimstone of Dürer.

The Eruption of Mt Vesuvius, which was painted in Naples in 1777, is virtuoso Volaire, a feast of light and counterpoint. Dominating the left two thirds of the painting is the raging, angry volcano, exploding like the Roman god of fire in a wild paroxysm against men who inquired too deeply into its secrets, spewing a fountain of rock and flame from its throat. Rivers of lava stream down its

heavy sides and collect in molten lakes at its base. In the right third of the painting the nearly full moon shines in serene contrast—passively, eternally—over the affairs of men, its light streaking the bay and pointing out the safe silhouettes of ships at anchor. It has, after all, witnessed many such outbursts of the god over the centuries. In the diagonal foreground, tiny figures from all stations of life flee across a bridge in various attitudes of terror, their hopes and aspirations ashed before the awesome power of nature. At the far right, a group of desperate suppliants drop before a shrine and beseech Gennaro, the martyred bishop and patron of Naples, for aid, the puny fire of their torches an ineffectual extravagance against escape from the fire of Vesuvius.

For sheer drama, few scenes can equal an aroused volcano. But Volaire is a master of the theater as well, and he spares no device in presenting his show. He casts light against dark, fire against water, firelight against moonlight, billowing smoke against sculpted cloud, frenzy against calm, an agitated mountain against the peaceful bosom of the bay, tiny, rational man against the feat of awesome, passionate nature. It is the apocalyptic scene of terror.

Other painters of the 18th century, notably Robert and Wright of Derby, also turned out the immensely popular scenes of Naples and Vesuvius that travelers took home like so many souvenirs of their Grand Tour, but only Volaire mastered the volcano so thoroughly that he became its official Boswell. Today these scenes are scattered in museums throughout the world and many a city can boast of its *Vesuvius*.

Pierre-Jacques Volaire (1727-before 1802), *The Eruption of Mt Vesuvius*, 1777, French. Oil on canvas. 135 × 226.1 cm. Courtesy of the North Carolina Museum of Art, Raleigh, North Carolina; purchased with funds from the Alcy C. Kendrick Bequest and the state of North Carolina, by exchange.

JAMA®

THE JOURNAL of the American Medical Association

December 7, 1984

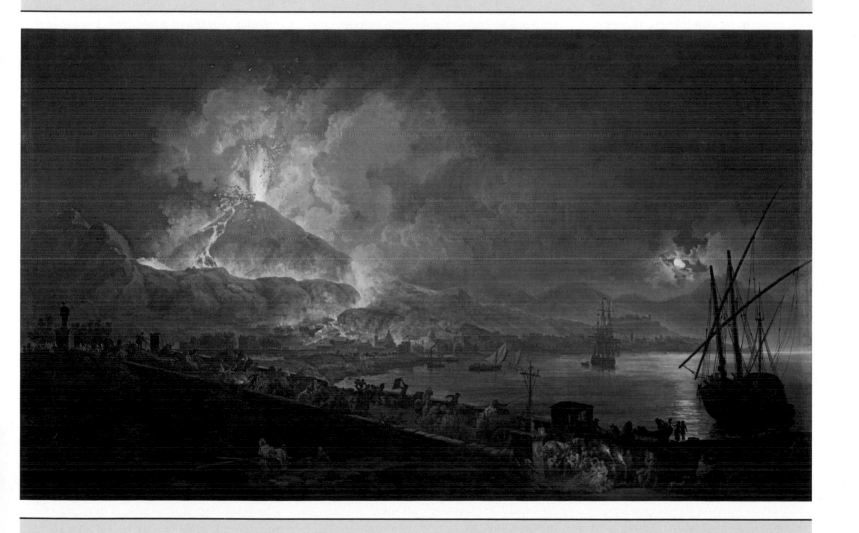

FRANÇOIS BOUCHER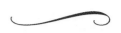

A Sleeping Baby

For more than 250 years the art of François Boucher (1703-1770) has suffered the vicissitudes of taste. Enormously popular during most of his lifetime, his paintings and drawings were the epitome of the rococo style favored by the court of Louis XV and especially by the king's young mistress, Madame de Pompadour. Playful, gay, sensual, delicate, even pretty, his works characterized the mood of the Paris aristocracy, at last released from the oppressiveness of the Versailles court by the death of Louis XIV. But toward the end of Boucher's life the mood changed again, and taste was converted to the austere, formal style of Neoclassicism. The French critic Diderot, who led the attack on Boucher, condemned him for his immoral choice of subject, often nude, dimpled goddesses, and complained that his cupids and cherubs were never doing anything useful such as "studying lessons, reading, writing or picking hemp." "What an abuse of talent! What a waste of time!" he swore on one occasion. "People of great taste, of severe and classical taste, will have nothing to do with him," he wrote on another occasion. After a visit to Boucher's studio in 1752, Sir Joshua Reynolds, the reigning English portraitist, remarked that much of his output was "hack-work." And more than 60 years after Boucher's death, the English landscapist John Constable wrote, "the climax of absurdity to which art may be carried…may be best seen in the works of Boucher." Only a century after his death did the Goncourt brothers of Paris bring him to favorable attention once again. But renewed favor has been slow to develop, and it is only in the past decade or so that interest in Boucher has been rekindled to the point of putting on a major exhibit of his drawings.

Boucher was born in Paris, the son of an embroidery designer. At age 17, he entered the studio of François Lemoyne and then worked as an illustrator to support himself. At 20, he won the prestigious Prix de Rome from the Académie but did not go to Rome until 1727 because of lack of funds. For the next four years he remained in Rome, where he admired greatly the works of Tiepolo. He was also influenced by the works of Veronese, Rubens, and Watteau. In 1733 he married 17-year-old Marie-Jeanne Buseau, who became his model for many a Venus. Boucher quickly became a protégé of Mme de Pompadour, who rewarded him with royal favors. In 1737 he became a professor

> *…infancy, which can never be described by the infant and only imagined by those who are beyond it…*

at the Académie; in 1752 he attained a long-coveted apartment in the Royal Palace of the Louvre; in 1755 he was made chief inspector of the king's Gobelins tapestry manufactory, and in 1765 he reached his pinnacle as director of the Académie and Chief Painter to the King. He died in Paris of "asthma" at age 66.

Boucher's output was enormous. By his own count, he did more than 10,000 drawings and 1000 paintings. Of the drawings, however, only about 1000 are known today, and one quarter of these are in North America. Boucher's subject matter was the idealized and make-believe world—the world as he and the royal court wished it to be. His models were most often his wife and three children. And his obsession, according to art historian Leo Bronstein, was the baby—innocent, artless, chubby, and pink—for infancy, which can never be described by the infant and only imagined by those who are beyond it, is the ultimate idealized world of the adult. Moreover, Boucher worked during the Age of Rationalism in France, and what could be farther removed from the rational man than the sleeping infant?

A Sleeping Baby is undoubtedly one of Boucher's own children. Clutching a dress full of flowers, it sleeps on in trusting abandon, unaware of the intrigues of the royal court on which his father's fortunes depended. The drawing is in typical rococo style. Its superb craftmanship is built entirely on a structure of curves and arabesques, from the perfect oval of the head to the graceful arcs of the chubby legs. In another setting the infant will become Cupid, asleep in his bower of bliss.

Drawing as a finished art form did not become recognized until about the mid-18th century, when it was finally accepted for exhibition at the Salon. Drawing may be said to be the most intimate of all art forms, for in a drawing, the artist is least able to disguise himself. The line, with all its subtle variations, is as personal as a signature. The contact between artist and viewer is direct, revealing, and truthful, without the veil afforded by the color and brushwork of a painting. Moreover, there is in a drawing a spontaneity that renders it truer to the artist's feelings and more honest than a finished painting often can be. A drawing may, in fact, be likened to a nude: it is a painting with its clothes off, an artist at his most revealing and at his most vulnerable.

François Boucher (1703-1770), *A Sleeping Baby*, nd, French. Black, red, and white chalk, green and yellow watercolor on pale buff paper. 23.1 × 29 cm. Sold by Christie's, London, England, December 9, 1982.

JAMA®

THE JOURNAL of the American Medical Association

December 21, 1984

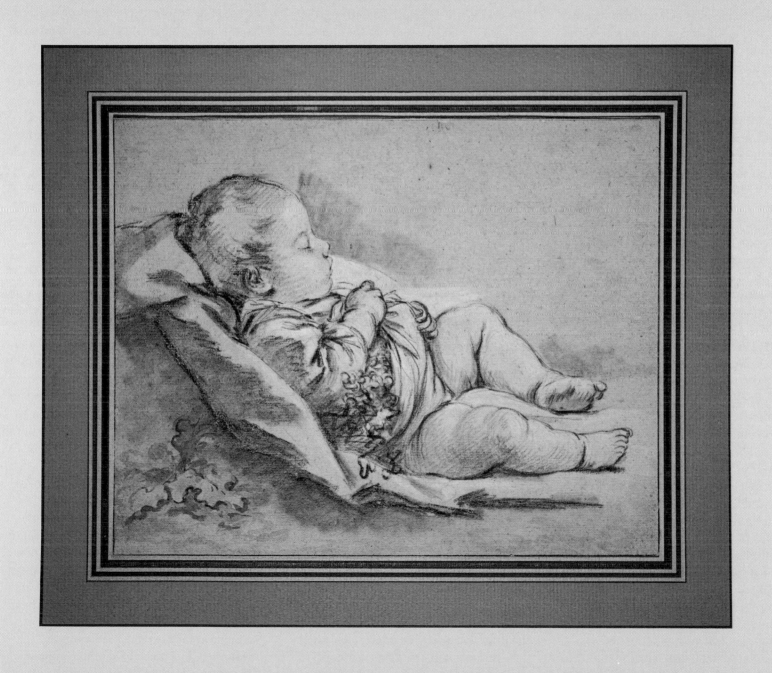

SIR JOHN LAVERY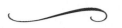

Sister Juliet

It is one of those ironic twists of life that the blessings of medicine have so often been yoked to the evils of war. Throughout history so closely linked are the advancements of medicine with the destruction of war that Hippocrates himself admonished young men who would be surgeons to "go to war." Nearly 25 centuries later little has changed.

In a 1984 photo-essay in *American Heritage*, picture editor Jane Colihan described some of the advances in medicine that have come from wars in which the United States has been involved. During the Spanish American War, for example, the number of deaths from tropical diseases, especially from malaria and yellow fever, was 14 times greater than those from combat. But after the war, during the occupation, yellow fever was eradicated from Havana for the first time, due largely to the work of Carlos Finlay, MD, Major Walter Reed, MD, and Major William Gorgas, MD. During World War I, new weapons technology in the form of shellfire caused the destructive and disfiguring shrapnel wound, and plastic and reconstructive surgery was born. When the heavily manured farmland battlefields of France and Belgium meant almost certain tetanus infection of wounds, an antitoxin was developed. And with the great number of wounded and dying on the battlefield from mustard gas and shellfire, the sorting method known as "triage" was developed.

Not the least of the benefits of World War I was the impetus given to the recognition of nursing as a profession. From the early efforts of Florence Nightingale during the Crimean War and of Clara Barton during the American Civil War, the United States developed a Nurses Corps made up only of graduate nurses, which served for the first time in World War I. The heroism of British nurse Edith Cavell became an inspiration to thousands of young women on both sides of the Atlantic. After nursing both German and Allied soldiers, Cavell was charged with helping British and French soldiers to escape, but she remained at her post and was executed by a German firing squad in 1915.

World War II brought methods for the large-scale collection and transport of whole blood, the development and use of dried plasma, and the recognition that shock must be treated immediately, right on the battlefield. Penicillin went into large-scale production as well and revolutionized the treatment of wound infection, pneumonia, meningitis, and venereal diseases. The development and widespread use of chlorophenothane (DDT) for the first time reduced the number of deaths from typhus.

> *"…all responsibility of living had been taken from you…"*

The Korean War saw the first use of Mobile Army Surgical Hospitals (MASH), where operating teams set up in the forward area to care directly for the wounded. The climate directed that new methods for treating frostbite be developed, and vascular surgery came into its own as a specialty by drastically reducing the number of amputations of injured limbs. Vietnam brought the use of helicopters to evacuate the wounded directly and rapidly from the place of injury to a place of definitive care, a system adapted today for use in emergency medical care for civilians. As spectacular as the advances of medicine during wartime have been, however, the price will always be unacceptably high.

It is ironic, too, that the beauties of painting should come out of the tragedies of war. The Irish painter Sir John Lavery (1856-1941), who was commissioned by the British government to chronicle the events of World War I, recognized this when he wrote in his autobiography years later that his war paintings "appeared to me totally uninspired and dull as dishwater…Instead of the grim harshness and horror of the scenes I had given charming color versions, as if painting a bank holiday on Hampstead Heath…I felt nothing of the stark reality, losing sight of my fellow men being blown to pieces in submarines or slowly choking to death in mud. I saw only new beauties of color and design." Regretting that he had been unable to go to the Front he said, the closest he came to the horrors of war was painting wounded soldiers in a London hospital and listening to their stories. Lavery had other insights into war, especially as to why men are so keen to enlist when war breaks out. Although 58 years old and a pacifist at heart, when war was declared in 1914 he joined the Artist's Rifles, a motley crew of painters, sculptors, actors, musicians, hairdressers, scene shifters, and the like, who drilled in the quadrangle of Burlington House in the heart of London. "It was a fine sensation," he wrote, "to feel that all responsibility of living had been taken from you, that all the worries of house and home had ceased to exist. You were walking on air to the tune of 'It's a long way to Tipperary,' and nothing mattered. The intoxication was complete for the time being."

Sister Juliet is one of Lavery's "sanitized" war paintings, done at war's end in 1918. It shows the drawing room of an elegant London house, probably that of Lady Juliet Duff, that has been requisitioned as a hospital for British officers. As was the custom in Europe during World War I, aristocratic ladies often volunteered to serve as nurses, and Lady Juliet herself is shown as such a nurse at the far right, reading to the wounded. In a scene of careful composition, the vertical lines of the high-ceilinged room, tall windows, upright piano, high dressing table, and tall bottles and vases contrast sharply with the horizontal flatness of the beds, emphasizing the helpless condition of the wounded men. The women's figures, both at oblique angles, suggest caring, com-

Continued on p. 213

JAMA®

December 28, 1984

THE JOURNAL of the American Medical Association

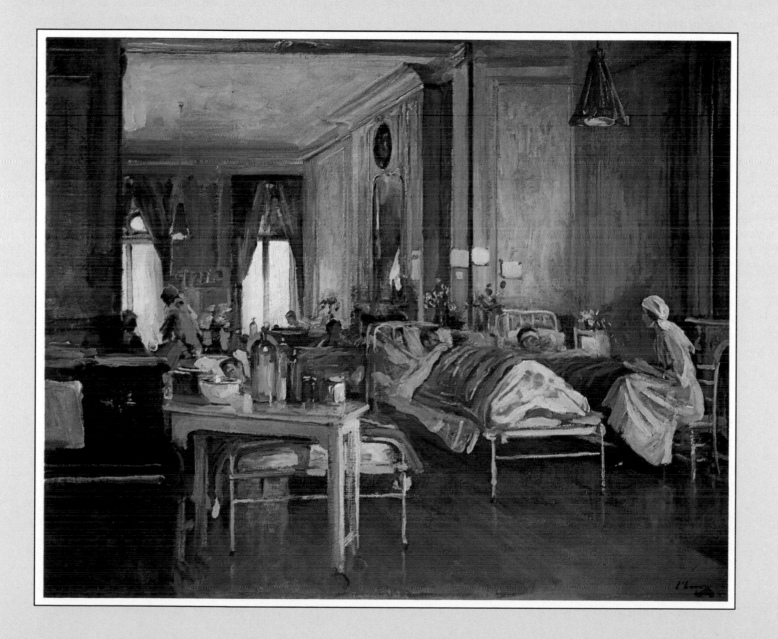

ANDREW WYETH

Winter, 1946

Until he was 28 years old, Andrew Wyeth (1917-   ), son of the painter N. C. Wyeth, was—in his own words—"just a clever watercolorist—lots of swish and swash." Then, in 1945, his father was killed when the car he was driving stalled on the railroad tracks near the family home in Chadds Ford, Pennsylvania. The event shook young Wyeth profoundly. It was, he said, the "real turning point" of his life. From that point on, watercolor was no longer able to carry his deep emotion, and he turned to tempera, a more steady, but also a more difficult, medium.

Winter, 1946 is the first tempera Wyeth did after his father's death. A young, adolescent boy, dressed in cast-off aviator's jacket and helmet and oversized boots, plunges headlong down a broad, brown hill. He is off balance and out of control, his gloveless hand flung out, his shadow following. He is about to cross a road made by the ruts of a vehicle—perhaps by his father's car—that has left its impression in the soft, spongy earth. Cold remnants of a past snow lie to

"It was me, at a loss— that hand drifting in air was my free soul, groping."

the left, along the fence. Behind him, the vast expanse of the hill rises, powerful and timeless, like the burial mound of a giant, preempting all but the tiniest portion of the sky. Of the boy, Wyeth said, "It was me, at a loss—that hand drifting in the air was my free soul, groping. Over on the other side of that hill was where my father was killed, and I was sick I'd never painted him. The hill finally became a portrait of him."

Wyeth's draftsmanship captures exquisitely the loneliness and disorientation that follows the death of someone close. At the same time, the principal lines of the composition express the ultimately prevailing strength of the survivor. For example, lines extended through the left leg and left arm of the boy

form a stable isosceles triangle, with the boy's shadow as its base. At the moment, the triangle is tilted forward in precarious balance, to be sure, but not so far that it will not, if left alone to follow its own laws of dynamics, return to the horizontal.

"People talk to me about the mood of melancholy in my pictures," Wyeth said. "I think the right word is not 'melancholy,' but 'thoughtful'…I prefer winter and fall, when you feel the bone structure in the landscape—the loneliness of it—the dead feeling of winter. Something waits beneath it—the whole story doesn't show. I think anything like that—which is contemplative, silent, shows a person alone—people always feel is sad. Is it because we've lost the art of being alone?"

Andrew Wyeth (1917-   ), *Winter, 1946*, 1946, American. Tempera. 79.7 × 121.9 cm. Courtesy of the North Carolina Museum of Art, Raleigh, North Carolina; purchased with funds from the state of North Carolina.

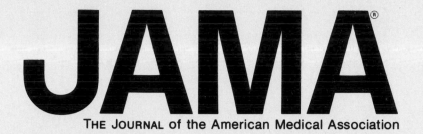

January 4, 1985

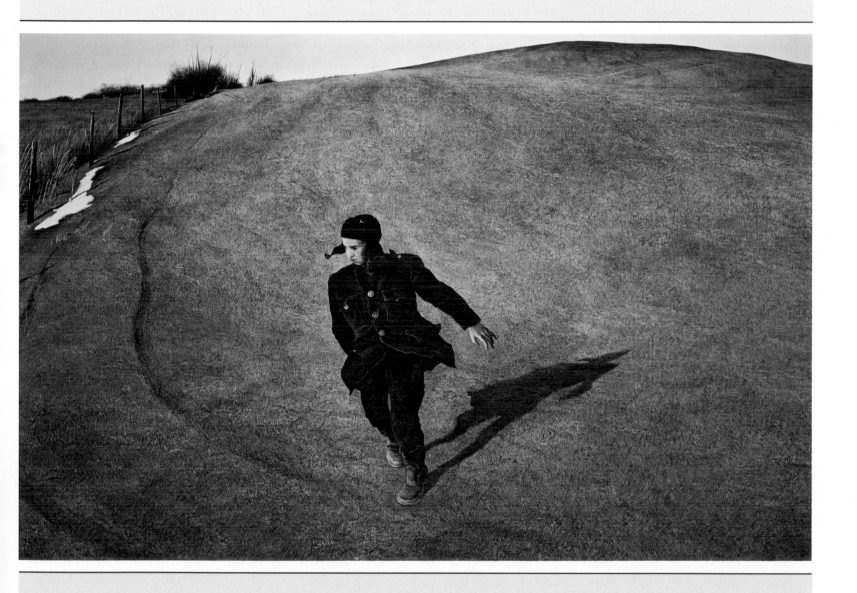

CANDIDO PORTINARI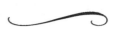

Coffee

Candido Portinari (1903-1962) is widely acclaimed as Brazil's most famous painter, and *Coffee* is called one of his most famous paintings. Born on a coffee plantation in the state of São Paulo, Portinari was the second of 12 children born to Italian immigrant parents. Later the family moved to the nearby town of Brodowski where one of the most memorable experiences of Portinari's life occurred when he was 8 years old: a group of itinerant painters allowed him to help paint stars on the ceiling of Santo Antonio's Church. After that there was never any question of the path he would follow.

At the age of 15 he entered the National School for Fine Arts in Rio de Janeiro, so poor that he could afford only the bathtub in a boardinghouse for a bed. He remained at the school for ten years, supporting himself largely by portrait commissions. In 1928, after developing into a somewhat academic painter, he won a *Prix de Voyage*, which allowed him three years' study and travel in Europe. During this time he deliberately painted little but observed much, especially in the museums of London and Paris. In Europe two more determining events of his life occurred: he discovered that he did not wish to be a portraitist and, paradoxically, he discovered the great depth of his Brazilian roots. "My strong desire," he said, "surging from deep inside my soul, is to be like Veronese, a painter of great scenes with many figures grouped in large compositions with diverse structures." The art he wished to create would be a "true Brazilian art." He returned to Brazil in 1931 and three years later began turning out the huge mural-like canvases for which he has become known. *Coffee* is among the earliest.

Coffee is, in a sense, the early fulfillment of that strong desire surging from deep inside his soul. It is a great scene, with many figures grouped in large compositions, and it has diverse structures. It is also true Brazilian art. The scene is simple and straightforward: women are picking coffee beans, men are moving coffee sacks, and a foreman, gun at his hip and spurs at his heels, is directing the operation. But the scene could be archetypal as well. With only minor changes, it could as easily be a scene of the Israelites building the pyramids, the women mixing straw and mud, the men hauling bricks, and the overseer, whip at his side, calling the pace. As one critic noted, Portinari's figures are not types, but prototypes.

> "I came from the waters of the sea/and was born on a coffee plantation/ of red soil…"

In *Coffee*, Portinari has achieved a remarkable wedding of form and content. The overall pattern of the painting is one of interlocking diagonal lines, suggesting the gridlock of poverty and oppression in which the workers are trapped. The precise rows of trees, blotting out even the horizon, suggest the tedium and endlessness of the labor; the harsh color contrast between muted green and reddish brown suggests the severity of the workers' lives.

Portinari's style has been called baroque, after the pattern of counterpoint one finds in a fugue. Thus, the deep red soil and the white-garbed figures form alternating bands of dark and light, one answering the other. The muscled forms of the men counterpoint the graceful figures of the women; only the figure of the foreman breaks the rhythm of the line. The ribbed bark of the tall palm tree at the corner of the grove is answered by the column of coffee sacks in left midground, while a ladder has its counterpoint in the smaller column of sacks outlining the foreman. The entire composition is anchored in place by the figure of the sitting woman in the left foreground, in which all of the contradictions of the painting are resolved.

Of his birth Portinari wrote, "I came from the waters of the sea/and was born on a coffee plantation/of red soil," referring to his parents' voyage from Italy across the Atlantic to Brazil and to his own birth on a coffee plantation. But he could as well have been referring to his birth as a painter, for only when he left Europe and returned to Brazil did his talent reveal itself in a painting of the red soil of a coffee plantation.

Portinari achieved international renown in 1952, when he was commissioned to do the War and Peace panels for the United Nations headquarters building in New York. The huge (280 square meter) murals were installed on the two front walls of the delegates' entry hall in 1957 with Secretary-General Dag Hammarskjöld presiding. Another mural can be seen in the Hispanic Society's reading room in the Library of Congress. All in all, 76 paintings of Portinari's total output of some 4000 works are believed to be in the United States, most of them in private collections.

Portinari died in Rio de Janeiro in 1962 of lead poisoning contracted from the pigments he used.

Candido Portinari (1903-1962), *Coffee*, 1935, Brazilian. Oil on canvas. 130 × 195 cm. Courtesy of Projeto Portinari, Rio de Janeiro, Brazil.

JAMA®

The Journal of the American Medical Association

January 11, 1985

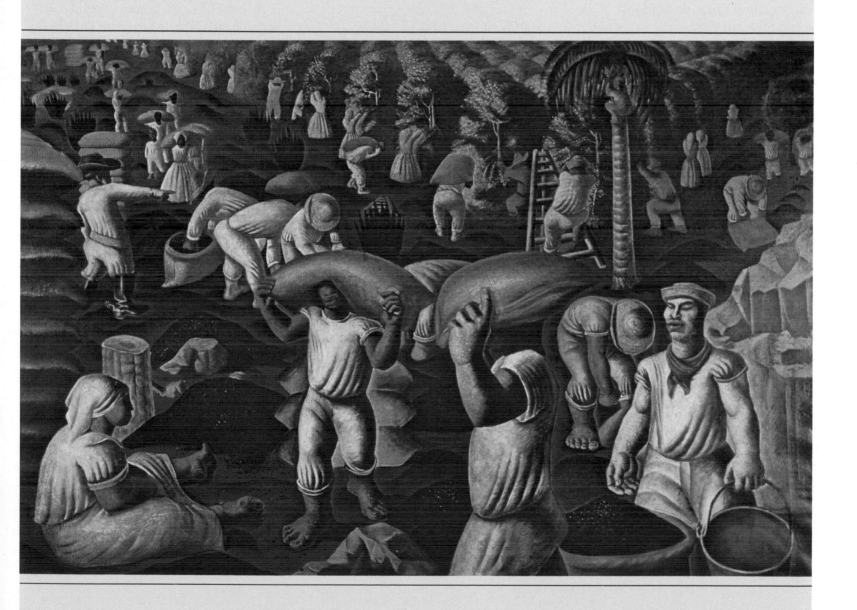

WALTER SICKERT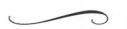

Ennui

When Virginia Woolf saw an exhibition of the paintings of the English Impressionist Walter Sickert (1860-1942) in London in 1933, she wrote that just as the novelist uses words to paint pictures, so did Sickert use his brush to paint words. No painting of his better demonstrates the truth of her statement than does *Ennui*. An English translation of the word *ennui* does not exist, but a dictionary is not needed to describe, indeed, to feel, the exquisite pain behind the word. Sickert has painted boredom, fatigue, tedium, life-weariness, disgust. He shows us two people whose lives no longer have a destination, whose spirits have withered in the desert.

Perhaps the closest English equivalent we have to ennui is what William McNamara describes in *The Art of Being Human* as "the noon-day devil." It is a kind of insidious despair, he says, that creeps up on one in the middle of things: the middle of the day, the middle of a job, the middle of winter, the middle of life. What once was fresh, new, and lyrical becomes stale, flat, and a dull routine. A more contemporary word might be simply "burn-out."

Sickert was in his mid-50s when he painted *Ennui*. At least five oil versions are known and there are many more drawings, all worked on over the five-year period between the war years of 1914 and 1918. The present version, the last, differs from the others in that it is smaller, the colors are

> *…two people whose lives no longer have a destination, whose spirits have withered in the desert.*

somewhat brighter, and a little more warmth has been added in the form of patterned wallpaper and table covering.

In typical Sickert style, the composition is tight, even dense, heightening both the mood and the ambiguity of the scene. For example, the actual relationship between the two figures is unstated. Whether it be that of father and daughter, husband and wife, or lover and mistress is not clear. But ambiguous though it is, it is clear that the relationship is a close, even symbiotic, one and that it is destructive to each. Sickert expresses this by overlapping the two figures and by placing them so close together that their bodies almost touch. Moreover, the closeness of the relationship is further emphasized by the placement of both heads on the same perpendicular line, while the torsos follow harmonious diagonal lines. An additional bond of unity between the two figures is created by the single bureau, whose diagonal lines lead directly to the figures. Yet by simply facing the figures in opposite directions, the woman turned to the wall with her eyes

closed and the man staring into space, each unable and unwilling to see the other, Sickert turns the relationship into a negative one. Despite their closeness there is a planetary distance between them. That the mere presence of the other has become a burden is shown by the obvious weariness of each body, the woman using the bureau to support her full weight, the man sagging heavily in the chair. At the same time a sense of the emptiness of each is conveyed by the huge, nearly bare table, which occupies most of the foreground. "It is all over with them…" Woolf wrote. "The accumulated weariness of innumerable days has discharged its burden on them."

Sickert, one of six children, was born in Munich to a Danish father and an English-Irish mother. When the boy was 8, the family moved permanently to London. In his teens he studied acting, a compromise between his own desire to study art like his father and his parents' wish that he study law. He acted professionally for a time and then, at the age of 21, entered the Slade School in London to begin a painting career that was to last 60 years. When he died suddenly at the age of 81, an unfinished painting was on his easel. He has been called "possibly the most important English painter since Turner."

Walter Sickert (1860-1942), *Ennui*, c 1918, English. Oil on canvas. 76 × 56 cm. Courtesy of the Ashmolean Museum, University of Oxford, England.

JAMA

THE JOURNAL of the American Medical Association

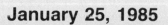

January 25, 1985

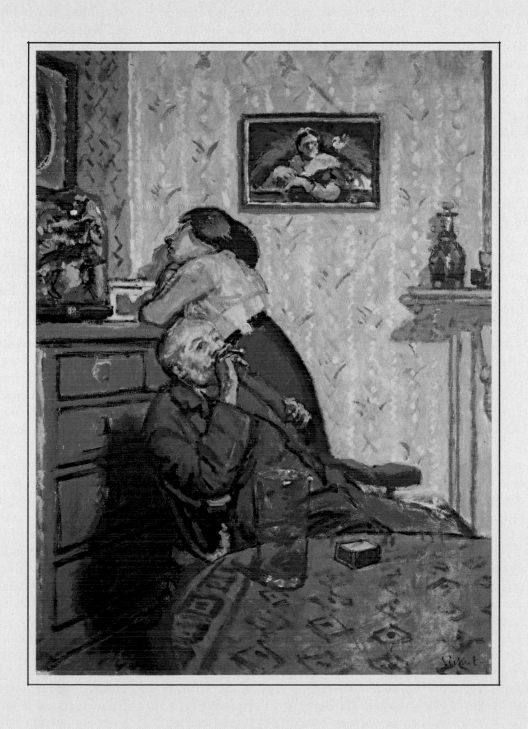

GRANT WOOD

Woman With Plant(s)

More than 40 years after his death, critics remained divided over Grant Wood (1891-1942); the American public, however, is not. As long ago as 1930 the public adopted Wood as its national spokesman and although enthusiasm has waxed and waned over more than 50 years, his *American Gothic*, that much-interpreted paean to the Iowa farmer and his spinster daughter, remains, along with *Mona Lisa*, one of the most parodied portraits ever painted. Yet as Wanda Corn notes in her introduction to a recent exhibition of Grant Wood paintings, the symbol survives while the name of its creator is almost unknown. This is not new for Wood. Before he was adopted as an instant national celebrity in the early 1930s, he had been painting, unknown outside his native Iowa, for two decades.

Wood was born a farmer's son, the second of three boys and one girl, just outside Anamosa, Iowa, a small town 25 miles north of Cedar Rapids. His father was Francis Maryville Wood, a hardworking, prosperous farmer, whose Quaker family had left Virginia and settled in Iowa at the close of the Civil War. His mother was Hattie Weaver, whose family had come from New York State and taken land near Anamosa at the same time. Hattie taught school in Anamosa, and both parents attended the local Presbyterian church, where Hattie played the organ and Francis taught Sunday school. Little distinguished Grant Wood's childhood as an Iowa farm boy—except that he liked to draw—until 1901. It was then that his father died suddenly at the age of 46; Grant was 10 years old. With her four children, the youngest 2 years old, Mrs Wood moved to Cedar Rapids, transplanting the family from the relatively provincial farm to a thriving city. Here, in Cedar Rapids, Grant would continue to live with his mother until she died in 1935, when Wood was 44.

Wood's attempts at education in the visual arts were so sporadic and apparently so poorly directed that he may be considered virtually self-taught. Immediately after graduating from high school, he spent two summers studying the decorative arts at the Minneapolis School of Design and Handicraft and Normal Art. During the winter of 1912 he attended a life-drawing class three nights a week as an unmatriculated student at the State University of Iowa (now University of Iowa) in Iowa City and taught on a provisional teacher's certificate at a one-room schoolhouse just outside Cedar Rapids. Between 1913 and 1916 he worked in Chicago as a metalsmith, designing jewelry, and attended night classes at the Art Institute

> *"My most useful reference book…is a Sears Roebuck catalogue…"*

of Chicago. He left Chicago precipitously in 1916, when he learned that his mother and sister were about to be evicted from their home in Cedar Rapids. For the next few years, after army service designing camouflage, he painted and taught art in the Cedar Rapids public high school system. From 1923 to 1924, on a year's leave of absence, he traveled in France and Italy and briefly attended classes at the Académie Julian in Paris. Finally, in 1925, he retired from teaching to devote himself exclusively to painting.

Until 1929 Wood's output consisted mainly of undistinguished, unabashedly sentimental paintings of the "picturesque"—streams, landscapes, trees, fountains, doorways—done in an Impressionist style. Then, in 1928, while visiting the Alte Pinakothek in Munich, he was impressed by the German and Flemish old masters—especially by paintings of Memling and Dürer—and felt that he had at last found what he was looking for. He would combine the methods and styles of the old masters with the everyday life and scenes of Cedar Rapids to create a peculiarly American type of painting, a type of painting that, in time, came to be known as "Regionalism." In a later interview with a newspaper reporter, Wood was to state: "I began to realize that there was real decoration in the rickrack braid on the aprons of the farmers' wives…My most useful reference book…is a Sears Roebuck catalogue… I discovered that in the very commonplace, in my native surroundings, were decorative adventures and that my only difficulty had been in taking them too much for granted."

Woman With Plant(s) is one of Wood's earliest paintings after his return from Munich, and it marks the beginning of his new style. The subject is his mother, now 70 years old. Like the subjects in Renaissance portraits, she holds her attribute in her hands, in this case the sturdy sansevieria plant, also known as snake plant or mother-in-law's tongue. Additional testimony to her gardening abilities is given by the begonia and geranium plants at her side. The Renaissance style is further emphasized by the miniature landscape in the background, in this case the Wapsipinicon Valley, where she had lived all her life. But even more to the Renaissance theme is the detail and character given the face and the hands, while the remainder of the painting—the sitter's costume, the landscape—is highly stylized. Moreover, like the old masters, Wood painted on composition board and used a glazing technique to give his colors depth.

Wood also displayed his considerable decorative talents in *Woman With Plant(s)*. The prominent pattern of golden rickrack on the apron is repeated in the yellow-green markings of the snake plant, for example. The soft, rounded forms of the woman are picked up in the brooch at her neckline, in the earrings, the plump begonia leaves, the treetops, the rolling hills, and the sails of the windmill. The river snaking its way through the fertile valley is repeated in the upright sansevieria and in the veins of the begonia

Continued on p. 213

JAMA®

THE JOURNAL of the American Medical Association

May 10, 1985

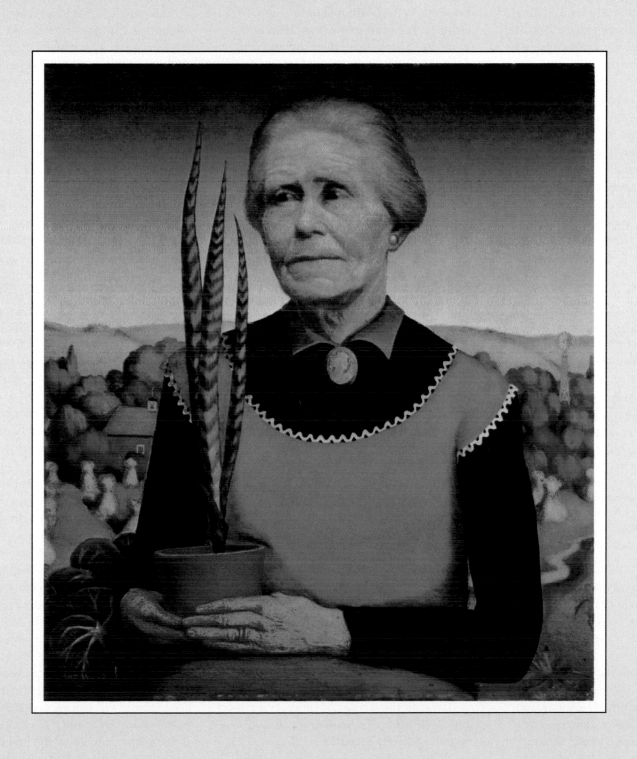

VINCENT VAN GOGH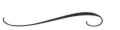

Irises

In early May 1889, Vincent van Gogh (1853-1890), painter, 36 years old, arrived in Saint-Rémy, a small town in the Midi of France, some 17 miles from Arles, where he had been living for the past 15 months. Immediately, as prearranged by his brother Theo, he voluntarily entered the hospital, a 12th-century Augustinian monastery converted to an asylum for the insane. The buildings were surrounded by gardens and grain fields, and Vincent hoped to paint them while he was interned.

The circumstances that led to van Gogh's decision to enter the asylum at Saint-Rémy had begun some four months earlier, when he and Gauguin were living in the famed "yellow house" in Arles. What happened there on the Sunday night of December 23, 1888, and Gauguin's precise involvement in the episode have never been made completely clear, but a week later the following item appeared in a local newspaper:

Last Sunday night at half past eleven a painter named Vincent van Gogh, a native of Holland, appeared at the maison de tolérance No. I, asked for a girl called Rachel, and handed her…his ear with these words: 'Keep this object like a treasure.' The police, informed of these events, which could only be the work of an unfortunate madman, looked the next morning for this individual, whom they found in bed with scarcely a sign of life. The poor man was taken to the hospital without delay.

Accounts of the immediate aftermath vary. One has van Gogh calmly asking the police for his pipe and tobacco and money box. Another states he was unconscious for three days. Nevertheless, within two weeks, he was discharged from the hospital in Arles, was back in his yellow house (without Gauguin, who had returned to Paris), and during the next ten days completed four works, one a portrait of Dr Felix Rey, the young physician who cared for him in the hospital, and probably the two self-portraits that show him with a bandaged head.

Van Gogh's recovery was short-lived, however. At the beginning of February he wrote to Theo that he was very tired and also that "There are moments when I am twisted by enthusiasm or madness or prophecy, like a Greek oracle on the tripod." Before the week was out he was returned to the hospital suffering from hallucinations and fears of being poisoned. Again, within ten days things were hopeful enough for van Gogh to return to the yellow house, although he took his meals and spent his nights at the hospital. This time, however, his neighbors were not pleased ("It seems that people here

> ## *"There are moments when I am twisted by enthusiasm or madness or prophecy…"*

have some superstition that makes them afraid of painting," Vincent wrote to Theo) and 30 of them petitioned the mayor that van Gogh either be returned to his family or be committed to a mental institution because he had, as they wrote:

for some time and on various occasions furnished proof of the fact that he does not dispose of his full mental faculties, that he indulges in excessive drinking after which he finds himself in such a state of excitement that he does not know what he says or what he does and that his instability inspires public fear for the residents of the sector, especially for the women and children.

Thus, on the last day of February a police officer closed the yellow house and returned van Gogh to the hospital.

Dr Rey explained to van Gogh that his difficulties were caused by his not eating enough nor at regular times, keeping himself going instead on coffee and alcohol. To Theo Vincent wrote, "I admit all that, but at the same time it is true that to attain the high yellow note that I attained last summer, I really had to be pretty well keyed up." Van Gogh preferred to blame his neighbors, remarking about the disquiet that had reigned all that winter in Arles, even quite apart from what had befallen him. "…business not too good, resources exhausted, people discouraged and…as you said, not content to remain spectators, and becoming nuisances from being out of work—if anybody can still make a joke or work fast, down they come on him." By mid-April van Gogh was hopeful again—enough to store the furniture from the yellow house, to sublet two rooms from Dr Rey, and to buy a new suit and six pairs of socks. Yet when it came to the reality of once more living alone and caring for himself, it was more than van Gogh could face. He wrote to Theo: "…I feel myself definitely incapable of starting once more to take a new studio and to remain there alone, either here in Arles or elsewhere …And thus I wish to remain interned provisionally for my own tranquility as well as for that of others."

The "provisional internment" of which van Gogh spoke was the asylum of Saint-Paul-de-Mansole in nearby Saint-Rémy-de-Provence. Here he hoped to stay for three or four months, living in the asylum but being granted privileges to work and paint outside. Later he reappraised his situation to say that he felt he needed a year. Thus it was that van Gogh arrived in Saint-Rémy on May 8, 1889, and left almost exactly a year later, on May 16, 1890, "cured," as his physician wrote in the official record. When he arrived and when he left, the irises and lilacs were in full bloom, and among the very first and last paintings van Gogh did at Saint-Rémy are irises, the first painting one of irises in their natural state of wild profusion, the last a painting of a bouquet confined in a vase.

Continued on p. 213

JAMA®

THE JOURNAL of the American Medical Association

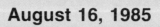

August 16, 1985

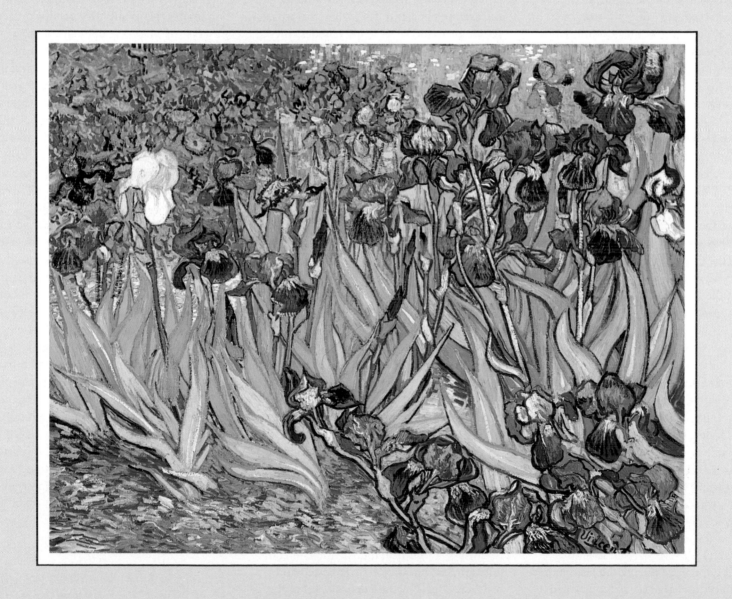

WILLIAM ADOLPHE BOUGUEREAU

La Grande Soeur

In the Paris of the 19th century what was or was not art was determined by the Salon. This was a huge, usually annual, exhibition of new paintings selected by a jury of academic painters because the works conformed to official standards of the Academy. Without acceptance by the Salon, an artist could hardly expect to sell his work, since the public looked to it as the absolute arbiter of taste and was unlikely to buy anything that had not been so approved.

It was natural, then, that a young artist who had public acclaim and financial security as his goals would chart his career carefully and work at it systematically. For example, he would graduate from the École des Beaux-Arts, the official art academy in Paris, and capture the Prix de Rome, which carried with it four years of additional study in Italy and the assurance of an exhibition at the Salon. He would become in time a teacher at the École des Beaux-Arts and collect medals and honors with further exhibits at the Salon: Medal Second Class by age 30, Medal First Class by age 32, and Chevalier of the Legion of Honor before age 35. By age 50, or shortly thereafter, he would be elected a member of the Institute, thereby making him part of the very jury that selected works for exhibition at the Salon, and before the age of 55 he would be awarded the Grand Medal of Honor for his cumulative successes. Along the way he will have garnered so many other awards and honors that no one will any longer think to question his taste or judge his work. He will have become French "official taste" itself.

Such was the career of William Adolphe Bouguereau (1825-1905). Such was his power and popularity during the last quarter of the 19th century that he virtually ruled the Salon. Ironically, that period is no longer remembered for Bouguereau's paintings, however, but for those of the very artists he systematically excluded from the Salon: Manet, the Impressionists, Cézanne. Cézanne, in fact, bitterly referred to the Salon as "le Salon de Bouguereau." Ironically, too, Bouguereau's reputation as an artist suffered a sharp decline at his death, just as Cézanne's began to rise. Only in the past decade or so has there been a modest revival of interest in Bouguereau.

Bouguereau was an assiduous and systematic worker, turning out some 700 completed canvases in his career. So programmed were his activities that he is reported to have

…promise given but consummation denied?

said at one point, "I lose five francs every time I piss." His subject matter followed the sentimental, pious, often mawkish taste of the day, and his canvases were characterized by a smooth, glossy, highly polished finish. So identified with him was this style that Degas referred disdainfully to any shiny canvas as being *bouguereauté* ("bouguerated").

The life-size *La Grande Soeur* is typical of Bouguereau's work during his early 50s, when he was at the height of his powers. The subject is calculated to appeal to bourgeois notions of the life of the "poor, but happy" peasants of France. All the virtues are implicit: care, concern, tenderness, love, harmony, cleanliness, modesty, "holy poverty," the family of many children. The execution is flawless, a technical tour de force in composition and line, perfectly balanced and brushed. The colors are delicate, yet at the same time strong and warm, and represent the complete spectrum—from violet, indigo, and blue-green to yellow and orange-red. In short, each part of the painting is perfect. Why, then, does such a painting, with all its technical beauty, leave the viewer with a sense of unease, of promise given but consummation denied?

It may be that while *La Grande Soeur* stimulates the intellect to an admiration and respect for Bouguereau's considerable talents, it fails to engage the emotions. Intuitively one feels, for example, that the Madonna-like young girl and the infant she dresses on her lap bear as much relation to actual French peasant life as the slick mini-dramas of television bear to real American life. Bouguereau has strained his talents through such a fine mesh of diligence that he has filtered out all the mystery. He has solved the formula of the painting, but he has lost the sacrament of the girl and the infant. In short, his very perfection has become an imperfection. In this case the whole is not greater than—or even equal to—the sum of its perfect parts; it is considerably less.

Bouguereau had a formidable talent, which he disciplined and directed well. He was industrious and was rewarded during his lifetime not only with medals and honors but with the high prices his paintings commanded. Today, there is once again interest. Yet for all his talent Bouguereau lacked that spark of genius that would have lit up the viewer's soul. Like Sisyphus, Bouguereau labored mightily. But he never succeeded in sending the rock crashing down the other side of the mountain.

William Adolphe Bouguereau (1825-1905), *La Grande Soeur*, 1877, French. Oil on canvas. 146 × 88.9 cm. Courtesy of Christie's, New York, New York (sold October 27, 1983).

JAMA®

THE JOURNAL of the American Medical Association

November 15, 1985

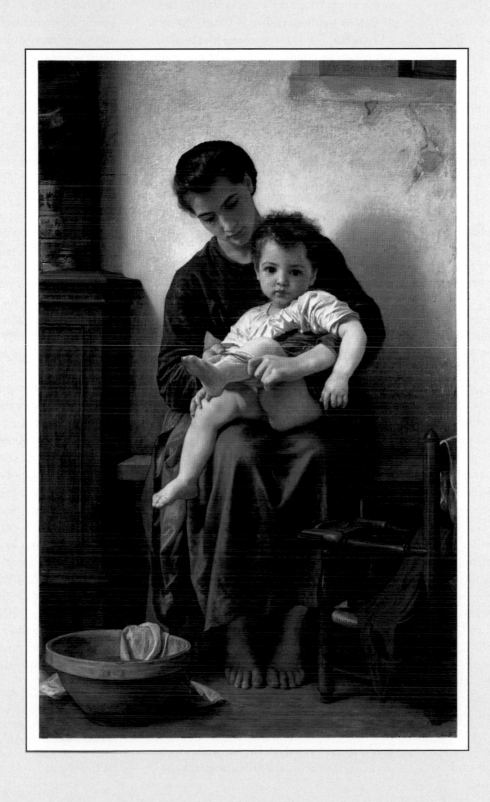

FRANCESCO DEL COSSA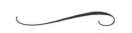

Saint Lucy

Francesco del Cossa (c 1435-1477), one of the leading painters of the northern Italian Renaissance, is remembered chiefly for two works. The first consists of three frescoes, completed in 1470 for the d'Este family of Ferrara for the Hall of the Months of the Schifanoia Palace. Disappointed with what Duke Borso paid him for the frescoes, Cossa shortly thereafter moved to Bologna. There, in 1474 or 1475, he executed a large altarpiece for the Griffoni Chapel in San Petronio. *Saint Lucy* is one of the panels of that altarpiece.

Originally, the Griffoni altarpiece consisted of five panels: in the center, a life-size, full-length painting of St Vincent Ferrer, a popular Spanish Dominican priest and preacher who had died in 1419 in France, and on either side paintings of St Peter and St John the Baptist, also full-length and life-size. Above St Peter and St John were life-size kneeling figures of St Florian, chosen probably because Florian was the Christian name of one of the members of the Griffoni family, and St Lucy, long one of the most popular saints in Italy and elsewhere. In the early 18th century, the altar was moved and subsequently dismantled. The separate panels may now be seen in London, Milan, and Washington, DC.

Through the centuries, St Lucy has been a rich source of legend and lore. Valid historical data confirm only that she lived during the third century, that she was associated with Syracuse, Sicily, and that she died at the beginning of the fourth century during the Diocletian persecution. As early as the fifth century, a Lucia cult was flourishing in Syracuse, and during the sixth and seventh centuries it spread to Rome, Ravenna, and Milan. By the end of the seventh century, St Lucy was being celebrated in England in prose and verse. The stories were based on the *acta* of St Lucy, which have been proved historically worthless, but these legendary accounts have persisted through the centuries.

According to one version, Lucy was a Christian descended from a noble and wealthy Syracuse family, who, as a girl, vowed her virginity to God and her wealth to the poor. When her pagan suitor learned of this, he denounced her to the governor as a Christian. She was sentenced to a brothel, but when the guards tried to take her there, she miraculously had become immovable. Four oxen, it was said, could not budge her. Next, she was sentenced to be burned to death, but the flames had no effect. Finally, she died when a sword or poniard was thrust through her throat.

> *...patroness of light and sight and protector against blindness...*

In the Middle Ages, perhaps because her name suggested *lux* or *lucem*, the Latin word for light, St Lucy was invoked as a protection against, or cure for, blindness and to the store of legends were added those concerning her extraordinary eyes. One version has them torn out at the time of her martyrdom, another has her presenting them to her unwanted suitor because she did not want to be tempted by his admiration for them. In each version her eyes are restored to her, more beautiful than before. Still another Lucy story says her life is a confusion with the legend of Lucina, the Roman goddess of childbirth, the Mother of Light, and the one who opens the eyes of newborns. According to that version, Christian vandals stole the jeweled eyes from a gigantic statue of Lucina, but when they tried to steal the statue as well it weighed so heavily that, like St Lucy, it could not be budged.

In ancient times, the Romans celebrated the Festival of Lucina on the shortest day of the year because it was she who rekindled the sun. From medieval times, St Lucy's feast has been celebrated on December 13, which, in the Julian calendar of the time, was the shortest day of the year. A popular folk saying was "Lucy-light, the shortest day and the longest night." Another folk practice predicted events of the coming 12 months according to what happened on each of the 12 days between the feast of St Lucy and Christmas. In Sweden, the custom of celebrating Lucia morning on December 13 arose in the 18th century and continues today. Because it is the longest and darkest night of the year, extra nourishment is needed and food and drink are served at dawn, by candlelight. In the 19th century a *Lucia*, a young girl dressed in white with a crown of flickering candles on her head, was chosen to serve the food, traditionally coffee, specially shaped saffron rolls, ginger biscuits, and *glögg*. More recently, it has become customary each December, when the Nobel prizes are awarded, for the winner of that year's prize in literature to crown the Lucia chosen to represent Stockholm.

St Lucy and her legends have frequently been a subject for artists. The earliest example is a sixth-century mosaic in Ravenna, where she is shown with the virgins Saints Crispina and Cecilia. In late medieval art she is first shown with attributes, most often portrayed by two eyes carried on a plate and a palm branch, the symbol of victory over death through martyrdom, in her hand. Occasionally she is shown with a lamp, its light suggesting the Latin derivation of her name, or a book, symbolizing the light that comes from truth. St Lucy was especially popular with artists of the Italian Renaissance, who, like Cossa, frequently portrayed her on altarpieces. It is perhaps her reputation as patroness of light and sight and protector against blindness that made her so appealing as a subject to painters.

JAMA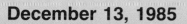

THE JOURNAL of the American Medical Association

December 13, 1985

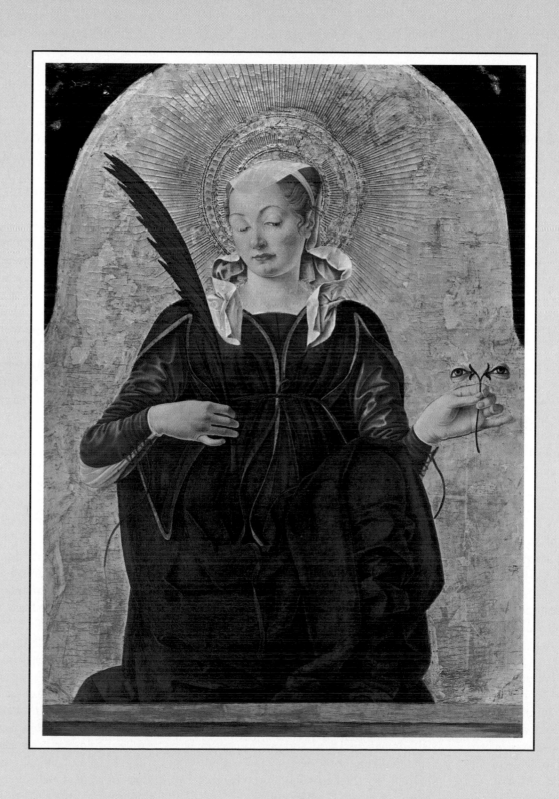

VINCENT VAN GOGH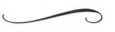

Madame Roulin and Her Baby

On the evening of Sunday, February 19, 1888, Vincent van Gogh (1853-1890), a would-be painter who had never sold anything and who had been receiving his entire financial support from his younger brother Theo for the past several years, left Paris on a train bound for the Midi, Provence. His specific destination was Arles, a town of 23,000 inhabitants situated on the Rhone some 760 kilometers south of Paris and 40 kilometers north of the Mediterranean. His health that winter had not been good. He had been drinking and smoking excessively, and he found the cold, darkness, fog, snow, and rain of the Paris winter intolerable. By going south he hoped for sun and warmth; more than ever, he wished to make a fresh start, yet another "new beginning" or, as he put it, "a rebirth."

Van Gogh's first sight of Arles at noon the next day did not augur well. Snow covered the ground; he was soon to learn what a mistral was—that violent, cold, dry, northerly wind that could blow hard for up to six weeks at a time and be emotionally unsettling. Moreover, the town itself, for all its Roman origins, was hardly picturesque. What he found was a mélange of Roman ruins and Gothic remnants, modern gas works and sprawling railroad yards, flatness and filthiness. But when the sun finally shone, van Gogh found that the colors of its landscape were like no others and that its women did indeed possess their fabled beauty of face, carriage, and costume.

At the age of 34, this newest inhabitant of Arles had nothing but a string of failures behind him, each of them a hoped-for "new beginning in life." He had been a clerk for an art dealer in The Hague, London, and Paris, a language teacher and lay preacher in England, a bookseller in Dordrecht, a theology student in Amsterdam, a self-proclaimed missionary to the poverty-stricken coal miners of the Borinage in Belgium, and an art student in Brussels and Antwerp. And throughout his life he expressed his desire to

be a doctor so that he could bring consolation to the poor and suffering. Not until 1880, only ten years before he died, had he discovered that painting was his real métier. Only two years before his death did he discover the sun-baked vistas of Arles.

In early December 1888, when he had been in Arles for some nine months, van Gogh wrote exultantly to his brother that he had "made portraits of a *whole family*… you know how I feel about this, how I feel in my element, and that it consoles me up to a certain point for not being a doctor." The family he spoke of consisted of 47-year-

> *…an attempt to bring light to darkness, to recreate himself yet again from the chaos he felt building within.*

old Joseph Roulin, the town's postmaster and his good friend, his 37-year-old wife Augustine-Alix, whom van Gogh was to paint more times than anyone save himself, their two boys, Armand, age 17, and Camille, age 11, and a 4-month-old baby, Marcelle. *Madame Roulin and Her Baby* is one of these portraits.

Van Gogh has chosen a curious, almost shocking pose for his models. One expects a more conventional scene—the infant cradled in its mother's arms or feeding at her breast, for example, and one expects to see tenderness, warmth, and security—all the qualities traditionally associated with maternal bonding. Instead, van Gogh has made the mother a secondary, shadowy figure. She is withdrawn, distanced, and pensive, as though contemplating some deep sorrow within herself. Her chief role is as a prop for the baby, which van Gogh has thrust forward,

almost out of the canvas. The infant stands uncertainly on her mother's lap, looking accusingly at the viewer, wondering, bewildered, dismayed, angry—as though it were van Gogh himself. The colors, too, are unconventional. The mother's face is green, while the large unrelieved background is an intense yellow. It has been slapped on hastily, except around the baby's head, where a carefully brushed halo effect may be seen.

What was van Gogh trying to express with this portrait? Although his temperament could accept the authority of no church, van Gogh was an intensely religious man. Yet he was unable to paint manifestly religious scenes. Twice that summer he had begun a Christ figure, only to scrape off the canvas through a profound sense of unworthiness. In September he had written to Theo, "I want to paint men and women with that something of the eternal which the halo used to symbolize, and which we seek to confer by the actual radiance and vibration of our colorings." And shortly after he did *Madame Roulin and Her Baby* he wrote, "Had I the strength to continue I would have done portraits of saints and saintly women from life who would have appeared as of another century, and they would be middle-class people of today and yet would be related to very primitive Christians." Additionally, van Gogh made this portrait in December. Christmas, always a time of great emotional significance for him, was approaching and Madame Roulin and baby Marcelle would have been a natural reminder of the Madonna and Child.

Again, Giovanni Bellini, the 15th-century Venetian painter, has a similar pose of a sad-faced Madonna supporting a standing, reluctant, sorrowing child. It was also the custom for Gothic and Renaissance painters to place religious subjects against a layered, brilliant gold-leaf background, an effect van Gogh has simulated with intense yellow and a palette knife. Finally, Renaissance painters underpainted their panels with *terra verde*

Continued on p. 214

JAMA

THE JOURNAL of the American Medical Association

December 27, 1985

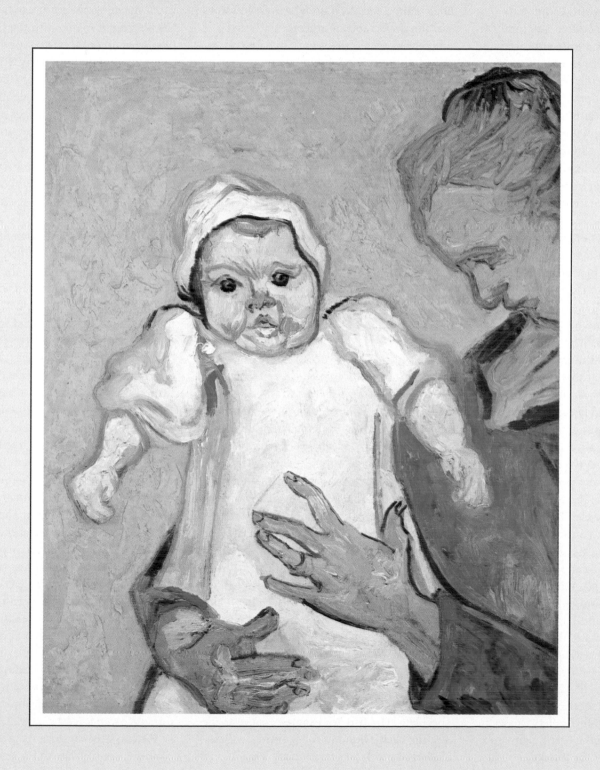

PABLO PICASSO ～

Composition for a Mardi Gras Ball

At the end of World War I, life in Europe seemed to come loose at its hinges. It swung crazily between a decade that had seen battlefields a train ride away and millions more dead in an epidemic of flu and a brand-new decade that promised everything to everyone—especially peace, prosperity, and eternal youth to anyone who could grab them. The capital of this giddy, frenetic world was Paris, where the beau monde marked off the seasons by fancy dress balls, costume parties, and masquerades. It was as though, having seen enough of wounded horses, dead riders, and young brides buried within days of chills and fever, the audience trooped en masse to another theater where a happier play was billed.

Though not the sun of this universe, Pablo Picasso (1881-1973) was nevertheless an important satellite, and he shone brilliantly wherever he went. Whether it be a fancy dress ball given by the Comte and Comtesse de Beaumont at their town house on rue Masseran on the occasion of Mardi Gras or a party on an old barge tethered in the Seine given by the young heirs to the Mark Cross fortune, Gerald and Sara Murphy, Picasso and Olga would be there. Olga saw to that. Also there would be such other guests as Stravinsky, Cocteau, Coco Chanel, Diaghilev, Blaise Cendrars, Léger, the Princesse de Polignac, and many others. To one of the Comte's parties Picasso came disguised as a matador. To another party he wore his new dinner jacket, made magnificent by the red, fringed bullfighter's cummerbund he wore beneath it.

Like Paris society, Picasso's life had also been turned topsy-turvy toward the end of the war. Approaching his 40th birthday, he left behind his bohemian lifestyle and a string of mistresses and married Olga Khoklova, a dancer with the Ballets Russes, daughter of a colonel in the czar's army, and member, albeit minor, of the Russian nobility. Gone forever were the days at Lavoir Bateau on Montmartre. He now lived on the fashionable rue La Boétie, at No. 23, an address Olga had picked. As if both to presage and to seal the respectable bourgeois life Picasso was now expected to live, a son, Paulo, was born in February 1921.

At age 40, Picasso was rich and famous and respectable. But he was worried, as he would be often in his life, about what to do next. Cubism was behind him. He had broken with Derain and with Braque. Apollinaire was dead. Yet the decade was in its springtime. For a while Picasso turned to a serene neoclassicism and then to still life. Neither apparently satisfied him for any

> *...in short, a counterpoint of flesh and spirit.*

length of time. As the decade wore on, Olga's social climbing, Picasso's dislike of imposed order, and his own isolation from his creative peers began to wear on him. Moreover, after the birth of Paulo, Olga's mental health began to deteriorate. Increasingly, Picasso put his anger and his rage into his painting. By the end of the decade, he was painting those violent distortions of the human anatomy, especially of female anatomy, that have often been used to label Picasso a misogynist.

Meanwhile, however, Picasso produced other works that, while not landmarks in his development, do mark events in his life and are pleasant to look at besides. *Composition for a Mardi Gras Ball*, for example, was painted especially for the Comte Étienne de Beaumont on the occasion of the fancy dress ball he gave at his home for Mardi Gras in 1923. Indeed, the "BAL" at the top center proclaims the occasion. For the rest, one can speculate. The fish, for example, suggests the sea; the background of the painting, with its slashes of black on grayish pink, suggests scintillating water—sun dancing on the tips of tiny waves.

The sign of the fish can also have many other meanings in art: It can be a symbol for the feeding of many, as in the Gospel story of the feeding of the five thousand, and is thus appropriate for a party, especially for one celebrating Mardi Gras (literally, "fat Tuesday"), the last day of plenty before Ash Wednesday heralds the beginning of the 40 days of fasting before Easter. In the Old Testament story of Jonah, the fish, probably a dolphin, is a symbol of the Easter Resurrection. The fish is also the symbol for the month of February, when the sun enters its sign in the zodiac. Although it is a movable feast and can occur in either February or March, Mardi Gras most often occurs in February. Finally, Neptune, the Roman god of the sea, is often portrayed with a dolphin and is identified by his trident, or three-pronged fork, here suggested by one of the feet of the figure on the left.

The two figures are, in fact, interesting in themselves. They can be seen as a man and woman in Mardi Gras costume, the man as Neptune, the woman as his wife, the sea nymph Amphitrite. Neptune's tiny head, which contrasts with the large fish-skeleton body and exaggerated trident legs, suggests enormous physical desire—at the expense of intellectual analysis—an attribute familiar to both Neptune and Picasso. The woman, on the other hand, is more elaborately costumed. She suggests Picasso's personal feeling toward women at this time and toward Olga in particular. Her larger head suggests rationalization, even scheming perhaps; her torso is all uterus. Most importantly, however, every inch of her exterior carries triangular projections like small, sharp teeth, or like the painful shards of her already fragmenting personality. Picasso found Olga still desirable, but increasingly difficult, even as early as 1923.

Picasso's colors suggest various other concepts appropriate to the occasion of Mardi Gras. The overall purplish cast, while recalling some of the colors of his Harlequin

Continued on p. 214

JAMA

THE JOURNAL of the American Medical Association

February 7, 1986

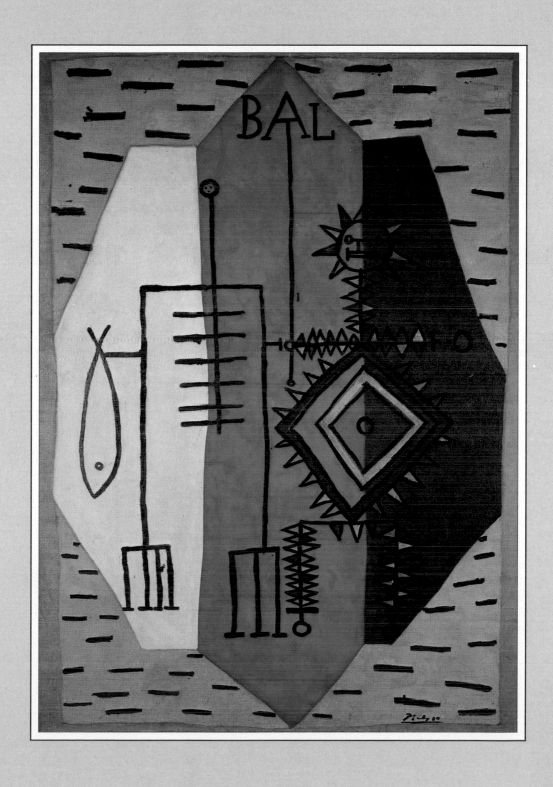

DIEGO RIVERA

Flower Day

Diego Rivera (1886-1957) is known primarily as a mural painter. He also did many easel pieces, however, of which Flower Day won the purchase prize of $1500 at the Pan-American Exhibition in Los Angeles in 1925.

Rivera was a man of paradox, whether in work, in love, in politics, or in religion; wherever he went controversy followed. He was a huge man—300 pounds, 6 feet—yet he moved with grace. He loved beauty, yet his friends called him "frog face" because of his protruding eyes. He could seem to be doing nothing for weeks and then work 18 hours a day, seven days a week, for weeks on end. He married many times, yet many times he neglected to marry. He was a member of the Communist party off and on and celebrated the anniversary of the Bolshevik revolution in the USSR, but he also painted murals for American capitalists. Henry and

...it is just this quiet joy in human life and its possibilities that Rivera was able to communicate.

Edsel Ford were his friends. He greatly loved the simple life of the Mexican peasant, but he was enthusiastic about American expressways, industrial machinery, and football ("joyous," he called it). He could paint the words "*Dios no exista*" and later announce that he was indeed a Roman Catholic. In short, neither facts nor the laws of logic seemed to trouble Rivera greatly. He had

the freedom of the child's mind, which can invent whatever it needs whenever it needs it.

Characteristically, *Flower Day* contains and reconciles many contradictions. It portrays the simple flower procession of the Indians. Yet, at the same time, the symbolism points to the ancient pagan fertility rites of spring as well as the Christian rite of Easter, traditionally observed on the first Sunday after the first full moon of spring. A strong stained-glass quality suggests reverence in the presence of the holy. And indeed, it is just this quiet joy in human life and its possibilities that Rivera was able to communicate. In each cycle of rebirth of the land and its inhabitants, we are in possession of hope.

Diego Rivera (1886-1957), *Flower Day*, 1925, Mexican. Oil on canvas. 120.6 × 147.3 cm. Courtesy of the Los Angeles County Museum of Art, Los Angeles, California; Los Angeles County Fund.

JAMA

THE JOURNAL of the American Medical Association

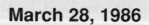

March 28, 1986

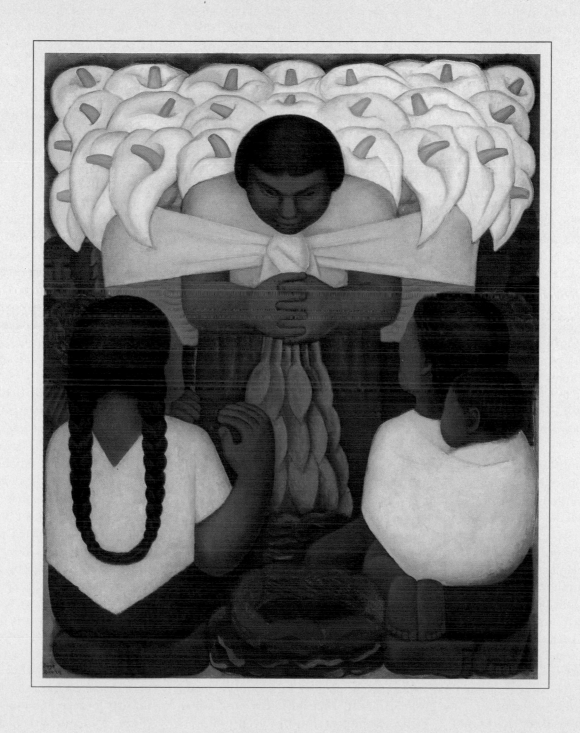

THOMAS EAKINS

The Agnew Clinic

Professor D. Hayes Agnew had spent more than a quarter of a century teaching anatomy and surgery to students at the University of Pennsylvania. He was, in the words of a biographer, "a quick but a precise operator and his use of instruments was light and graceful." During the Civil War, he became something of an expert on gunshot wounds, and he was the chief surgeon attending President Garfield when he was assassinated in 1881. He devised a new procedure for separating webbed fingers, as well as many new surgical instruments, among them an instrument for compressing bleeding intercostal vessels. Among his publications was the three-volume work *The Principles and Practice of Surgery*. Much beloved by his students, he was especially noted for his physical stamina, his equanimity, his soundness of judgment, and the clarity of his teaching. Now, in 1889, at the age of 70, Agnew was about to become professor emeritus of surgery and his students wished to honor him. Thomas Eakins (1844-1916) was commissioned to paint his portrait, which was to be presented to the school at the May 1 commencement only three months away.

Eakins took the commission; it was one of his few. The agreed-on fee, to be raised by subscription from the 25 members of the three classes at the school, was $750. Eakins, however, had another idea. Fourteen years earlier, he had painted the portrait of another eminent Philadelphia surgeon, Dr Samuel D. Gross. He had shown Gross not as a conventional single figure, but life-size, in the surgical amphitheater, surrounded by students and assistants, performing an actual surgical procedure. He would do the same for Dr Agnew, except that he would make the painting even larger (Gross' portrait was 8 feet high by 6 ½ feet wide), with more figures, including—in spite of the short time available—a likeness of every student who had commissioned the painting. Like Agnew, who at times would dissect for 12 to 18 hours

a day, Eakins worked from early morning until evening, catnapping on the floor in front of the canvas when he could not go on. Even the frame was carved by Eakins, with the Latin words for "D. Hayes Agnew, MD, the most experienced surgeon, the clearest writer and teacher, the most venerated and beloved man." But he finished on time and the painting, nearly 6 feet by 11 feet, was accepted by Dr S. Weir Mitchell on behalf of the trustees of the University of Pennsylvania at its unveiling at the commencement on May 1, 1889. It became known as *The Agnew Clinic*.

> *...as the buxom country girl glowing with good health attends a woman little older than herself who has lost a breast.*

The scene is the university's surgical amphitheater. Agnew has just completed a mammectomy and has stepped away from the table, much as Eakins himself may have stepped back to reflect on his painting. He is perhaps expounding on a detail of the procedure or pointing out the necessity for meticulous hemostasis in wound closure, or perhaps even recalling the gloomy future this young woman faces should she survive the risks of the surgery itself, such as bleeding and infection. Agnew's assistant, Dr J. William White, who would succeed him as professor of surgery, closes. Dr Joseph Leidy II, his arm across the patient's legs, sponges blood from her chest, while the intern, Dr Ellwood Kirby, administers ether by the open-drop method. An unidentified nurse, holding a tray for instruments, completes the group in the pit. Above them, in four tiers, rise the

students in varying attitudes of attention (a student in the top row, for example, catches up on some of the sleep he probably missed the night before). At the right edge of the painting is a likeness of Eakins, painted by one of his former students, now Mrs Eakins. Whispering to him is Dr Fred H. Milliken.

Fourteen years had elapsed since *The Gross Clinic*. But in that short time, great advances had been made in the practice of surgery, some of which are noted in *The Agnew Clinic*. Most obvious is that neither patient nor physician any longer wears street clothes. Each is appropriately gowned or draped. Still, however, the surgeons wear neither masks nor gloves. The amphitheater is artificially lighted, not only giving greater control over illumination but permitting a more flexible operating schedule as well. Gross, for example, operated under natural light from a skylight and confined his surgery to the hours between 11 AM and 3 PM. Finally, a female nurse is present, assisting with an instrument tray.

Other comparisons between the two paintings may also be made. Whereas the format of *The Gross Clinic* is vertical and the picture area somewhat smaller, here the format is horizontal, emphasizing the posture of the patient, and the picture area is greater. Gross dominated the first painting by being the apex of a triangle of figures. Here Agnew is off to the side, isolated, and at the lowest part of the painting. Indeed, one could make two separate paintings by drawing a vertical line through the empty space in front of Agnew, the left portion becoming a single-figure portrait of Agnew, the right portion a painting of a surgical procedure. But the drama of the situation would be lost. With Agnew at the far left of the circular pit, he becomes an eccentrically placed axis that imparts force and motion to the action in the pit. Moreover, diagonals from the upper left of the painting point to the scalpel in his left hand (Agnew was ambidextrous), while the diagonal balustrade on the right leads

Continued on p. 215

JAMA®

May 23/30, 1986

THE JOURNAL of the American Medical Association

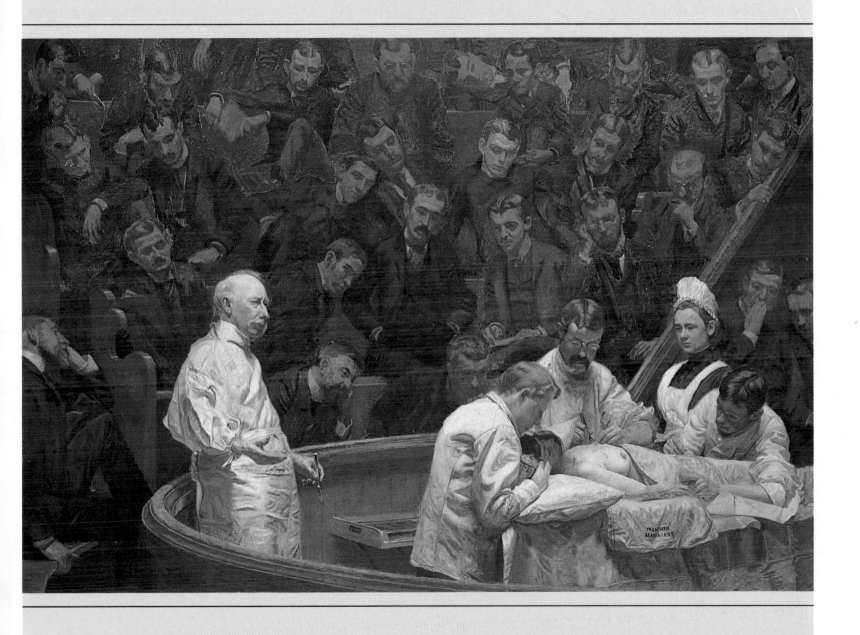

GIOVANNI BATTISTA GAULLI

St Joseph and the Infant Christ

Giovanni Battista Gaulli (1639-1709), called Baciccio after the Genoese diminutive of his baptismal name, was a man who enjoyed the favor of several popes and nearly all of the cardinals of the church—a not inconsiderable feat for 17th-century Rome. Alexander VII was so charmed by the young Genoese that he gave orders that Baciccio was to be given access to him at any time, entering by way of the secret stair, if necessary. Baciccio was to paint the portraits of all seven popes he knew, from Alexander VII to Clement XI, and, as his biographer Pascoli notes, "of all the cardinals, of all the important people who lived during his time and who came to Rome."

Good fortune had not always smiled on Baciccio, however. Born in Genoa in 1639, while he was still in his teens he lost his entire family to the plague: mother, father, and ten brothers and sisters. Moreover, toward the end of his life Baciccio lost a son under tragic circumstances—some accounts say suicide, while others say a distraught Baciccio attempted suicide and had to be confined for a time. Yet he had a natural gift for attracting the attention of well-placed persons, and it served him well. Accounts of the time describe him as "eager, lively, and full of ginger." As an orphan in Genoa, he had come to the attention of the ambassador to Rome of the Republic of Genoa. Some say he hid in the ambassador's galley as it was about to weigh anchor for Rome. Once in Rome he came to the attention of the great sculptor-architect Bernini and became his protegé.

> *...the point, as T.S. Eliot says, at which time touches eternity.*

With Bernini as his mentor it was but an easy step to papal and aristocratic Rome.

The high period of Baciccio's work came in the years between 1672 and 1685, when he was in his mid-30s to mid-40s. It was during this period that he did the frescoes for the ceiling of Il Gesù, the mother church of the Jesuit order in Rome, and the work for which today he is most well known. During this period he also did many oils, most of which have disappeared, but of which *St Joseph and the Infant Christ* survives. Typical of Baciccio's work, the colors are warm, the mood joyful, the occasion a single, frozen instant. The draperies are as deeply carved as a Bernini statue and yet the air currents about them are still vibrating. It is work of a kind that caused a Spanish critic to call Baciccio a "Bernini in paint."

St Joseph and the Infant Christ is the title by which this painting is commonly known. Yet on close inspection one may begin to ask questions about certain discrepancies that come to mind. Christ, for example, was 30 years old when Joseph died, yet this man, with his balding scalp, thinning hair, and flowing white beard, is already aged. He surely will not live 30 years more. Nor are his hands those of a workman, a carpenter. Finally, the background suggests that the setting is a temple, whereas for such a tender scene with Joseph and the child the setting might more appropriately be a manger. With this in mind, it is suggested that perhaps the man is not intended to be Joseph but Simeon, who was in the temple at the time of the rite of purification and who took the child in his arms, saying that this was what he had waited for, that now he could die in peace. The painting could perhaps more properly be called *Simeon and the Infant Christ* or, simply, *Nunc Dimittis*, for Simeon's words on that occasion. Be that as it may, a title does not a painting make. The reality remains that of a man's joy when he holds a child in his arms.

Baciccio had the ability to catch—and thus to prolong, even to infinity—that half-glimpsed, fleeting moment that is the present—the point, as T. S. Eliot says, at which time touches eternity. Baciccio is able to preserve the lost moments of daily life and to remind us that they have in fact never ended. Like the language of the child, Baciccio's painting has no past or future tense. It is all present, like the joy of Joseph, or Simeon, or any man who has ever gazed at his newborn in his arms.

Giovanni Battista Gaulli (1639-1709), *St Joseph and the Infant Christ*, c 1670-1685, Genoese. Oil on canvas. 127 × 97.2 cm. Courtesy of the Norton Simon Foundation, Pasadena, California.

JAMA®

THE JOURNAL of the American Medical Association

June 13, 1986

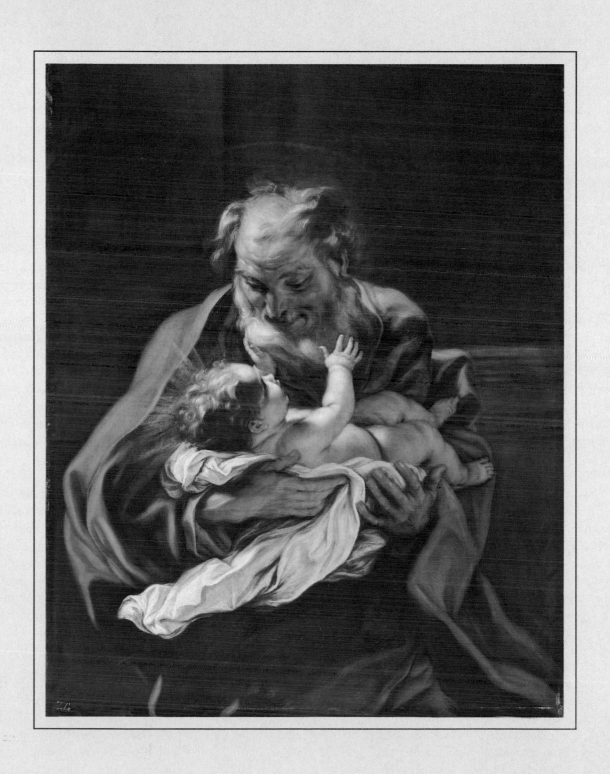

CLAUDE MONET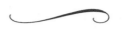

Wild Poppies

The Franco-Prussian War of 1870 dispersed the little band of painters that had been converging regularly on the Café Guerbois in Paris. Here, with 38-year-old Manet as a kind of unofficial leader, the small group had met informally, usually on Thursday evenings, and discussed, always passionately, sometimes noisily, their opinions on art. As yet, the term Impressionist did not exist and the company was known among their few followers as the Batignolles group, after the street address of the café. Among the youngest were Renoir and Claude Monet (1840-1926); Bazille was younger by a year. Cézanne and Sisley were 31, Degas was 36, and Pissarro, at 39, was the oldest. The outbreak of the war in July brought the meetings to an end.

Renoir, refusing a staff commission, was drafted into the army and sent to the Pyrenees to train horses. There he became gravely ill with dysentery. Bazille joined the crack infantry unit, the Zouaves, and was killed in November. Cézanne hid out from both the draft and his father, living with his mistress in L'Estaque. Degas enlisted in the infantry (where it was discovered that his right eye was almost blind), while Pissarro went first to Brittany and then to England with his family. Sisley, being English, was not eligible for the draft. Monet, meanwhile, fled to England leaving behind his bride of two months, Camille, and 3-year-old son, Jean. Together, Monet and Pissarro worked in London, and Monet later went to Holland. In December 1871, at the age of 31, Monet returned to France, where he rented a house for himself, Camille, and Jean at Argenteuil. He would remain here until 1878, in one of the longest settled periods of his life to that time. Here, nearly all of the Café Guerbois friends would join Monet at one time or another. Here would be born Impressionism.

Until 1851, Argenteuil had been a small (population 4000), pastoral town some 27 kilometers down the Seine from Paris, noted chiefly for its wine and the ruins of its seventh-century abbey (whence its 12th-century prioress, Héloîse, eloped with the theologian Abélard down its main boulevard). The townspeople also mined gypsum and made plaster (from which plaster of paris received its name). With the coming of the railroad, which shortened the distance from Paris to 11 kilometers and the time to 15 minutes, Argenteuil became a sprawling suburb undergoing the throes of industrialization and recreational use by Parisians. When Monet arrived, the orchards, gardens, and vineyards remained, but now they might be neighbored by a tannery, a tallow factory,

> *…that summer of 1873 was a profusion of brilliant colors and sparkling canvases…*

a lace factory, a dye factory, or a starch factory. There were also iron works and gas works. A proposed oil refinery was voted down. Moreover, from the new sewer system in Paris, organic waste was dumped into the Seine at a point just above Argenteuil on its way to the Channel. Nevertheless, Argenteuil was the sailing capital of Paris and the location of many a wealthy Parisian's pied-à-terre and a popular spot for their Sunday outings.

In Argenteuil, securely married, free of the draft, and close to an evening at the Café Guerbois, Monet was prolific. To this period, which saw both the dawn and the high noon of Impressionism, belongs *Wild Poppies*, which Monet painted during his second summer in Argenteuil, when he and Renoir worked together, often setting up their easels before the same motif. For Monet that summer of 1873 was a profusion of brilliant colors and sparkling canvases as he painted the gardens, flowers, and fields of Argenteuil.

The design of the painting is simple. Midway across the canvas, a row of poplar trees on the ridge of a hill divides the scene into sky above and earth below. The sky is a transitional sky, with white clouds drifting apart to unveil the blue. The ground is dappled with multiple shades of green. The grasses are tall and accentuated by a hedge of yellow-green at the center of the painting. To the left, poppies are sprinkled across the meadow like drops of blood—as indeed real blood would mingle with poppies in the fields not too many years and too many miles hence—while to the poppies' left yellow goldenrod blooms. Coming over the crest of the hill are a woman and a child setting out on a walk across the meadow, the woman's closed parasol tucked in her arm. Near the bottom of the painting another woman walks through the grass carrying her open parasol, while a young boy picks poppies beside her. His hatband reflects the red of the poppies, while the pink roof of a house in the background fastens the eye back on the woman and boy. Both women and both children were probably modeled by Camille and their son Jean. It is interesting to note that, in the lower figures, Jean's features are painted in, whereas Camille's face is blank.

Although he had occasionally exhibited at the annual Salon, most often Monet's works were rejected. In the same summer that *Wild Poppies* was painted, Monet, Pissarro, Sisley, and Renoir were therefore planning a society of artists who would exhibit independently. This group, known as the *Société anonyme coopérative des artistes, sculpteurs, graveurs, etc*, was chartered in December 1873 and held its first exhibit in April 1874 at Nadar's, a vacant photographer's shop in Paris. Thirty members participated. *Wild Poppies* was probably among the paintings Monet exhibited. Ridicule, mockery, and sarcasm in the public press were extreme and the name *Impressionist* was first used to describe the painters. Total receipts of the show were 360 francs. Sisley received the most, 100 francs.

Continued on p. 215

JAMA®

The Journal of the American Medical Association

July 18, 1986

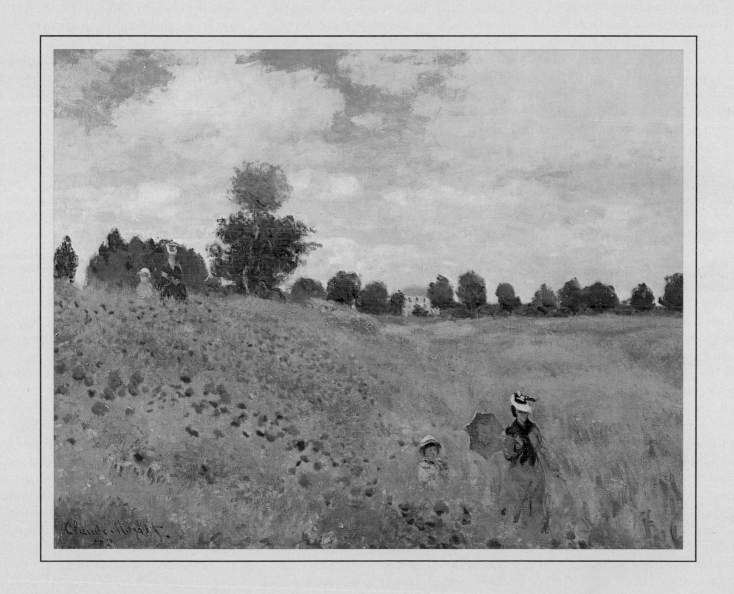

ÉDOUARD MANET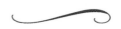

Le Bon Bock

Throughout his life, the urbane, witty, sophisticated Édouard Manet (1832-1883) had but two desires: to paint sincere works and to obtain the approval of the public and the critics at the official Salon. That the two desires should prove irreconcilable left him bewildered and, finally, embittered. His beginnings were auspicious enough; he gained an honorable mention and warm praise at the Salon of 1861, when he was 29. Such good favor was short-lived, however. In subsequent Salons, he was either rejected by the jury or, if he did exhibit, ridiculed and lampooned by the public and the press. The climax came in the Salon of 1865, when Manet scandalized everyone by exhibiting his *Olympia* and *Christ Mocked by the Soldiers*. And the depths of humiliation were perhaps reached the following year when Manet, hearing himself congratulated roundly as he entered the Salon, rushed to the M's only to find that the well-wishers had confused him with Monet. Years later, recalling this incident, Monet said, "How bitter it must have been for one whose sensitivity was always bared to the quick as his was!"

Manet, for his part, remained puzzled by the hostility his paintings aroused. Unlike his Impressionist colleagues, he did not consider himself a revolutionary. In the scientific spirit of the times, Manet wished only to paint the truth as he saw it, to be the pure researcher. And truth as he saw it lay not in the subject matter of the painting, but in the record of light and its various gradations as it is transmitted to the retina of the artist and thence through his hand to the canvas. Manet was, in fact, indifferent to subject matter. In itself, he considered it value free. The real subject was not the object "out there," but light as it is reflected by that object. What this light happened to reveal was quite beside the point. The point was light; how well the artist painted this light was what should be judged. But neither the critics nor the public saw it this way. The object "out there" mattered and mattered a

great deal. Accustomed as they were to the warmed-over academic styles and subjects presented year after year at the Salon, the viewers wanted nothing more than to spend an easy Sunday afternoon looking at pretty pictures. They did not want to be shocked into reconsidering the world about them. Thus, they were horrified to see a well-known Paris prostitute stretched out nude on her couch and scandalized to see their Christ in the guise of a Paris locksmith.

With *Le Bon Bock* (*The Good Beer*), which Manet exhibited at the Salon of 1873, the story was different, however. Here was a

> *...he is perhaps unaware that* le bon bock *could be one of his problems as well as one of his pleasures.*

good Parisian engaged in that most innocent of Parisian pleasures, a good beer. Manet and the public were at last in accord. Manet received from the critics the praise he coveted. Ironically, however, his Impressionist friends were less than pleased. *Le Bon Bock* was not true Manet, they felt. It lacked vigor and originality. It was more like the old masters, in particular like Frans Hals. And, indeed, Manet had the previous winter been in Haarlem, where he had studied the portraits of Hals. But his friends went even further, deciding that *Le Bon Bock* proved that one could be successful only if one compromised his principles. Henceforth they would boycott the Salon and instead have their own independent exhibits. When the first of these opened the following year, Manet refused to join his friends, pointing to his success with *Le Bon Bock*. To Monet and Renoir he said, "Why don't you stay with me [at the Salon]? You can see very well that I am on the right

track." To Manet's refusal to exhibit with the Impressionists Degas retorted that Manet was more vain than intelligent. But Manet preferred to be loyal to the Salon, which, however, had not been and would not be very loyal to him. And, now that he had the approval of the public, he had not the approval of his friends.

Whereas Manet had affronted the public when he had painted an ordinary locksmith as Christ, now he pleased the public by painting an ordinary Frenchman engaged in an ordinary occupation: sitting in the café at the end of the day. The model for *Le Bon Bock* was the engraver Emile Bellot. He is seated at a table in the Café Guerbois on the Grande rue des Batignolles, where Manet and his friends would meet in the evenings to discuss their work. Manet, who needed more than 60 sittings for this portrait, shows the corpulent engraver as a bon vivant who is especially adept at indulging the senses. His generous paunch, his rosy cheeks, and his red nose bespeak a man who in his lifetime has tippled too many "good beers." Sitting contentedly in the warmth of the café and drowsily mulling over the day, he is perhaps unaware that *le bon bock* could be one of his problems as well as one of his pleasures.

After his success with *Le Bon Bock* in 1873, Manet was not to have another success at the Salon until 1881. Even so, the second-class medal he was awarded came largely through the connivance of a friend who was influential with the jury. Not much mattered any longer to Manet, however, for by the end of that year he was fatally ill with tabes dorsalis.

Today, Manet is recognized as pivotal in the progression of painting from the Giottos of the 13th century to the modern abstraction of the 20th century. By his insistence that it is light and not the scene before the painter that is the chief actor in the drama of the canvas, he paved the way to a future where the scene would disappear altogether. Where once viewers looked *through* a painting to see a part of the world, they would, in the

Continued on p. 215

JAMA®

September 19, 1986

The Journal of the American Medical Association

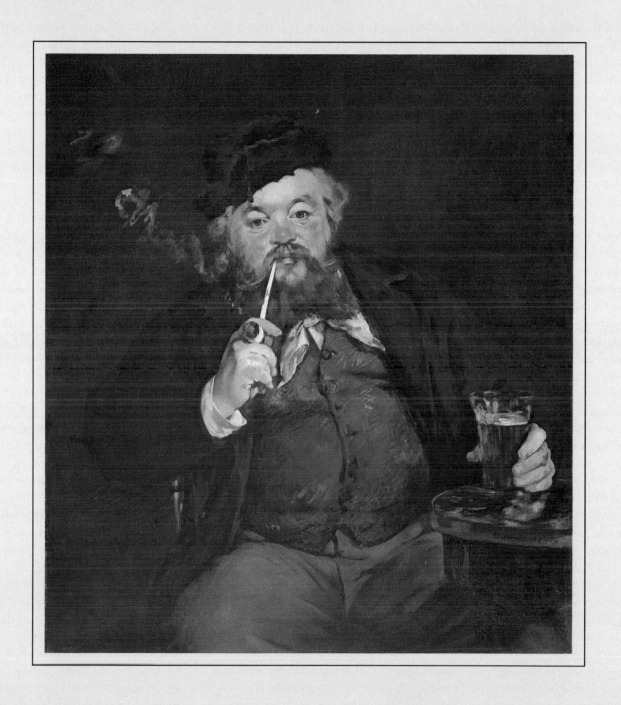

GIOVANNI FRANCESCO BARBIERI (IL GUERCINO)

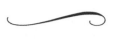

St Luke Displaying a Painting of the Virgin

As remote as the relationship may at first seem, medicine and painting have an association with each other that extends back many centuries. In the medieval guild system, for example, painters and apothecaries belonged to the same professional group, the guild of St Luke. On the basis of a reference in St Paul's letter to the Colossians ("Luke, the beloved physician, and Demas, greet you" [Colossians 4:14]), Luke has traditionally been assumed to have been a physician. How and why the legend grew that he was also a painter is unknown, but numerous portraits of the Virgin or of the Virgin and Child supposedly painted by Luke can still be found today. It was only natural, then, that painters should sooner or later portray this popular legend about their patron in their own works.

Beginning with the Netherlandish painters of the 15th and 16th centuries, St Luke painting the Virgin becomes a standard theme for artists, the most famous portrayal being one done by the Flemish painter van der Weyden. Such paintings were often presented by the artist to his guild. They may show the Virgin alone or holding the infant. The painting may be a simple studio portrait or an elaborate rendering of the Virgin in clouds, as the artist might imagine her to appear in a vision. The painter may show Luke standing before the easel or he might portray him kneeling as he paints. The theme became especially popular in counter-Reformation art and gradually spread southward where it was taken up by Italian artists. One such example, from northern Italy, is *St Luke Displaying a Painting of the Virgin*, done by Giovanni Francesco Barbieri (1591-1666) when he was 61 years old.

Barbieri, better known as *Il Guercino* because of his squint (Italian *guercio*: one-eyed, squinting), was born in the small northern Italian town of Cento, near Bologna. His father, Andrea Barbieri, drove a cart and regularly supplied the painters Carracci with wood. Guercino first came to public attention at age 8, when he painted a picture of the Virgin on his house. At the age of 16, he was apprenticed to Genarri, a minor artist of Cento. (One of Genarri's sons, a painter and a surgeon, was later to marry one of Guercino's sisters.) Less than ten years later, Guercino had his own studio in Cento and had begun teaching. Lodovico Carracci remarked at that time of Guercino's "felicity of invention, fine draughtsmanship, and

> *...Luke is the patron of both physicians and artists.*

happy coloring. He amazes every one who sees his works." When the Cardinal-Archbishop Ludovisi of Bologna became Pope Gregory XV in 1621, he took Guercino to Rome with him, where Guercino did the famous *Aurora* ceiling fresco for his palace. Gregory XV's reign was short, however, and in 1623 Guercino was back in Cento. He remained working there for almost 20 years, until his rival, Reni, died in Bologna. In 1642, Guercino moved to Bologna, becoming its undisputed master until his death in 1666, at the age of 75.

Guercino's Roman years are important in that his painting began to undergo a gradual change in style. Under the influence of the Carracci brothers and the canons of public taste (in other words, the marketplace), Guercino's style changed from freewheeling, emotional, dynamic baroque, and full of tension, to the more static, serene, balanced, less exciting classical style, stable and eternal. It is to these later, classical years that *St Luke Displaying a Painting of the Virgin* belongs. Guercino was in his early 60s and living in Bologna when he painted it.

In the 17th century, one of the most famous paintings of the Virgin ascribed to Luke was found in Bologna. It is this painting that Guercino reproduces in his work. For his model of Luke, Guercino used a fellow townsman, Aurelio Zaneletti, who had commissioned the piece. It is dusk, and Luke gestures to the painting he has just finished. He invites us also to admire it, while an angel gazes in awe. On a table at the right are Luke's attributes as one of the four Evangelists: the inkpot and quill, the book and the ox. The pen and the book signify Luke's authorship of the third Gospel as well as of the Acts of the Apostles. The ox is one of the four marvelous beasts described in Ezekiel and in Revelation that are used to signify the four Evangelists. The ox is chosen for Luke because it is a symbol of sacrifice, and Luke opens his Gospel with the account of Zechariah sacrificing in the temple. Usually the ox is winged, but here Guercino exercises artistic license to attach the wings to the angel instead.

St Luke Displaying a Painting of the Virgin has that "felicity of invention, fine draughtsmanship, and happy coloring" by which Lodovico Carracci characterized his townsman. Verticals, diagonals, horizontals, and color all combine to make a whole. The painting itself may be seen as two separate portraits, one of the Virgin's picture, the other of Luke, bound together by the diagonals of the angel's body and the right arm and hand of Luke. Verticals—the edge of the frame, the table leg, the pillar, the Child, and the Virgin—and horizontals—again, the frame itself, the tabletop, the book, the ox, and the angel's left wing—are also united by diagonals—Luke's torso and limbs, the angel's torso and right leg, the easel, the bench, and the frame of the Virgin's painting. Moreover, the shape of the tower in the right background echoes the shape of the Virgin's canvas, while the reds, blues, oranges and greens answer back and forth. This is not the

Continued on p. 215

JAMA

The Journal of the American Medical Association

October 10, 1986

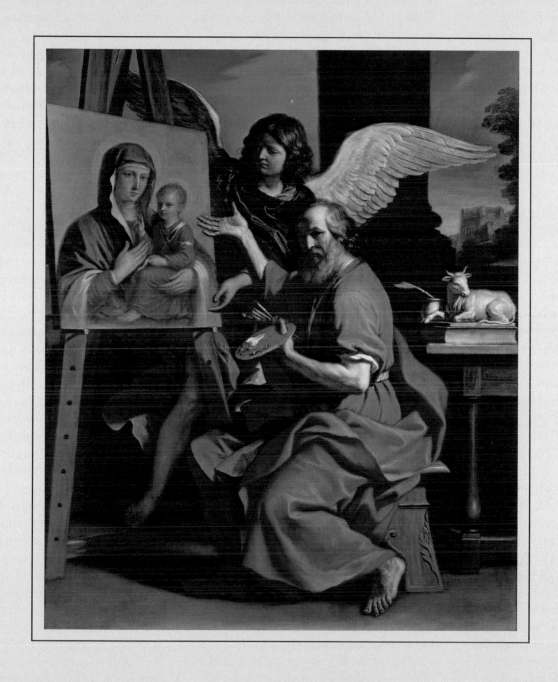

MARSDEN HARTLEY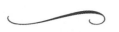

The Aero

All his life, Marsden Hartley (1877-1943), one of the pioneers of modern art in America, was a lonely man with a restless spirit. For more than 30 years, he traveled widely on two continents, never staying longer than ten months in the same lodgings. In his search for what he called the truth in art, he changed his style almost as often as his locale, progressing through all the art movements of his time: Academic Realism, Impressionism, Neo-Impressionism, Postimpressionism, Analytic and Synthetic Cubism, Fauvism, Symbolism, and, finally, Expressionism. He was also influenced by as many artists, including Ryder, Matisse, Picasso, Cézanne, Kandinsky, and Marc, and writers, including Thoreau, Emerson, Francis Thompson, and Emily Dickinson.

Hartley, christened Edmund, was the youngest of nine children, and the only boy, born to Eliza Jane (Horbury) and Thomas Hartley, a cotton spinner in the factory town of Lewiston, Maine. Four of the children died in childhood, and Hartley's mother died when he was 8. When the boy was 12, his father remarried (Martha Marsden) and moved to Cleveland, leaving Hartley behind with a married sister. Of these childhood years Hartley later said he recalled little, except that they were "vast with terror and surprise." At age 15, he dropped out of school to work in a shoe factory in Auburn, Maine, and the following year he rejoined his father and stepmother in Cleveland, working as a messenger and office boy in a marble quarry. At age 19, he began weekly painting lessons in Cleveland, and two years later he received a scholarship to the Cleveland School of Art. Thereafter, his fortunes progressed rapidly. He was awarded a five-year stipend of $450 per year, three times what he had made as an office boy, to study art in New York.

Despite his father's prediction that he would end as a failure, Hartley enrolled in the New York School of Art. He was 22 and on his way. For the next five years, his life assumed a rhythm of art study in New York during the winter and nature study in Maine during the summer. Influenced by Emerson, he developed further his own deeply mystical and intuitive leanings and, briefly, considered abandoning art for the priesthood. But when his stipend ran out at the end of 1904, Hartley supported himself by working as an extra in the theater and was also introduced to the homosexual community of Philadelphia. He renewed contact with his father and stepmother, who were again living in Maine, and he replaced the Edmund in his name with Marsden, his stepmother's maiden name.

> *…he at last had found the means of expressing the vision of truth that was uniquely his.*

The next decisive point in Hartley's life came in 1909, when he was 32. Alfred Stieglitz gave him his first one-man show at the 291 Gallery and became his staunch supporter. Although the show was a financial failure, it made him a part of the Stieglitz circle and led to a second show in 1912, and from that to the funds for his first trip to Europe. In April 1912, Hartley left for Paris. Though Hartley frequented the avant-garde artist cafés of Paris—the Dôme, the Rotonde—and even the salon of Gertrude Stein and her brother Leo, Parisian society had only a slight effect on him. More compatible with his ideas on art was the German circle that gathered at the Restaurant Thomas on the Boulevard Raspail. It was here that he met the sculptor Arnold Rönnebeck, an officer in the German army, and his cousin, the 24-year-old Karl von Freyburg. Hartley found he much preferred the mystical-intuitive orientation of the German circle to the logic and rationality of the French circle.

In January 1913, he made a brief trip to Berlin and was so enthusiastic about the city that he vowed to return there to live, and in May he did so.

Hartley was happy in Berlin. Here he could satisfy two conflicting needs: being part of a crowd, yet retaining solitude and anonymity. In a city such as Berlin, he said, one could "be common" and not attract attention. He was also greatly taken with the colorful pageantry of the military: the daily parades, the waving banners, the footmen, and the splendidly uniformed officers on horseback. Moreover, his friends Rönnebeck and von Freyburg, the latter himself now a lieutenant in uniform, were there. Together, the three of them formed what Hartley described as a "beautiful triangle." Von Freyburg he called "the one idol of my imaginative life." It was in this setting of pre-World War I Berlin that Hartley's style underwent a major change and he began one of his best known series, the military paintings. In them he was able to resolve his mystical leanings and his love of the military. Though he denied that there was any hidden symbolism in the paintings, but only things that he had "observed casually from day to day," the paintings are emblazoned with a colorful heraldry of circles, squares, triangles, crosses, numbers, letters, and stars. Many can be read as homage to von Freyburg, while others evoke the pomp and ceremony of a tense prewar Berlin. Brilliantly colored and crowded with forms, they are, said Georgia O'Keeffe, like "a brass band playing in a small closet." To this period belongs *The Aero*.

On October 17, 1913, the German navy's newest and largest dirigible, the zeppelin L-II, exploded in midair and burned as it was being tested at the aerodrome just outside Berlin. All 28 men aboard were killed. It has been suggested that The Aero commemorates the disaster. According to newspaper accounts, the airship was flying at an altitude of about 180 meters when three shattering explosions set it afire and caused it to fall as a blazing

Continued on p. 215

JAMA®

The Journal of the American Medical Association

November 7, 1986

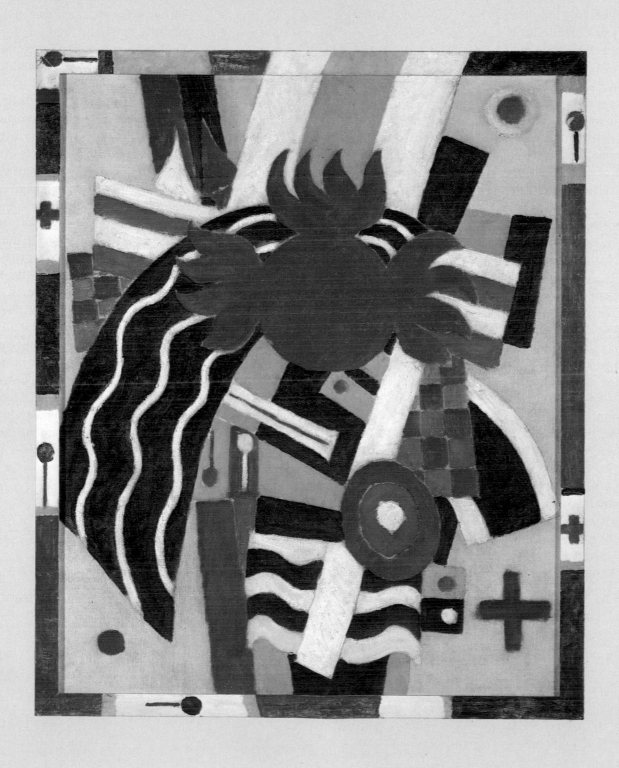

CLAUDE MONET

Snow at Argenteuil

When the Franco-Prussian War broke out in the summer of 1870, Claude Monet (1840-1926) was working in Le Havre. With him were the 23-year-old Camille (née Doncieux), his bride of less than three weeks, and the couple's 3-year-old son, Jean. In September, with France losing the war, Monet fled to England and then to Holland, leaving Camille and Jean in France. Only in December 1871, ten months after the war had ended and six months after the rebellious Paris Commune had been quashed, did Monet return. With Camille and Jean he settled in Argenteuil.

In the decade of the 1870s, postwar Argenteuil was a booming suburb of Paris, collecting itself around its railway station and two bridges. An easy afternoon's round trip from Paris by river, rail, or road, its fields, orchards, and rural vineyards were rapidly disappearing to developers, and new houses and industry were supplanting them at an alarming rate. On Sundays it was the Parisian's pleasure palace, with boating in the Seine, a decent local wine, and walks in the poppy fields. Here, in this part-industrial, part-rural suburb, Monet, Camille, and Jean would remain for six years, Monet's longest settled period since boyhood. He would produce more than 170 paintings, almost half his total output until then. From this hybrid of bustle and idyll would be born the painting that is today called Impressionism.

According to art historian Paul Tucker, some of Monet's most beautiful Argenteuil

To him the snow was what a cadenza is to a soloist.

works, nearly two dozen in all, are not the sparkling sunlit garden works we are familiar with, but scenes of the winter of 1874/1875. Here, with light coming from the subdued sun and reflecting off snowy roofs and ground, Monet could push his theories and methods to the limit. To him the snow was what a cadenza is to a soloist. It demanded all the virtuosity of his repertoire. It is to this winter of 1874/1875 that *Snow at Argenteuil* belongs. It reminds one of those heavy, wet falls of rain and snow that might surprise spring on its way to April, or perhaps catch a late October unawares.

Even though he himself lived in one of the new houses built by the developers, in *Snow at Argenteuil* Monet chooses mostly to ignore the scars on the land left by the speculators. Yet he does document one of the signs of the progress in Argenteuil, a new road. At the time Monet painted *Snow at Argenteuil* he was living near the railway bridge. The scene is behind his house, where the new road, prominent in the foreground, had just been built to provide better access to the railway station. The time is late afternoon and the viewer looks westward. In the

sky faint tinges of pink express the hidden sunset. On the road, pedestrians protected by umbrellas pick their way to the center of town. Snow falls lightly, hushing the land and restoring its innocence. Only the smoke drifting above the chimney suggests an intrusion.

But it was not documenting the new road that interested Monet in Argenteuil. Whether he was painting snow, a sunrise through a mist, a haystack in summer, a cathedral in Rouen, or even a steam engine in a railway station, Monet's subject was always the same: light. But not just any light at any time: it had to be the exact light that was reflected in time in the instant he saw it. It had to be the impression of the moment. That moment of light may have passed like a breath, but to Monet it contained eternity. In *Snow at Argenteuil* this moment is as fleeting as a snowflake, but he has fixed it on the canvas as it was then and will never be again.

In painting the light of Argenteuil as it was reflected from its shrinking rural landscape and growing industrial wound, Monet knew that one cannot possess light, or time, or beauty any more than one can possess a snowflake. One can only look—and sometimes, like Monet, try to make a painting.

Claude Monet (1840-1926), *Snow at Argenteuil*, c 1874, French. Oil on canvas. 54.6 × 73.8 cm. Courtesy of the Museum of Fine Arts, Boston, Massachusetts; bequest of Anna Perkins Rogers.

JAMA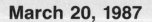

The Journal of the American Medical Association

March 20, 1987

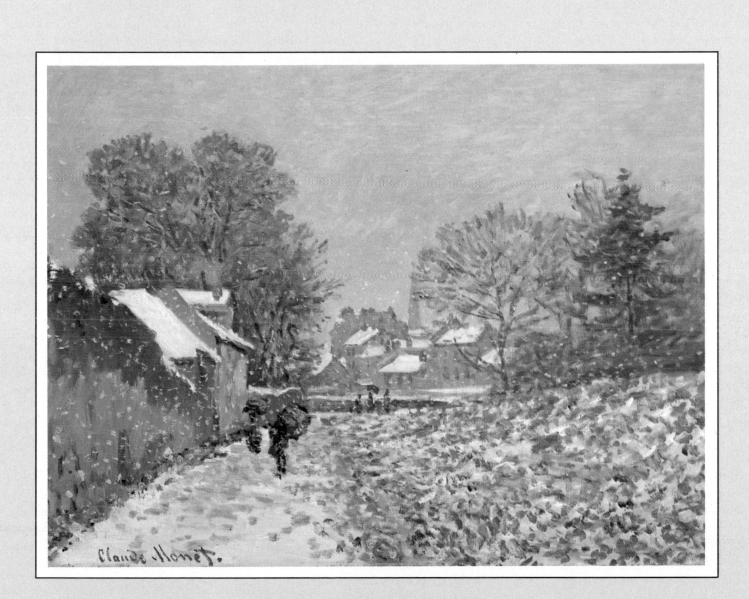

ANDREW WYETH

Battleground

On September 11, 1777, the American Army, with some 8000 Continentals and 3000 militiamen under General George Washington, and the British army, with 13,000 British and Hessian soldiers under General William Howe, met and clashed in south-eastern Pennsylvania on the banks of the Brandywine Creek. Washington's army was centered at Chads Ford, a narrow crossing of the Brandywine on the road to Philadelphia, while right and left flanks protected other fords upstream and downstream. The battle raged from morning till early afternoon, when Howe's army suprised Washington's army by surrounding its right flank, threatening to cut it off. The Americans fought them off until sunset, then withdrew; in the meantime the British easily crossed the Brandywine at Chads Ford. According to one, later, eyewitness account, the Brandywine ran "red with blood and was damned with bodies." Howe lost 500 men in the encounter, Washington 1000. Howe and his men went on to winter in Philadelphia, Washington and his men to Valley Forge. *Battleground* is Chads (now Chadds) Ford as seen by Andrew Wyeth (1917-   ) two centuries later.

Wyeth, who was born in Chadds Ford and received his early and only training from his father, the popular illustrator N.C. Wyeth, is undeniably the best-known painter living in the United States today. And, while professional critics have had skirmishes of their own from time to time over whether Wyeth is a "real" artist or, like his father, primarily an illustrator, it does not seem to matter to the public. A Wyeth painting always commands an audience. Like primers for those who are learning a new language, Wyeth's paintings speak plainly, in words of one syllable that anyone can understand, and his vocabulary is neither fancy nor esoteric. He paints mostly with nouns—solid words like

man, house, hill, river, ruts—and qualifies them with only the most familiar of adjectives—earth words like *brown, blue, fawn, white*. His plot is as spare as a Shaker room, his colors as somber as a Shaker's dress, and his meaning as simple and as gifting as a Shaker hymn. A Wyeth is constructed to last.

In *Battleground*, as in all of Wyeth's paintings, the nouns have also proper names and personal histories. The man, for example, is the Wyeth family's longtime friend and neighbor, George Heebner. Mr Heebner, a former chemist, is also a cabinetmaker and has restored the buildings shown midground

> *Wyeth's paintings speak plainly, in words of one syllable that anyone can understand…*

to their pre-Revolutionary state. The house, which witnessed the battle at Chads Ford, is the Wyeths' own. To the right is its mill and race of turbulent Brandywine water. The story goes that the 18th-century owner ground glass as well as wheat into the flour that he supplied to the British army. The long, low building with only its roof visible is a shed, open at the front, and the building on the left is the granary. It was behind the granary, so another story goes, that two Hessian soldiers were killed during the Battle of the Brandywine. Beyond the building, almost consuming the sky, are the hills overlooking the Brandywine, covered with their winter stubble of trees and brush.

But most arresting, and to some the most significant part of the painting, are the wheel

ruts that are frozen into the ground like the orbits of atoms, or the paths of stars, or the crossings and connections and parallels of human lives. They, together with the placement of the central figure off the geometric center of the painting, create in the viewer a dynamic tension that seeks resolution. The sense of tension is heightened when one realizes that, whereas the wheels both enter and leave at the right of the painting, the man is, in fact, walking in the opposite direction, away from them, out of the painting. Yet there is the sense that he is not so much leaving something as going forward toward something else. Finally, on the mostly tawny canvas, there is the single note of blue, startling and singular as a robin's egg in a cache of straw. The blue is, in a sense, the "loose end" that Wyeth is so fond of, until one realizes that it is the cap alone that connects the man to the buildings he has restored. He is a bridge over two centuries of American history.

Wyeth's worlds are often austere and wintry, places where the skeletons of things may be seen. Yet his worlds are not dead; they only slumber in order to renew themselves. They express the interiority of life, where one may withdraw to regroup one's forces to fight again. *Battleground* is Wyeth's portrait of a man and his milieu. It is a well-ordered and harmonious world; the battlefield is peaceful, the buildings are solid, the houses are lasting, and the rivers and hills have been there from the beginning. It is a world of hope where trees will leaf, rivers will thaw, and robins will be heard again.

Andrew Wyeth (1917-   ), *Battleground*, 1981, American. Tempera on panel. 125.7 × 115.9 cm. Courtesy of the Nelson-Atkins Museum of Art, Kansas City, Missouri; gift of Enid and Crosby Kemper Foundation in memory of Jerome H. Scott, Jr.

JAMA

The Journal of the American Medical Association

November 6, 1987

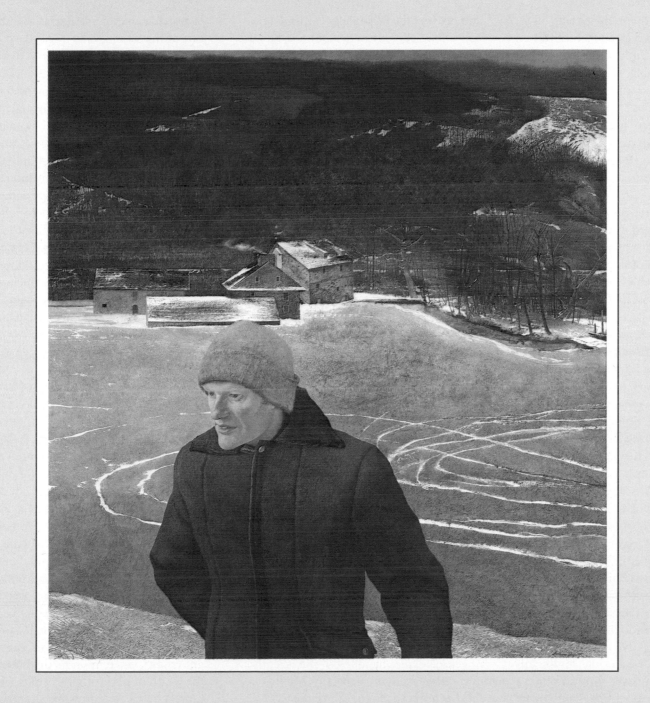

FRA ANGELICO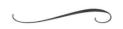

The Healing of Palladia by Saint Cosmas and Saint Damian

Enriched by trade with the Orient, an active export market, and a business acumen worthy of a 20th-century stockbroker, the city-republic of Florence entered the 15th century like a queen arrayed in gold of Ophir. Cosimo, "the Elder," and Lorenzo, "the Magnificent," were her consorts. Her sons would be princes over all the earth and would make her name forever remembered. From them would come a renovation of Western civilization, called *rinascimento* by the Florentines and known as the Renaissance by the rest of the world. It was a time of rediscovery of the ancient and the invention of the new, and no area would be untouched. Sons of Florence established dynasties in language, literature, art, philosophy, commerce, banking, and preaching and also in such things as politics, intrigue, murder, and monopolies. It was for others to discover the world. Florentines had discovered themselves and they were, in short, full of themselves. A Florentine nobleman may have had to be wary of his relatives, but he could well cast an arrogant eye over the rest of mankind.

Sometime around the beginning of the 15th century, probably between 1400 and 1402, in the hills of Tuscany just outside Florence, a boy was born, Guido, son of the farmer Pietro. Probably sometime between 1417 and 1423, when he was in his late teens or early 20s, Guido joined the strict and austere Observantine branch of the Dominican Order of Friars Preachers in nearby Fiesole, taking the name Fra Giovanni. He also vowed himself to lifelong observance of poverty, chastity, and obedience and received holy orders. Meanwhile, his life followed the general monastic formula of *ora et labora*, which, in the case of the Dominicans, meant prayer, meditation, reading, performing works of mercy, and preaching against heresy. For Fra Giovanni, however, *ora et labora* had but a single rubric: the painting of pictures that would praise God

and instruct the faithful. By the time Fra Giovanni died, only in his mid-50s, he was known as the "finest master in the art of painting in Italy." In a poem written by a fellow Dominican, he was referred to as "John the angelic painter…no less in repute than Giotto or Cimabue." Today, we know him as simply Fra Angelico (1387-1455). It is enough.

One of the major developments in Angelico's artistic life came when he was in his late 30s and early 40s. The Fiesole Dominicans moved from the Tuscany countryside to Florence, where they took

> "…figures more delicate or more judiciously arranged can hardly be conceived."

over the decaying buildings of the monastery of San Marco. Aided by contributions from Cosimo, the structures were redesigned and rebuilt, and paintings for the church and convent, their public areas as well as the monks' cells, were requested from Fra Angelico and his assistants. Best known of these is the larger than life-size panel for the high altar. Here, in a painting rich in color and in symbols, the Madonna sits with the Child before a gold-brocaded curtain. On either side of the throne are four standing angels, while fanning out to left and right are six standing saints. Kneeling on an ornate Turkish carpet, which serves to demonstrate Angelico's expert handling of the recently introduced rules of perspective, are two third-century Christian saints, the twin brothers Cosmas and Damian. Surrounding the altar was a series of eight or nine smaller paintings, collectively called the *predella*. Small (each *predelle* was about 30 cm high and 45 cm wide), the *predella* was intended

to provide an edifying narrative of the life of one of the saints of the large altarpiece. For his *predella*, Fra Angelico chose to illustrate the lives of Cosmas and Damian, important in Florence because they were the patrons of the Medici and were renowned for their works of mercy. Both physicians (and patrons of physicians), their lives were a mother lode of legend for the painter. Not only did they perform miraculous cures, including the first limb transplantation, but they withstood various attempts by the emperor Diocletian to murder them, events lending themselves to a dramatic and colorful presentation. Less dramatic, but not less miraculous perhaps, the brothers took no fees for their services.

The Healing of Palladia by Saint Cosmas and Saint Damian is one of the panels, now in Washington, DC, of the *predella* of the San Marco altarpiece. Here, in an arrangement similar to the frames of a modern comic strip, we have the story of Palladia and the physicians as it was told in the *Golden Legend*, a book of Christian devotion published in the 13th century. Palladia, a wealthy woman, had gone to numerous physicians in search of a cure for a mysterious illness. Not only was she not cured, but soon she had used up almost all her wealth. At last she found the brothers Cosmas and Damian, who visited her and gave her a potion that cured her (left). Grateful for the return of her health, she offered a gift to Damian, who, according to his promise to take no fees, refused it. Palladia, however, became angry, and Damian was finally forced to accept her gift (right), whereupon he then incurred the wrath of his brother Cosmas. Cosmas, however, had a vision while sleeping and was directed to forgive his brother, which he did. (One may be quite certain that it is Damian who is shown accepting the gift when one recalls that the *predella* was commissioned by Cosimo.)

196

Continued on p. 215

JAMA®

The Journal of the American Medical Association

November 20, 1987

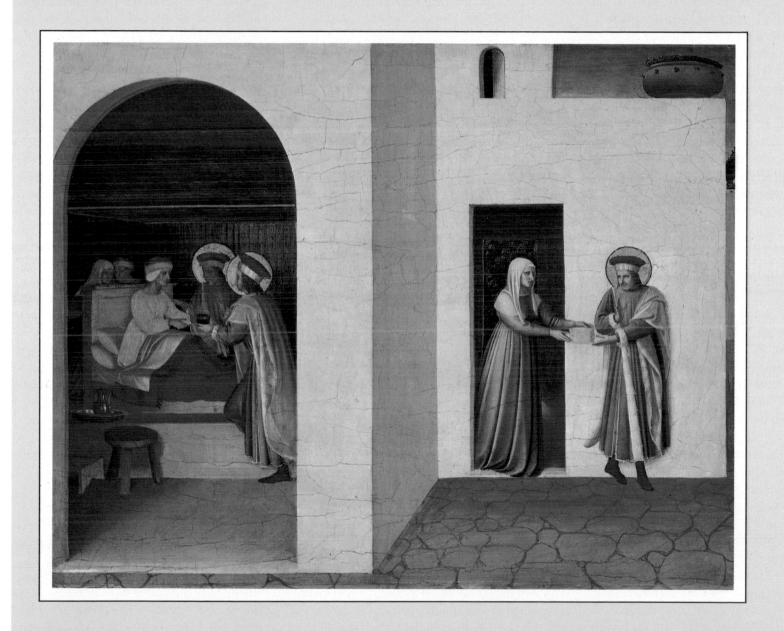

EDVARD MUNCH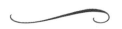

The Sick Child

Two hundred years ago, in Europe, no disease was as common or as feared as pulmonary tuberculosis. Its causative agent and mode of transmission were unknown and treatment was deemed hopeless. Based on the observation that "consumption" often killed several members of the same family, usually in childhood or young adulthood, it was widely believed that heredity, in the form of "weak lungs," played a major role. Moreover, the disease seemed to have a predilection not only for the young but for the gifted—for the youthful genius, the poet, the beautiful maiden. Although by mid-century the epidemic slowly began to abate, the first hard evidence that the disease was less a mystery to be suffered and more a problem to be solved came only in 1882. Robert Koch, a German physician and bacteriologist, demonstrated that a bacillus present in tubercular lesions produced the same disease when transferred to animals. For this, Koch would be awarded the Nobel Prize in Medicine and Physiology in 1905.

Meanwhile, in Norway, where, in 1880, the annual mortality from tuberculosis still stood at 300 per 100,000 population, the 17-year-old Edvard Munch (1863-1944), who was destined to become Norway's greatest painter, entered the School of Design in Kristiania (now Oslo) to begin his studies. The son of a physician, he was the second of five children and scion of a greatly respected Norwegian family, well known in intellectual circles. But this gave small solace to Munch. Throughout his life, he would remember his childhood as an unrelieved horror of sickness and for the loss of everyone on whom he had come to depend. He recalled how, at age 5, at Christmas, he had stood with his 6-year-old sister Sophie and his younger siblings at the bedside of their mother while Sophie sang "Silent Night" and the mother kissed each child in turn. Shortly thereafter, the children learned that their mother was dead, of consumption.

Throughout his boyhood, Munch was himself often ill and feverish, but as he entered his teens it was his closest friend and companion, his sister Sophie, who took to the sofa and the blankets and the pillows. In 1877, when she was 15 and Munch 14, Sophie succumbed to the mysterious tuberculosis. Her death left an imprint on Munch that he was able to bear only by eventually transforming the experience into art. This seminal painting became *The Sick Child*, which Munch completed in 1886, when he was only 23. Successive versions of the same painting would appear throughout his life at

> *...but her body is as light, as transparent, and as fragile as the dust that is left when a butterfly dies.*

roughly ten-year intervals, so that Sophie's death runs through Munch's life like the leitmotif of a grand opera. He was well into his 60s when he completed his last version.

The year Munch began his first version of *The Sick Child*, 1885, he had spent a brief period in Paris, where he was greatly taken with the work of van Gogh. And, like his Dutch contemporary, Munch yearned to create a masterpiece, one that would convey not just a likeness of the subject, but an entirely new art that would put emotion and mood on the canvas in the form of the colors and shapes he would choose. "Perhaps some other painter can depict chamber pots under a bed better than I can," Munch said. "But put a sensitive, suffering young girl into the bed, a girl consumptively beautiful with a blue-white skin turning yellow in the blue shadow—and her hands! Can't you imagine them? Yes, that would be a real accomplishment, painting such hands, showing how

tired they are as they rest on the blanket, fiddle with the sheet, and fold back the blanket seam. It's a white blanket: can't you see it? Some day, I shall paint just such a picture. And then imagine light breaking into the room with spots of sun on the dark walls. Oh, that will be so remarkably beautiful—so simple and peaceful."

The motif of *The Sick Child*—illness, invalidism, death—was rather common in paintings of Munch's time. Some artists romanticized the theme, others became melodramatic (as, for example, did Munch's teacher and colleague, Christian Krohg, when he placed a fading rose in his dying sister's hand). For Munch, however, such an overpowering theme as death and dying had to be stated not only simply, with strong shapes and somber colors, but honestly, as he himself had actually felt it in boyhood. He had to paint not only the familiar, mundane colors and shapes of illness, such as the water glass, the spoon, the medicine bottle, the pillow, and the heavy coverlet, but also the less-defined shapes and more muted colors of isolation, loneliness, helplessness, anger—even guilt.

For Munch, his honesty lay precisely in simplicity. He painted only two figures, a woman and a girl. The woman is old and drab and bowed and her body is as heavy as grief itself, pushing down, like a rock. The girl is young and vibrant and on fire with life, but her body is as light, as transparent, and as fragile as the dust that is left when a butterfly dies. Moreover, each of the women is isolated in her own world and time, separate from the other, and would remain so imprisoned, except that Munch then takes their hands and places them in the very center of the canvas where they reach out to join each other. Munch's people have become, as he would later say (in an uncanny echo of van Gogh's words to his brother), "living people, who breathe and feel and suffer and love. People [will] understand the holy quality about them and bare their heads before them as if in church.

Continued on p. 216

JAMA®

December 11, 1987

The Journal of the American Medical Association

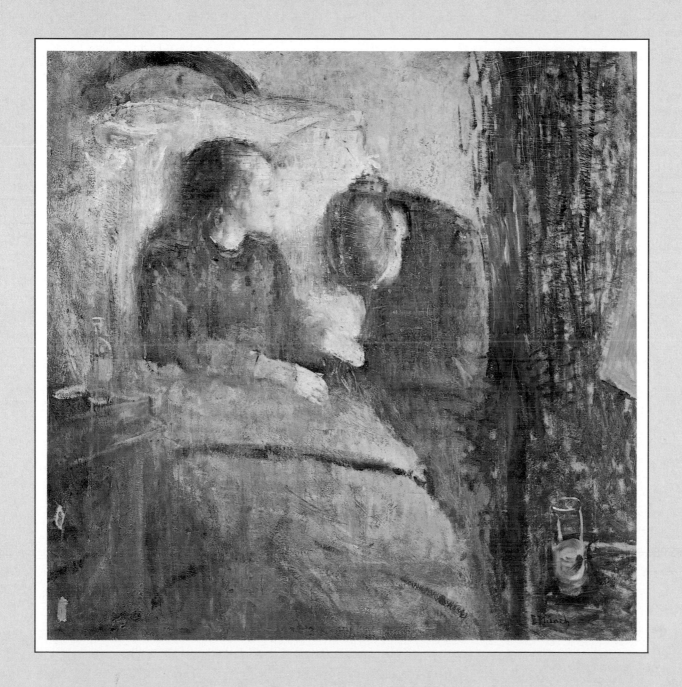

BIBLIOGRAPHY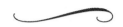

Arnheim R: *The power of the center: a study of composition in the visual arts,* Berkeley, Calif, 1982, University of California Press.

Baigell M: *A concise history of American painting and sculpture,* New York, 1984, Harper & Row.

Baigell M: *Dictionary of American art,* New York, 1982, Harper & Row.

Baudelaire C: *Art in Paris, 1845-1862: salons and other exhibitions reviewed by Charles Baudelaire,* ed 2, Oxford, England, 1981, Phaidon Press (Translated by Mayne J).

Berenson B: *The Italian painters of the Renaissance,* Ithaca, NY, 1980, Cornell University Press.

Berger J: *The success and failure of Picasso,* New York, 1980, Pantheon Books.

Boyle RJ: *American impressionism,* Boston, 1974, New York Graphic Society.

Brettell RR, McCullagh SF: *Degas in The Art Institute of Chicago,* New York, 1984, Harry N Abrams.

Broude N, ed: *Seurat in perspective,* Englewood Cliffs, NJ, 1978, Prentice-Hall.

Cachin F, Moffett CS, Bareau JW: *Manet 1832-1883,* exhibition catalogue, New York, 1983, Harry N Abrams.

Canaday J: *Late Gothic to High Renaissance painters: an authoritative survey of the great Western painters from Giotto through Jan Brueghel,* New York, 1972, WW Norton.

Canaday J: *Baroque painters: an authoritative survey of the great Western painters from Caravaggio through Goya,* New York, 1972, WW Norton.

Canaday J: *Neoclassic to post-impressionist painters: an authoritative survey of the great Western painters from John Trumbull through Cézanne,* New York, 1972, WW Norton.

Canaday J: *The lives of the painters, IV: plates and index,* New York, 1969, WW Norton.

Carey J: *The horse's mouth,* New York, 1965, Harper & Row.

Clark K: *Civilisation: a personal view,* New York, 1969, Harper & Row.

Clark K: *Landscape into art,* New York, 1979, Harper & Row.

Clark K: *The nude: a study in ideal form,* AW Mellon Lectures in the Fine Arts, National Gallery of Art, Washington, DC: 2; Bollingen Series XXXV:2, Garden City, NY, 1956, Doubleday Anchor Books.

Cohen JM, Cohen MJ: *The Penguin dictionary of quotations,* 1976, Penguin Books.

Corn WM: *The art of Andrew Wyeth,* San Francisco, 1973, The Fine Arts Museums of San Francisco.

de Beauvoir S: *The second sex,* New York, 1970, Bantam Books (Translated by Parshley HM).

Delacroix E; Wellington H, ed: *The journal of Eugène Delacroix,* Ithaca, NY, 1980, Cornell University Press (Translated by Norton L).

Doesschate Chu PT, ed: *Courbet in perspective,* Englewood Cliffs, NJ, 1977, Prentice-Hall.

Edgerton SY Jr: *The Renaissance rediscovery of linear perspective,* New York, 1976, Harper & Row.

Eggum A: *Edvard Munch: paintings, sketches, and studies,* New York, 1984, Clarkson N Potter (Translated by Christophersen R).

Eitner L: *Neoclassicism and romanticism, 1750-1850: sources and documents, I, enlightenment/revolution,* Englewood Cliffs, NJ, 1970, Prentice-Hall.

Eitner L: *Neoclassicism and romanticism, 1750-1850: sources and documents, II, restoration/twilight of humanism,* Englewood Cliffs, NJ, 1970, Prentice-Hall.

Eliot TS: *Four quartets,* London, 1949, Faber and Faber.

Enggass R, Brown J: *Italy and Spain, 1600-1750: sources and documents,* Englewood Cliffs, NJ, 1970, Prentice-Hall.

Ferguson G: *Signs & symbols in Christian art,* London, 1982, Oxford University Press.

Fifield W: *Modigliani,* New York, 1976, William Morrow.

Freedberg SJ: *Painting in Italy: 1500-1600,* ed 2, Penguin Books.

Fromentin E; Gerson H, ed: *The masters of past time: Dutch and Flemish painting from Van Eyck to Rembrandt,* Ithaca, NY, 1981, Cornell University Press.

Fry R, *Cézanne,* a study of his development, London, 1927, L & V Woolfe.

Gardner H; de la Croix H, Tansey RG, eds: *Gardner's art through the ages,* ed 6, New York, 1975, Harcourt Brace Jovanovich.

Gedo MM: *Picasso: art as autobiography,* Chicago, 1980, The University of Chicago Press.

Gedo JE: *Portraits of the artist: psychoanalysis of creativity and its vicissitudes,* New York, 1983, The Guilford Press.

Gerdts WH: *American impressionism,* Seattle, 1980, The Henry Art Gallery; University of Washington.

Gerdts WH: *The art of healing: medicine and science in American art,* Birmingham, Ala, 1981, The Birmingham Museum of Art.

Gilbert CE: *Italian art, 1400-1500: sources and documents,* Englewood Cliffs, NJ, 1980, Prentice-Hall.

Goldwater R, Treves M, eds: *Artists on art: from the XIV to the XX century,* 1972, New York, Pantheon Books.

Gombrich EH: *Art and illusion: a study in the psychology of pictorial representation,* AW Mellon Lectures in the Fine Arts, National Gallery of Art, Washington, DC: 5, Bollingen Series XXXV:5, Princeton, NJ, 1972, Princeton University Press.

Goodrich L: *Thomas Eakins,* 2 vols, Cambridge, Mass, 1982, Harvard University Press.

Gordon R, Forge A: *The last flowers of Manet,* New York, 1986, Harry N Abrams (Translated by Howard R).

Grun B: *The timetables of history: a horizontal linkage of people and events. Based on Werner Stein's Kulturfahrplan,* New York, 1975, Simon and Schuster.

Hall J: *Dictionary of subjects & symbols in art,* ed 2, New York, 1979, Harper & Row.

Hamilton GH: *Painting and sculpture in Europe: 1880-1940,* ed 3, 1984, Penguin Books.

Harris AS, Nochlin L: *Women artists: 1550-1950,* exhibition catalogue, New York, 1981, Alfred A Knopf.

Hauser A: *The social history of art, I: Prehistoric, Ancient-Oriental, Greece and Rome, Middle Ages; II: Renaissance, Mannerism, Baroque; III: Rococo, Classicism, Romanticism; IV: Naturalism, Impressionism, the Film Age,* New York, 1951, Vintage Books (Translated by Godman S).

Henri R: *The art spirit,* Philadelphia, 1960, JB Lippincott.

Hilton T: *Picasso,* New York, 1975, Oxford University Press.

Hodin JP: *Edvard Munch,* New York, 1972, Oxford University Press.

Holt EG, ed: *A documentary history of art, III: from the classicists to the impressionists: art and architecture in the 19th century,* Garden City, NY, 1966, Anchor Books.

Holt EG, ed: *A documentary history of art, II: Michelangelo and the mannerists; the baroque and the eighteenth century,* Garden City, NY, 1958, Doubleday Anchor Books.

Holt EG, ed: *A documentary history of art, I: the Middle Ages and the Renaissance,* Garden City, NY, 1957, Doubleday Anchor Books.

Hoopes DF: *The American impressionists,* New York, 1977, Watson-Guptill.

Horne HP: *Botticelli: painter of Florence,* Princeton, NJ, 1980, Princeton University Press.

Hughes R: *The shock of the new,* New York, 1982, Alfred A Knopf.

Hulsker J: *The complete van Gogh: paintings, drawings, sketches,* New York, 1980, Harry N Abrams.

Janson HW, Janson DJ: *History of art: a survey of the major visual arts from the dawn of history to the present day,* ed 2, New York, 1980, Harry N Abrams.

Jung CG et al: *Man and his symbols,* Garden City, NY, 1983, Doubleday.

Kahr MM: *Dutch painting in the seventeenth century,* New York, 1982, Harper & Row.

Kandinsky W: *Concerning the spiritual in art,* New York, 1977, Dover (Translated by Sadler MTH).

Kinder H, Hilgemann W: *The Anchor atlas of world history, I: from the Stone Age to the eve of the French Revolution,* Garden City, NY, 1974, Anchor Press/Doubleday (Translated by Menze EA).

Kinder H, Hilgemann W: *The Anchor atlas of world history, II: from the French Revolution to the American bicentennial.* Garden City, NY, 1978, Anchor Press/Doubleday (Translated by Menze EA).

Letheve J: *Daily life of French artists in the nineteenth century,* New York, 1972, Praeger (Translated by Paddon HE).

Larousse dictionary of painters, New York, 1981, Larousse.

Levey M: *A concise history of painting: from Giotto to Cézanne,* New York, 1968, Oxford University Press.

Levey M: *A history of Western art,* New York, 1968, Oxford University Press.

Loran E: *Cézanne's composition: analysis of his form with diagrams and photographs of his motifs,* ed 3, Berkeley, Calif, 1963, University of California Press.

McCoubrey JW: *American art, 1700-1960: sources and documents,* Englewood Cliffs, NJ, 1965, Prentice-Hall.

McNamara W: *The art of being human,* Garden City, NY, 1967, Echo Books.

Mann C: *Modigliani,* New York, 1980, Oxford University Press.

Maritain J: *Creative intuition in art and poetry,* AW Mellon Lectures in the Fine Arts, National Gallery of Art, Washington, DC:1, Bollingen Series XXXV:1, Princeton, NJ, 1977, Princeton University Press.

Maxon J: *The Art Institute of Chicago,* New York, 1970, Harry N Abrams.

Murray P, Murray L: *A dictionary of art and artists,* ed 4, 1977, Penguin Books.

Newman JH. *The idea of a university: defined and illustrated,* Westminster, Md, 1973, Christian Classics.

Nochlin L: *Impressionism and post-impressionism, 1874-1904: sources and documents,* Englewood Cliffs, NJ, 1966, Prentice-Hall.

Nochlin L: *Realism,* 1978, Penguin Books.

Nochlin L: *Realism and tradition in art, 1848-1900: sources and documents,* Englewood Cliffs, NJ, 1966, Prentice-Hall.

Panofsky E: *Early Netherlandish painting: its origins and character; I, text; II, plates,* Charles Eliot Norton Lectures: 1947-1948, New York, 1971, Harper & Row.

Panofsky E: *The life and art of Albrecht Dürer,* ed 4, Princeton, NJ, 1971, Princeton University Press.

Pater WH: *The Renaissance: studies in art and poetry,* Chicago, 1977, Academy Press.

Penrose R: *Picasso: his life and work,* ed 3, Berkeley, Calif, 1981, University of California Press.

Pool P: *Impressionism,* New York, 1967, Oxford University Press.

Read H: *A concise history of modern painting,* ed 2, New York, 1974, Oxford University Press.

Rewald J: *The history of impressionism,* ed 4, New York, 1973, The Museum of Modern Art.

Rewald J: *Post-impressionism: from van Gogh to Gauguin,* ed 3, New York, 1978, The Museum of Modern Art.

Richardson EP: *A short history of painting in America: the story of 450 years,* New York, 1963, Thomas Y Crowell.

Rosenblum R, Janson HW: *19th-century art,* New York, 1984, Harry N Abrams.

Ruskin A, adaptor: *17th & 18th century art,* New York, nd, McGraw-Hill.

Ruskin J; Evans J, ed: *The lamp of beauty: writings on art by John Ruskin,* Ithaca, NY, 1980, Cornell University Press.

Schiff G, ed: *Picasso in perspective,* Englewood Cliffs, NJ, 1976, Prentice-Hall.

Schneider L, ed: *Giotto in perspective,* Englewood Cliffs, NJ, 1974, Prentice-Hall.

Shikes RE, Harper P: *Pissarro: his life and work,* New York, 1980, Horizon Press.

Soyer R: *Diary of an artist,* Washington, DC, 1977, New Republic Books.

Stein G: *The autobiography of Alice B Toklas,* New York, nd, Vintage Books.

van Gogh V: *The complete letters of Vincent van Gogh: with reproductions of all the drawings in the correspondence,* 3 vols, ed 2, 1978, Boston, New York Graphic Society.

Varnedoe K: *Northern light: realism and symbolism in Scandinavian painting, 1880-1910,* ed 2, Brooklyn, NY, 1982, The Brooklyn Museum.

Vasari G: *The lives of the artists,* 1965, Penguin Books (Translated and edited by Bull G).

Venturi L: *History of art criticism,* rev ed, New York, 1964, EP Dutton (Translated by Marriott C).

Vlaminck M: *Dangerous corner,* London, 1961, Elek Books (Translated by Roth M).

Vollard A: *Cézanne,* New York, 1984, Dover (Translated by Van Doren HL).

Vollard A: *Degas: an intimate portrait,* New York, 1986, Dover (Translated by Weaver RT).

Weil S: *Waiting for God,* New York, 1973, Harper & Row (Translated by Craufurd E).

White BE, ed: *Impressionism in perspective,* Englewood Cliffs, NJ, 1978, Prentice-Hall.

Williams WC: *Autobiography of William Carlos Williams,* New York, 1967, New Directions.

Wilmerding J et al: *American light: the luminist movement, 1850-1875,* exhibition catalogue, Washington, DC, 1980, National Gallery of Art.

Wise S, ed: European portraits, 1600-1900. In *The Art Institute of Chicago,* exhibition catalogue, Chicago, 1978, The Art Institute of Chicago.

Wittkower R, Wittkower M: *Born under Saturn: the character and conduct of artists: a documented history from antiquity to the French Revolution,* New York, 1969, WW Norton.

Wölfflin H: *Principles of art history: the problem of the development of style in later art,* New York, 1950, Dover (Translated by Hottinger MD).

continued from p. 60

FREDERICK LEIGHTON

Leighton went on to become a baronet, Sir Frederick, in 1866, President of the Royal Academy, as predicted, in 1878, and a baron, Lord Leighton of Stretton, in 1896, on the day before he died. Although he awakened at 5 o'clock one morning in excruciating pain from what was apparently a myocardial infarction, he sat on the edge of the bed until 7 o'clock before summoning his valet; like Newman's gentleman, he did not wish to cause any disturbance. Leighton died two days later after receiving chloroform to ease the pain. He is buried in St Paul's, London, one of the last of the Victorians.

Frederick Leighton (1830-1896), *Miss May Sartoris*, c 1860, English. Oil on canvas. 152.1 × 90.2 cm. Courtesy of the Kimbell Art Museum, Fort Worth, Texas.

continued from p. 62

ROBERT HENRI

or the physician, such as Henri's brother, or even the artist and teacher, Henri himself. To be successful, all must be keen observers and sensitive and intuitive students of the human personality. Above all, each must have the unshakeable belief that behind the facade of every human person always lies a surprise. It is their task—whether physician, gambler, or artist—to discover that unique quality.

Robert Henri (1865-1929), *Snow in New York*, 1902, American. Oil on canvas. 81.3 × 65.5 cm. Courtesy of the National Gallery of Art, Washington, DC; Chester Dale Collection, 1954. © 1995 The Board of Trustees of the National Gallery of Art.

continued from p. 66

EDVARD MUNCH

bring not only spiritual death, despair, to the man but physical death to herself in the act of giving birth. Finally, the third woman is the resigned woman, the woman who has suffered, has known pain, and has become wise. It is tempting to relate Munch's women to the eternal feminine of the Norse legends—Sieglinda, Fricka/Brynhilde, Erda—as did Wagner in his Ring Cycle, for example. These legends were, after all, the stuff of Munch's own Norwegian soul. His uncle was the distinguished historian Peter Andreas Munch, author of a most popular compilation of Nordic legends.

As firmly as Munch is identified with Symbolism, however, in color as well as theme, it was line that he considered most important. Here again, the very spareness of the line gives it its eloquence. Take away the voluptuous color and there remains an ascetic structure of bold horizontals (the garden wall) and determined diagonals (the bridge railings), as well as lesser supporting diagonals (the right slopes of the roofs, the hems of the dresses), all converging at the right edge of the painting just opposite the top of the wall.

Munch once said to a friend: "It is no fun to grow old, neither is it to die. We have really no great choice." Munch died on the afternoon of January 23, 1944, at the age of 80. He was, indirectly at least, a casualty of the war. On December 19, 1943, saboteurs had blown up the Filipstad Quay in Oslo, and the windows at Ekely, Munch's home in the suburbs, were blown in. He walked about restlessly in his garden and caught cold, which aggravated a lung ailment. He died six weeks later, but not before he had completed one last painting, a self-portrait depicting himself walking in the winter of his garden. The painting is entitled *Explosion in the Neighborhood*, 1944.

Edvard Munch (1863-1944), *Girls on the Jetty*, 1904, Norwegian. Oil on canvas. 80.5 × 69.3 cm. Courtesy of the Kimbell Art Museum, Fort Worth, Texas.

continued from p. 68

FRANK WESTON BENSON

Benson portrait to those in the Whistler work is almost too striking to mention.

But now the "personal" artist takes over again; this time it is the sitter who lends her reality to this intimate and mysterious moment between two people that Benson has been able to catch and to fasten to a piece of canvas. For example, the casual hairdo is somehow not in keeping with the elegance of the gown. Again, one is struck by the surprisingly large ears in one who is otherwise so delicate looking. But most distressing is the red nose, an incongruous detail, for if the sitter had forgotten to remedy it with a dusting of powder, surely the artist could have brushed it out with oils. Yet these are the very details that establish a time, a place, an identity, and an action for the sitter. Is it difficult to imagine, for example, that just beyond our view there sit garden shears, gloves, a basket of freshly cut flowers, and a large-brimmed hat hastily removed just moments earlier (though with brim not quite large enough to have kept the June sun from the tip of her nose)? The impression of delicacy and even fragility remains, but it covers a core of Yankee steel.

Writing in 1908, Minna Smith called *Portrait in White* a "first-rank work. Here is an ancestress," she said, "for some Salem-descended person of the future to hang on the wall of some Pacific palace of the twenty-first century, and say with just pride, 'Such was a gentlewoman of the olden day and such was the fashion of painting her grace and firmness, her delicacy and strength of character, her dependableness and alert vivacity of mind and figure, and, too, her intuitive big eyes and her diaphanous, billowing gown.'" Smith may have been a good critic, but fortunately for us, her prophetic gifts were somewhat less. Perhaps other portraits of Mrs. Benson do hang in a "Pacific palace," but for the moment this one is for all to share, the more important because it is no longer only a portrait of a New England artist's wife by her 19th-century Impressionist husband; it has become in itself a portrait of a time of innocence we can now experience in no other way.

Frank Weston Benson (1862-1951), *Portrait in White*, 1889, American. Oil on canvas. 122.2 × 97 cm. Courtesy of the National Gallery of Art, Washington, DC; gift of Sylvia Benson Lawson, 1977. © 1995 The Board of Trustees of the National Gallery of Art.

continued from p. 74

FREDERICK CARL FRIESEKE

Impressionists. Frieseke uses the device to demonstrate his virtuosity with color. The brilliant parasol expands like a cadenza into circles of cadmiums—reds, oranges, and yellows—broken only by pauses of mauve and brief accents of blue. Overall, the viewer sees little but color, the shapes dissolving into the light. It is as though the sun has been shattered into a million shards and that its pieces have come to earth as flowers or hats or garden walls, or the molten residue of a yellow lawn.

For all his scathing references to Impressionism as so much confectionery, Joyce Cary's Gully Jimson should have the last word; he came closer than he knew to the soul of painting when he called it "a sort of colored music in the mind." He also understood the creative soul: it is always starting with a clean canvas, he said, not forgiving the past, but forgetting the past. "Because it's true," he said, "It's a new world with every heart beat. The sun rises seventy-five times a minute."

---

continued from p. 76

CLAUDE MONET

But new battles were shaping for Monet, and, as befitted the size of his obsession, they were to be cosmic battles. The contest was between him and the sun; his work was always at the mercy of its daily circuit. Moreover, as each summer passed its solstice, Monet's spirits, too, began their descent. In 1890, when he had begun his "series" paintings, he wrote, "...at this time of year [October] the sun goes down so fast that I can't follow it. I've come to move so slowly that I'm in despair." Another time, when he was painting his "poplar series," he wrote that he had exactly seven minutes to work on a leaf before the light was so changed that he had to move on to the next canvas. Indeed, so obsessed with pure color did Monet become, and so desperately did he wish to reach essences, that he confessed he wished almost that he had been born blind; then he could see the world as he wished to see it—not as individual objects, but as patterns of colors only, colors for which there would not even be names. "What does the subject matter!" he said. "One instant, one aspect of nature contains it all." He echoes William Blake, who likewise knew that one can find "...a World in a grain of sand,...a Heaven in a wild flower,...Eternity in an hour."

Mme Hoschedé, whom Monet married in 1891, died in 1911 at Giverny, where they had lived since 1883. Monet lived on at his beloved Giverny until 1926, painting over and over again its Japanese bridge and lily pond formed from the specially diverted Epte branch of the Seine. Poignantly, for one who had such an eye, he died nearly blind, but working to the end. It is true, as Seiberling commented in her essay on these last works: vision is more than a matter of the eye.

---

continued from p. 78

WINSLOW HOMER

the nearest in a long, strong beat, the second in a broken rhythm, dotted strongly from the right by the white sails of the ship. To the left the pattern is repeated, but pianissimo, and in a different key, pale green. The left pattern is also reversed; it is the first breaker whose rhythm is dotted by the left ship. The ships, afterthoughts as they first seem to be, serve other functions as well. Diagonally, their extended lines meet in an exact right angle at the red ribbon on the girl's head; extended at a slightly different slope the lines will meet at the group of boys just to the right of the girl (who are in the exact middle of the painting), once again at a 90-degree angle. Vertically extended, the ships serve as a frame to the main group of children.

Homer was a man with a divided past. His life was a statement with two independent clauses, separated by a trip to Tynemouth, England, at age 43. The two parts stand in contrast to each other as oil to water and yet in complement to each other as male to female. As an artist he matured slowly and unseen, but thoroughly and completely, much as the embryo does. Only when he was 45 did he emerge, full-term, the Homer we most often think of today: the watercolorist, the chronicler of man's struggle with the sea (in a word, the universe), and the recluse of Prout's Neck, Maine.

But it is the early Homer, the Homer of the first clause that we are interested in here.

Perhaps *Beach Scene* is the conjunction that joins the two halves of his art. Perhaps, in these late oils, done just as he was switching to watercolor, as well as to different subjects, children were so often chosen because, in a country still scarred after so recent a war, these little ones, not born until after the war, were the only whole people.

There can be other meanings, too. As he neared 40 and remained unmarried, Homer was to show the first signs of that reclusiveness, even alienation, that was to seclude him eventually at Prout's Neck. Perhaps the Alice figure of *Beach Scene* is a hint of this sense of his no longer belonging, just as the girl is too old for the sunbonnetted girls, too young for the boys, but most important, completely isolated by her own manner. Why, for example, doesn't she have a beach costume? Why doesn't she at least take off her shoes and stockings? Can't she? Or won't she? Yet Homer shows her to be very involved in the group if not by her costume, then at least by the fact that the next wave is going to get her shoes very wet right to the tops. In this sense she echoes Homer in that he did not wish to adopt other painter's methods. He was self-taught, just as he wished. It is also about this time that Homer stopped painting his scenes of women in fashionable dress and turned exclusively to adult masculine subjects. (Homer himself had a reputation as a dapper dresser.) Does *Beach Scene*, with its wistful little girl dressed so stylishly and yet so improperly represent the final, wistful reconciliation of the feminine and masculine in Homer's nature?

No matter. By the time Homer would be embarked on the second half of his career, painting what most call his "typical work," these same children could, ironically, again be his adult models: the boys, the fishermen battling the sea in boats, the sunbonnetted girls among the group of women, and fiancées standing on a hill near the coast guard station counting off the fishing boats as they come in one by one. And Alice? She, too, would be there, apart, T. S. Eliot's Our Lady of the Promontory, perhaps, praying home her husband from the "sea's lips."

And Henry James? In the end he had to admit, "there is nevertheless something one likes about him. What is it?"

Indeed, who asks, or needs to?

continued from p. 82

WALT KUHN

of such "hot" colors. Perhaps he was trying to define planes or to see structure in a casually dumped basket of squash. Perhaps, like Cézanne, he was trying to see nature "in terms of the cylinder, the sphere and the cone." Or perhaps these autumn fruits represent the harvest of his life. No matter what, however, he had again produced his "one fine painting."

Like his powerful acrobats whose tensed muscles just barely conceal explosive action, there is in this apparently still picture the same tension and power. It is, in fact, not a static painting at all, but one in which the fruits have only paused in their tumbling, barred only temporarily from further action by the massive pumpkin in the foreground. A finger-touch more of pressure on the basket will unbalance the structure just enough to dislodge the pumpkin right out of the painting into our laps, followed no doubt by a cascade of squash.

Walt Kuhn held his last show in 1948 in New York. He died the following summer of a perforated ulcer, leaving a legacy to American art of not only the richness of the Armory Show, but his own personal bequest of not one but many fine paintings. When asked one day in the latter part of his life how his work was going, he answered, "I have more or less arrived at the point where I can make my brushes carry out my instructions." A modest assessment, indeed, but who could wish for more?

Walt Kuhn (1877-1949), *Pumpkins*, 1941, American. Canvas. 101.6 × 127.7 cm. Courtesy of the National Gallery of Art, Washington, DC; gift of the Avalon Foundation, 1968. © 1995 The Board of Trustees of the National Gallery of Art.

continued from p. 84

ALFRED SISLEY

continues to rise in a graceful arc until it rests our eye on the solid house on the far right amid the trees. A reprise of triangles, curves, and color can be found in the snow patterns on the ground.

But, like a line of melody, a painting must also move; that is to say, it must compel us to

follow. Whether it be the flicker of a smile about to break across a face in a portrait, or the foam on the waves in a seascape, or the bending of trees in a landscape, the movement must be there. For Sisley the movement was the sky. Sky was not backdrop; it *was* the action. "The sky has planes like the earth," said Sisley "…I insist on this part of the landscape because I should like you to understand fully the importance I attach to it." Look at Sisley's painting long enough—the clouds, the light, the snow on the ground. Soon it becomes evident that his clouds are moving, and even in what direction they head. But again, like music, there is another kind of movement in his painting, less obvious, but there, nevertheless, and that is the movement of time. Whereas music actually measures time as it is passing, Sisley's painting stops and even compresses time: past, present, and even future are seen as a single instant. Monet presents us with an instant of light on a haystack, but it is only that single moment and nothing more. Sisley, on the other hand, also gives us an instant, but within it is an entire day: night, morning, midday, even the approaching evening.

And here is Sisley's deception: Superficially his work may recall a 17th-century Dutch street scene, with all its bewitching architectural intricacy, or a Constable landscape with its solid reassurance, or the fluttery brushstroke and vibrant colors of the Impressionists. He is this, but more. He has removed not an instant *from* time, he has put time *into* an instant. That is to be the true Impressionist. He was, as Roger Fry calls him, no "mere recorder," but "a great imaginative artist."

Alfred Sisley (1839-1899), *Early Snow at Louveciennes*, c 1870, British (worked in France). Oil on canvas. 54.8 × 73.8 cm. Courtesy of the Museum of Fine Arts, Boston, Massachusetts; bequest of John T. Spaulding.

continued from p. 86

ÉDOUARD MANET

ings are among his most appealing in their very artlessness and in the immediacy with which they confront the viewer. They do nothing; they simply are. And true to his engaging manner, Manet made a present of

this still life with the three roses to a mysterious "Mme X" on the occasion of the New Year. It is not known who this Madame X was, nor whether she accepted the gift.

Early in 1883 Manet was finally confined to bed. In April, after much discussion among his physicians, his left leg was amputated because of gangrene. Again, for Manet, it was too late. He died ten days later, on April 30, aged 52 years.

Édouard Manet (1832-1883), *Flowers in a Crystal Vase*, c 1882, French. Oil on canvas. 32.6 × 24.3 cm. Courtesy of the National Gallery of Art, Washington, DC; Ailsa Mellon Bruce Collection, 1970. © 1995 The Board of Trustees of the National Gallery of Art.

continued from p. 88

CAMILLE PISSARRO

of the path. For example, the area to the left of the path is larger and so are the objects. However, the large tree on the left is effectively balanced by the tree on the right near the man because, although smaller, it is more compact and placed farther into the distance. The weight of the left tree is also lessened by the blossoms, which lift it to the sky, and by the diagonal tree adjacent, which pulls it to the right.

The two figures also maintain an equilibrium. The bent back of the woman, which is parallel to the horizon, has a powerful earth pull. She is ballast for the tree, whose blossoms would seem to make it rise like a balloon. The man, meanwhile, being almost vertical, is counterpoise for the form of the woman. He is reiterated in the tree next to him and in the vertical poplar in the far distance so that trees and humans on either side of the path are in perfect balance. This unity of earth and peasant is clinched by tree branches that arch over each figure in the exact contour of each back.

It was to be two years yet before the Impressionists were to hold their famous first independent exhibition and many years before they were to be critically acclaimed or even financially well-off. Nevertheless, the springtime was upon them. The year was at the morn; their world was dew-pearled.

Camille Pissarro (1830-1903), *Orchard in Bloom, Louveciennes*, 1872, French. Oil on canvas. 45.1 ×

continued from p. 90

HENRY BACON

his journalist's instinct was true in selecting the significant event.

As a painter Bacon is not highly regarded today. His composition and drawing are rated highly, but his scenes have a certain artificiality about them that, while they nonetheless charm, lack staying power. At best, they are pleasant; they do not offend. At worst, they lack the personal, the urgent, the something that compels us to respond with more than a nod of general acceptance. Their slickness, vividness, and permanence is that of a Madison Avenue piece. They are "portraits of manners."

Likewise, in composition Bacon is quite correct. The composition is decidedly angular, with the severe lines of the mast, the awning support, the boom, the rail, the slatted benches, the deck boards, and the rigging carefully relieved by the paired half circles of the deck chair and davits and the full circles of quoits, the plate, and the tea biscuit. One cannot fault the natural postures of the bodies, especially those of the two men, one with left leg crossed behind, the other with left leg crossed over. Nor is the exquisite detail lacking: the half-peeled orange in the reclining woman's right hand, the meerschaum in her husband's hand, the ruby on his left fifth finger. Ship's direction is also stated, not only by the woman's blowing veil and engine smoke, but most emphatically by the converging of all the lines and the massing of the weight at a point on the right edge of the canvas. Still, there remains a frozen quality about the painting. The lines and shapes lack a point of tension. It is a constructed painting, with posed people. But there is charm, and most of all, nostalgia.

Bacon died in Cairo in 1912, still the traveler, still the expatriate. The place he considered home is perhaps indicated by the last sentence of the 19-word obituary carried on page 11 of the *New York Times* from March 14: "Boston papers please copy." If the Times had noted his profession (which it did not),

it might have read, "Died yesterday, Cairo, age 75, Henry Bacon, the consummate illustrator, the journalist with an eye."

Henry Bacon (1837-1912), *On Shipboard*, 1877, American. Oil on canvas. 48.9 × 72.3 cm. Courtesy of the Museum of Fine Arts, Boston, Massachusetts; gift of Mrs Edward Livingston Davis.

continued from p. 92

ARTIST UNKNOWN

These represent holes made in the vellum by a kind of spiked wheel, or divider, which the monk would run down the edge to indicate the spacing between lines. This leaf, for example, has 38 lines.

Bede himself, commonly called the "Venerable," was a seventh-century English Benedictine from the Abbey of Jarrow. He was a warm and gentle man, well liked and an excellent and prolific writer on many topics, including history, biography, and grammar; he contributed greatly to the development of the English language. His best known work is probably the *Ecclesiastical History of the English Nation*, completed in 731. He died at Jarrow in 735, after a rapidly worsening "tightness of breath," but not until he had completed his own dictation to a young scribe, Wilbert. Appropriately, the work was a translation into English of the Gospel of St John. At his scribe's persistent urging he completed the work, the final sentence only moments before he died.

Artist unknown, *Saint John Dictating to the Venerable Bede*, c 1140, Austrian. Pen with brown and red ink, with color washes on vellum. 35.2 × 23.5 cm. Courtesy of the National Gallery of Art, Washington, DC; Rosenwald Collection, 1950. © 1995 The Board of Trustees of the National Gallery of Art.

continued from p. 94

MAURICE UTRILLO

and heavy pigment of the palette knife, too, suggest an impatience that could be triggered in a moment into violence. And the painting is brutal in the way it pulls in the viewer's eye and then bounces it from wall to wall, from one side of the street to the other, before it is

allowed to escape over the chimneys and into the sky. On this street there is no repose, only sullen houses, shuttered like Utrillo's soul.

And yet there is more. There is the energy and vigor of a spirit not yet domesticated. There is passion, but it is tethered by the artist's discipline. The tree does resemble those of Pissarro, but instead of being old and arthritic, it sizzles with electricity. Most of the power, however, comes from the fact that, for the duration of the painting, at least, Utrillo unshutters his soul and speaks honestly and directly, like the unguarded remark of a child who has not yet reached the age of circumlocution.

Such is the legend of Utrillo, only a quarter of a century after his death. There remain for facts his thousands of paintings. But even they, like the legend, continue to grow in number; especially for those paintings done in his later years, when he repeated himself from picture postcards, one cannot always separate the authentic Utrillo from the fabricated Utrillo. The strangest part of the story, however, is that whereas the father of Suzanne Valadon's son remains unknown, the father of Utrillo the painter is known: He is the physician who suggested that Suzanne find something to occupy her teenaged alcoholic son's interest—perhaps painting—since he knew her to be something of a painter herself.

Maurice Utrillo (1883-1955), *Rue Cortot, Montmartre*, 1909, French. Oil on cardboard. 45.7 × 33.6 cm. Courtesy of the National Gallery of Art, Washington, DC; Ailsa Mellon Bruce Collection, 1970. © 1995 The Board of Trustees of the National Gallery of Art.

continued from p. 96

SIR WILLIAM BEECHEY

picked up, in shape as well as in color, in the sister's slipper, repeated in her sash, and, finally, echoed in the orange-red in the upper left corner. From here the spectrum returns across the upper sky to end at its blue-violet margin on the right.

The grouping of the figures, while arranged to give unity to a difficult group of four, also bears a closer look. By allying so closely the brother and sister at the left, Beechey in effect changes a foursome into an easier threesome grouping. He then allots each child its own inviolable picture space, so that it would

continued from p. 205

almost be possible to cut the canvas apart and give each child a finished portrait: the boy-girl, a three-quarter length in the circular frame previously mentioned, the baby, her portrait in an equilateral triangle, which has its apex at the midpoint of the large portrait, and the oldest girl, a full-length in a rectangular frame bounded by the right edge of the canvas and left border of her skirt.

Although generally praising him, contemporary critics faulted Beechey on several counts, noting that his portraits lacked grace and his males power and that his draperies were flimsy. And while *The Oddie Children* does suggest some of this artificiality, it is immediately forgotten in the exquisite coloring, in the skillful composition, but most of all, in the ageless charm that is a child's by birthright and that Beechey has somehow allowed the children to retain. The Oddie children, growing up at the tag end of the 18th century, have long since grown old and died. As for Beechey's children, they have not changed much in 200 years. We could run into one or another of them tomorrow—or perhaps we have one of them with us right now.

Sir William Beechey (1753-1839), *The Oddie Children*, 1789, British. Oil on canvas. 183 × 182.5 cm. Courtesy of the North Carolina Museum of Art, Raleigh; purchased with funds from the state of North Carolina.

---

continued from p. 98

PIERRE AUGUSTE RENOIR

Structurally the composition is built on two strong lines, a horizontal that follows the bottom of the picture frame and lip of the vase and a vertical that drops down from the ribbon supporting the picture on the wall to intersect it and to mark Renoir's painting in thirds. The wide range of textures is also striking: the satiny table scarf, the rough leather book bindings, flower petals, paper, bamboo, feathers, porcelain, wood, metal, and ribbon. And finally, there are the shapes: ovals, circles, rectangles, curves, straight lines, and arabesques, all increasing the sensuous qualities of the painting. One wonders what Renoir thought of this painting. If he found

it somewhat clumsy, he was probably not dismayed. "God, the King of artists," he said, "was clumsy."

Pierre Auguste Renoir (1841-1919), *Still Life With Bouquet*, 1871, French. Oil on canvas. 73.2 × 58.9 cm. Courtesy of The Museum of Fine Arts, Houston, Texas; Robert Lee Blaffer Memorial Collection, gift of Sarah Campbell Blaffer.

---

continued from p. 104

CHARLES DEMUTH

gray intersecting beams, like theater spotlights, reflecting that Williams was also a playwright; and the "art," the fact that he was a painter as well. Curiously, Demuth does not indicate that this poet-playwright-painter was also a physician, unless he relies on the title of the poem to say it: "The Great Figure."

To the patient observer, the portrait will reveal even more. Depending on how one looks at it, the figure 5 is either receding into the background in tightening circles of sound, like echoes, or it is screaming toward us with increasing intensity until it reaches its ultimate pitch, in a kind of visual Doppler effect. Either way, the painting has sound and rhythm the same as a poem or a fire engine has sound and rhythm. It also has motion. If one includes the arch in the upper right-hand corner as part of the belly of a giant 5, then the 5 becomes the rim of a vortex that rushes in tightening eddies toward its center, sucking the viewer with it into the vacuum of night and the city. Interestingly, Williams had proclaimed his artist's "manifesto" in an essay entitled "Vortex," with which Demuth may well have been familiar.

Demuth's poster portraits of the 1920s are often said to have culminated in the pop art of the 1960s—the sterile rows of Campbell's soup cans, Marilyn Monroes, and the arid LOVE motifs. On the other hand, Demuth's *Figure 5* could just as well have come from some monastery of the Middle Ages, where it would have been an illuminated number in a medieval manuscript, except that the curlicues of nature's vines and flowers have been unbent into the lines and circles of the city's light and noise. Demuth himself, however, would not have liked such description. Words cannot explain a painting—it is only the eyes that can understand, he said. "They [paintings] are the final, the *nth*

whoopee of sight…'Look at that!' is all that can be said."

In October 1935, Demuth died suddenly after returning from one of his trips to New York City. The cause of death was never certain—whether as the result of diabetic coma or of insulin shock or even influenza was never determined—but Williams noted that Demuth always was careless about his insulin. His mother, "Augusta the iron-clad" as Demuth was fond of calling her, a widow since 1911 and now childless as well, lived on in the family home for another eight years. When she died unexpectedly in 1943, it was discovered that she had kept everything just as she had always kept it for Charles, even to his rubbers on the floor. In fact, there was even the tray for his insulin syringe with its fresh towel, changed each week, just as she had arranged it during his life.

Charles Demuth (1883-1935), *The Figure 5 in Gold*, 1928, American. Oil on composition board. 91.4 × 75.6 cm. Courtesy of The Metropolitan Museum of Art, New York, New York; Alfred Stieglitz Collection, 1949. © 1979 by The Metropolitan Museum of Art.

---

continued from p. 108

EASTMAN JOHNSON

and surprisingly vigorous, for by the date of the painting, Brown would have been in his late 70s.

Grandfather James epitomized the 19th-century American dream. Less than 70 years earlier, in 1800, his father, Alexander, his mother, and one brother, William, had arrived in Baltimore from Belfast and opened an import business; their capital consisted of some Irish linen, a few chairs, and some eight-day clocks. James, then 11 years old, and his two older brothers, John and George, were left behind in England; they were sent for only two years later. Meanwhile, business prospered, and father Alexander was not only importing linens, but had joined to them the export of cotton and tobacco. Soon the father and his four sons owned a shipping business and had also entered the international banking field in Baltimore as the firm of Alexander Brown and Sons. The eldest son, William, was dispatched to Liverpool, John to Philadelphia, and James to New York City and Boston, all to open branches of the family business. George remained in Baltimore, where he helped found the Baltimore & Ohio passenger railroad and became its first treasurer. Alexander in the meantime had become one of America's first millionaires (at his death less than 35 years after his arrival from Belfast, his estate was put at $2 million).

Few people have lived like the Brown family, and thus Johnson's painting is interesting for its rich, historically accurate background. What it also does, however, in its portrayal of the intimate exchanges among the three people in front of their own hearth, is to make legitimate, at least this once, the universal human urge to peek into other people's living rooms.

Eastman Johnson (1824-1906), *The Brown Family*, 1869, American. Oil on paper mounted on canvas. 59.3 × 72.4 cm. Courtesy of the National Gallery of Art, Washington, DC; gift of David Edward Finley and Margaret Eustis Finley, 1978. © 1995 The Board of Trustees of the National Gallery of Art.

---

continued from p. 110

VINCENT VAN GOGH

growth. *Sad and yet gentle, but clear and intelligent—this is how one ought to paint many portraits.*

To Gauguin he wrote (although the letter was apparently never sent): "Meanwhile I have a portrait of Dr. Gachet with the heart-broken expression of our time."

Portrait of Dr Gachet is one of two paintings van Gogh did of the physician. The other, which hangs in the Louvre, is similar, except that the coat is without buttons and there are no books on the table. Gachet sits, hunched over the table, the weight of his head supported by his clenched hand. The eyes are not focused on anything, unless it be his own inner pain. The facial muscles are slack, the lips slightly parted, as if speaking or not speaking were all the same. Behind him rise blue hills, like great mounds weighing on his blue shoulders, and beyond that is an indefinite sky, a blue that is neither night nor day. In sharp, almost violent contrast, a red and green table with yellow books intrudes at the lower left. Almost dead center is a glass with a sprig of foxglove.

Van Gogh has laid out on the canvas, though in a restrained and even subtle

manner, a description of the curtained world of the melancholic that is more telling than any textbook description. He emphasizes the prison of the depressed by making Gachet, the hills, and the sky all a continuum of blue. The lines are wavy and tentative. In contrast is the vivid, almost painful intrusion of color in the foreground, the lines clear-cut and decisive; this is the "rest of the world" that Gachet has been cut off from. Still, a bit of hope remains, no matter how small. Between the two worlds, the monotonal blue world of the sorrowing Gachet and the brilliant, vivid, clearly defined colorful world of the "others," van Gogh maintains a connection by placing Gachet's open hand on the table. Thus, Gachet is at once hopeless but hopeful, not yet completely isolated. How fundamental was this small symbol of hope is illustrated by the circumstances of van Gogh's suicide a few weeks later, for although it was he who made the decision to shoot himself, he nevertheless left the decision about his dying to someone else.

Finally, there is the matter of the two yellow books on the table. While they may serve simply to reflect the sitter's reading preference, just as the foxglove denotes his profession, and to provide a note of color, they may also be a subtle suggestion of the symbiotic, and eventually tragic, relationship that existed between Vincent and Theo. (Theo was to become insane and die within six months of Vincent's death.) The two books are the novels *Manette Salomon* and *Germinie Lacerteux* by Edmond and Jules de Goncourt, brothers who worked in such close collaboration that they were even able to keep the same diary. Vincent's recurring wish was that he and Theo could work as one, and their long correspondence suggests the diary of the de Goncourt brothers. It is also interesting to recall that when this painting was done, Theo had recently married, and Vincent commented in his letter to his sister Wil that Gachet was something like another brother. In this same connection, yellow is often considered to represent a wish for a new beginning, and while Vincent's recent arrival in Auvers-sur-Oise was another fresh start, it should also be noted that in that same letter to Wil, he referred to Gachet's hands as being the hands of an obstetrician, again, perhaps, a wish for a rebirth.

During the little more than two months van Gogh was to live in Auvers-sur-Oise, he

did 150 drawings, sketches, and oils, many of them his most famous works. He wrote to Wil:

What impassions me most…is the portrait, the modern portrait. I seek it in color, and surely I am not the only one to seek it in the direction. I should like—mind you, far be it from me to say that I shall be able to do it, although this is what I am aiming at—I should like to paint portraits which would appear after a century to the people living then as apparitions. By which I mean that I do not endeavor to achieve this by a photographic resemblance, but by means of our impassioned expressions—that is to say, using our knowledge of and our modern taste for color as a means of arriving at the expression and intensification of the character.

Almost prophetically, he wrote in his next letter: "There are modern heads which people will go on looking at for a long time to come, and which perhaps they will mourn over after a hundred years."

Vincent van Gogh (1853-1890), *Portrait of Dr Gachet*, 1890, Dutch. Oil on canvas. 66 × 57 cm. Courtesy of Christie's, New York, New York; sold May 15, 1990.

---

continued from p. 112

ARSHILE GORKY

Under Aerodynamic Limitations. When the murals were criticized for being "too modern," one critic defended them, saying, "It is dangerous to ride in an old-fashioned airplane. It is inappropriate to wait and buy one's ticket surrounded by old-fashioned murals. One of the great mysteries of modern life is the enthusiasm for streamlined trains, automobiles and airplanes shown by people who at the same time are timid when confronted by equally modern painting." Gorky also did murals for the Aviation Building at the 1939 New York World's Fair and for Ben Marden's Riviera at Fort Lee, New Jersey. All have been lost, with the exception of two of the ten Newark Airport panels just recently located— the victim of remodeling, reallocations of space, and 14 layers of paint. The Aviation Building and the Riviera have been demolished and with them, presumably, the murals.

In 1941 Gorky married for the second time, happily, and by 1945 the couple had two daughters. In 1941 he also organized and

continued from p. 207

taught a course in camouflage for the war effort. Perhaps it is not entirely accidental that he should have done so, for if camouflage is the art of concealment by taking on one's surrounding colors so as to escape injury, then Gorky was a master of it in his own life, constantly adopting poses and shifting facts to suit the occasion. But Gorky could not lay concealed for long. In January 1946 his studio in Connecticut burned, and less than a month later, he had surgery for cancer. Then, in a remarkable recovery, he followed this with two and a half years of his most creative work. "The secret [of creativity]," he wrote to his nephew at this time, "is to throw yourself into the water of life again and again, not to hang back, no reservations, risk everything, but above all strike out boldly with all you have." In a single summer he completed 292 drawings. But, in June 1948, while a passenger in an automobile driven by a friend, Gorky suffered neck injuries and paralysis of his painting arm. He ended his life less than a month later, on July 21, 1948, by hanging. On his easel was left a canvas entitled *Last Painting*.

Gorky's death had the shock of a full stop in a lyrical line of a beautiful melody. He died, not of cancer nor of auto injuries, but as his dealer Levy might have put it, of "unrequited art." The gap between his art and public appreciation of it was simply too great for him to bear.

Arshile Gorky (1905-1948), The Artist and His Mother, c 1926-1936, Armenian. Oil on canvas. 152.3 ¥ 127 cm. Courtesy of the National Gallery of Art, Washington, DC; Ailsa Mellon Bruce Collection, 1979. © 1995 The Board of Trustees of the National Gallery of Art.

continued from p. 116

WILLIAM MCGREGOR PAXTON

the year Paxton made his painting, one could call "as far as Minneapolis, Omaha, Kansas City, and the eastern portion of the Indian Territory." The busiest number in Boston was Haymarket 391, at that time the number of the Massachusetts General Hospital.

William McGregor Paxton (1869-1941), *The Girl at the Telephone*, 1905, American. Oil on canvas. 72.5 ×

49 cm. Courtesy of Galleries Maurice Sternberg, Chicago, Illinois.

continued from p. 118

DAVID TENIERS THE YOUNGER

throughout *Tavern Scene*, but brought to its greatest brilliance in the clothes of the cardplayers. Teniers had another trick up his sleeve as well, and that was the silvery tone he was able to give his colors. Again, it is evident in the almost pewter-like luster or iridescence of *Tavern Scene*, but this beautiful silver tint is also isolated in the smoke in the fireplace in the background and in the lazy spiral that rises from the man's pipe in the foreground.

David Teniers the Younger may be, as some say, only a minor member of the great nobility of Flemish painting, and his genre scenes may have grown trite, but many a minor nobleman can provide pleasant company, and what is now trite can once have been fresh and even novel. One hundred years after Teniers' death, William Blake, for one, could speak of "Rembrandt & Teniers," "Rafael & Michael Angelo" as being equally worthy of study. Yesterday's fashion is perhaps today's triteness—and tomorrow's discovery.

David Teniers the Younger (1610-1690), *Tavern Scene*, 1658, Flemish. Oil on panel. 48.7 × 68.7 cm. Courtesy of the National Gallery of Art, Washington, DC; gift of Robert H. and Clarice Smith, 1975. © 1995 The Board of Trustees of the National Gallery of Art.

continued from p. 120

GERARD TER BORCH

or a clever double entendre? Ter Borch, like the expert teller of a joke, has said everything, but explained nothing. *The Suitor's Visit* remains a jewel of the 17th century, a cameo of elegance and manners.

Gerard Ter Borch (1617-1681), *The Suitor's Visit*, c 1658, Dutch. Oil on canvas. 80 × 75.3 cm. Courtesy of the National Gallery of Art, Washington, DC; Andrew W. Mellon Collection, 1937. © 1995 The Board of Trustees of the National Gallery of Art.

continued from p. 122

JOHN SLOAN

living, living. It makes starving, living. It makes worry, it makes trouble, it makes a life that would be barren of everything—living. It brings life to life."

Sloan died in Hanover, New Hampshire, on September 8, 1951, age 80, ten days after undergoing surgery for cancer.

John Sloan (1871-1951), *The Lafayette*, 1928, American. Oil on canvas. 77.5 × 91.8 cm. Courtesy of The Metropolitan Museum of Art, New York, New York; gift of friends of John Sloan, 1928. © 1980 by The Metropolitan Museum of Art.

continued from p. 124

BERTHE MORISOT

courage to begin it...I drag myself about aimlessly, and I say 20 times a day that I am tired of everything. This is how my life goes. I am ashamed of being so weak-minded, but what can I do?" At the same time, she is looking forward to her visit with Edma in Lorient "to do something worthwhile." In late June, Berthe went to Lorient and that "something worthwhile" was the portrait of Edma at an open window. She was told it was a masterpiece, and it was exhibited at the Salon of 1870, where, however, she found it skied, that is, "hung so high that it is impossible to judge it."

Although the portrait is the occasion of the sisters' reunion, Berthe paints Edma in a heavy, pensive mood. Her body curves to the chair in a state of lassitude, as she absently fingers a fan, unmindful of the brilliant summer day outside and the neighbor women's activity in the windows across the street. And on what does Edma muse? On her marriage? On the child she carries? The career she has relinquished? Berthe has too much of the middle-class breeding to violate her sister's thoughts. She also has too much artistic finesse. Instead, she leaves us with the mystery, to ponder ourselves.

Berthe Morisot's paintings are much like she herself has been described: at once refined and elegant, subtle, reserved, and understated. They would never shout; instead, they whisper. Nor do they ever intrude; rather, they insinuate themselves quietly into our affections. In a crowded gallery they could easily be overlooked, but some mysterious quality draws us back to look again, more closely. Thus disarmed, we willingly succumb to their quiet charm, their subtle design, and exquisite color. She does not paint answers, of course, only questions. That is why, more than a hundred years later, we are still looking at the paintings of Berthe Morisot. They are sacraments of the human spirit.

Berthe Morisot (1841-1895), *The Artist's Sister at a Window*, 1869, French. Canvas. 54.8 × 46.3 cm. Courtesy of the National Gallery of Art, Washington, DC; Ailsa Mellon Bruce Collection, 1970. © 1995 The Board of Trustees of the National Gallery of Art.

continued from p. 126

EDWARD HAYTLEY

But it is not necessary to know the names of the various persons in the painting to appreciate Haytley's conversation piece. It is enough to see the important figure in the foreground to know that this is the Squire and that these are his family, his friends, his park, his Greco-Roman statuary and architecture, his "sacred pool," his cows, his sheep, his swans, even his fish. Haytley reinforces the feeling of satisfaction and contentment that inheres in this idyllic domestic scene by his carefully planned asymmetry and converging lines, but lines that are balanced by the ever-so-faint suggestions of curves in the hedges and hills beyond. Nothing is left to chance. The right side of the pool leads boldly to the center of the painting, just beyond the swans. It forms one leg of a triangular frame for the Squire, his niece and mistress of the manor, and the wife of his friend, who are profiled against the reflecting pool. Extended, the line pulls us directly to the neoclassical temple, above which it is intersected by a line extended along the left side of the pool. The other figures, placed along the sides of the pool as they are, are foils to the main interest of the painting, the Squire and his new temple. Such placement accentuates the line. Even the niece, though she is in the center of the main group of three, is subservient to the main interest, seated, as she is, and calling additional attention to the temple by painting it. Counterpoise to the compact weight of the temple on the left is provided by the cows

and sheep spread over the hills to the right. Finally, the whole composition is fastened to the canvas by well-placed trees and shrubs and billowy clouds.

Today we might look on such a squire with the faintest air of disapprobation at his sense of self-importance and pride in social class. On the other hand, we must also admit to at least a dollop of envy at such a scene. It is the clean, well-ordered, tranquil life of an 18th-century Lord of the Manor. Squire James, through the medium of the artist Haytley, has taken care to preserve it for us.

Edward Haytley (flourished, 1740-1761), *The Brockman Family and Friends at Beachborough Manor*, c 1743-1746, British. Oil on canvas. 52.7 × 65 cm. Courtesy of the National Gallery of Victoria, Melbourne, Australia; Everard Studley Miller Bequest, 1963.

continued from p. 128

PIERRE AUGUSTE RENOIR

without the falseness of cosmetics that attracted him. "What I like is skin," he said, "a young girl's skin that is pink and shows that she has a good circulation." Or perhaps it was because they reflected his philosophy of life. Children are unpredictable, as Renoir was unpredictable; they live totally in the present, as did Renoir. They do not fight life; they go where it carries them. They go along with the current, like a cork in a stream, as Renoir did. But in the last analysis, perhaps what attracted and challenged Renoir was that children have the same two qualities that Renoir himself said all art must have: They are indescribable and they are inimitable.

Pierre Auguste Renoir (1841-1919), *Child With Brown Hair*, 1887-1888. 11.8 × 10.2 cm; *Young Girl Reading*, c 1888. 15.6 × 11.2 cm; *Child With Blonde Hair*, 1895-1900. 9.7 × 8.5 cm. French. Canvas. Courtesy of the National Gallery of Art, Washington, DC; Ailsa Mellon Bruce Collection, 1970. © 1995 The Board of Trustees of the National Gallery of Art.

continued from p. 132

EUGÈNE DELACROIX

heroic proportions and difficult access, escaping to Champrosay where he unwound

and refreshed himself before a small easel and a simple crystal vase of flowers. It is also easy to imagine that at times such as these he especially liked to recall the vivid colors of his Moroccan trip, taken just a year earlier. In the colors of the bouquet, for example, perhaps there is hidden a sultan's robe. Or again, perhaps we may see in the dahlias, the lupin, the carnation, a yellow caftan, a purplish burnoose, an orange turban, or, in the green leaves, the sleeve of a pasha. They were all memories Delacroix carried home with him and recorded in his journal. His vase of flowers is a simple color essay on Morocco.

Delacroix died in Paris of tuberculous laryngitis. He left 1000 paintings, 2000 watercolors and pastels, and 9000 drawings, as well as lithographs. In his obituary Baudelaire called him "a volcanic crater artistically concealed behind bouquets of flowers." His friend Theophile Silvestre wrote: "Thus died, almost with a smile, on August 13, 1863, that painter of great race, Ferdinand-Victor-Eugène Delacroix, who had a sun in his head and storms in his heart; who for 40 years played upon the keyboard of human passions, and whose brush—grandiose, terrible, or suave—passed from saints to warriors, from warriors to lovers, from lovers to tigers, and from tigers to flowers."

Eugène Delacroix (1798-1863), *Vase of Flowers*, 1833, French. Oil on canvas. 57.7 × 48.8 cm. Courtesy of the National Gallery of Scotland, Edinburgh, Scotland.

continued from p. 134

CAMILLE PISSARRO

in short, one of unremitting toil and hardship, with little to show beyond the barest subsistence, but it is nonetheless a life to be cherished, as Pissarro cherishes it.

Pissarro's personality was as complex and as subtle as the autumn palette of *The Farm*. He was a bourgeois who called himself a "proletarian without overalls." He was a socialist and a philosophic anarchist, once watched by the police for his reading tastes. He was Jewish, patriarchal, and white-bearded, looking like Abraham, or a prophet. He was humble, wise, and mild-mannered, but proud, dogged, and single-minded when it came to work. A sense of achievement alternated with

continued from p. 209

a sense of discouragement. Doubts about his work persisted throughout his life. In his 60s he was still writing: "There are moments when I ask myself whether I really have talent…In fact I often doubt it." In his last letter, to his son, written in September 1903 when he was 73 years old, he said of his painting, "We are far from being understood—quite far—even by our friends." Yet he still kept to a rigid work schedule and had already completed 57 oils and gouaches in the first nine months of that year. Two months later he was dead of septicemia secondary to an abscess of the prostate gland. His physician was a homeopath who, his son complained, had "*never* even raised the blanket to see the condition of his patient."

Camille Pissarro (1830-1903), *The Farm (La Ferme)*, 1879. French. Oil on canvas. 58.4 × 69.8 cm. Gift of the L. C. and Margaret Walker Foundation; Muskegon Museum of Art, Muskegon, Michigan.

---

continued from p. 136

AMEDEO MODIGLIANI

Italian Madonna. She holds a baby, but the bond between them is missing. The emphasis of the painting is on the woman's eyes, her neck, and her hands. Instead of looking at the baby, which would be the conventional pose, the woman confronts the viewer, directly and boldly, her gaze penetrating deeply. Her eyes are almost accusing, but in the end the expression is more sad and knowing, as though she had come into possession of a secret, primal knowledge. She is like the victim of some mysterious tragedy who has become detached and spiritual, withdrawing herself beyond any further vulnerability. The long, graceful neck, which links the small, oval, elegant head with the more rounded maternal body, is accentuated by its frame of blue scarf and red collar. It is the bridge between the cerebral and the visceral and emphasizes the tensions that exist between the spiritual and the physical, between reason and passion. It is a tension strangely reconciled in a woman with a baby on her lap. The hands are loosely clasped, just barely supporting the baby, resignedly, as one holds another's parcel. The colors are

cool and remote, like the sitter, except for the accent of red. The skin tones, on the other hand, are ocher—reddish earth color—which reinforces the relationship of the body of the woman to the earth, to sexual love, and to physical nourishment of the baby. The line is graceful, curving, and feminine, but also creates a tension. The long, vertical body of the woman, for example, is broken by the diagonal line of the dark, squat, swaddled body of the baby. The downward thrust of the baby's cap provides an opposite diagonal across the woman's body. A minor note is sounded by the scarf that is askew over the bosom; it matches the slight irregularity of the face and also echoes the curve of the braid that has escaped from its coil. As a subject of the painting, the baby is almost an afterthought. Yet it is essential to the harmony of the painting, not only, as above, to the harmony of line, but also to the harmony of the sitter. The baby explains the sitter.

The myth of Modigliani the painter has become mixed with that of Modigliani the man. But in the paintings themselves, later in the sculpture, and again in the paintings, there is no such confusion. He sends back echoes of his compatriots Botticelli, Duccio, and Parmigianino, of Cézanne and Lautrec, of the sculptor Brancusi, and of primitive Africa and Oceania. But the melody is always Modigliani.

Amedeo Modigliani (1884-1920), *Gypsy Woman With Baby*, 1919, Italian. Oil on canvas. 115.9 × 73 cm. Courtesy of the National Gallery of Art, Washington, DC; Chester Dale Collection, 1963. © 1995 The Board of Trustees of the National Gallery of Art.

---

continued from p. 138

SANDRO BOTTICELLI

taught to him by Lippi, the picture space is shallow. The triangular figure group, denoting stability and calm, is placed in the front plane, right "up against the eye," as one writer phrases it. What little depth there is is achieved by an architectural frame, in this case fluted pilasters and Corinthian columns. In the background, enclosed in the frame of the portico, is an elemental landscape with miniature cypress trees, recalling the *hortus conclusus*, or enclosed garden, a device often used in earlier paintings of the Virgin, especially those of the Annunciation, to sym-

bolize her intact state. To emphasize the figures even more, they are disproportionately large in relation to the background and are placed in the center; indeed, the Virgin's chin and the baby's left hand are on dead center. A note of disparity is introduced by the relative sizes of the two figures, the Virgin being slender and fragile, the Child robust and chubby, almost too much for the Virgin to bear. The pose is three-quarters. In keeping with the new Florentine Renaissance spirit, the three-quarter pose had become popular because it revealed more about the character and emotions of the subject than did the closed-off, full profile pose common in the earlier years of the century. Typically again, according to tradition the lighting is from the left, with the Virgin's face partially lit from below by reflected light from the Child. The painting has a genre, or everyday, contemporary life, aspect in the richly colored and richly textured robes of the Virgin in that they are more likely to be worn by a well-born Florentine lady of the upper middle class than by a humble maiden from Galilee. But the Child's drape is again conventional, its grape-purple color learned from Lippi and symbolizing the Passion. In contrast to the rich material tones, the flesh is waxy and bloodless, the Madonna's face especially looking as though chiseled from marble, giving the pair an ethereal, otherworldly look.

But it is in line that Botticelli has few peers. The coarse rhythms of the columns contrast with the finer rhythms of the cypresses. The severe vertical lines of the pilasters contrast with the softer vertical rhythms of the red tunic. Likewise, the linear rhythm of the horizontal drapery folds across the thighs accentuate the vertical rhythm of the falling folds of the left sleeve, and to a lesser extent, the right. Most important, however, is the strong bonding between mother and child, and the compositional and dramatic means used to attain this unity. The two figures gaze intently into each other's eyes, the two heads in harmony along parallel lines, one upturned, the other down-turned. The close harmony of the two figures is again seen in the parallel of the Child's right arm resting on the Virgin's left hand. The other two hands, both pointing downward, are likewise parallel. Additionally, the Virgin's right hand parallels the Child's right leg, the index finger shaping itself to the right leg and the crooked little finger counterpointing the bend of the left knee. The paradox of the painting is in the Child, who looks older and wiser than the mother. Yet gravely, trustingly, he questions her. The tragedy is in her sorrowful reply, for she has no answer. "You might think," says Pater, "that the sorrow in her face was at the thought of the whole long day of love yet to come."

Three hundred years ago, Vasari thought that Botticelli painted with such great beauty as to "put envy to shame." In this generation Berenson found him "never pretty, scarcely ever charming or even attractive." But it is Pater who, in 1870, found the kernel. There is, he said, "a blending in him of a sympathy for humanity in its uncertain condition… with his consciousness of the shadow upon it of the great things from which it shrinks."

Sandro Botticelli (1444-1510), *Madonna and Child*, c 1470, Florentine. Tempera on panel. 76 × 55.5 cm. Courtesy of the National Gallery of Art, Washington, DC; Andrew W. Mellon Collection, 1937. © 1995 The Board of Trustees of the National Gallery of Art.

continued from p. 140

GABRIEL METSU

that of mother or chaperone, but of procuress. The procuress was a most popular subject of 17th-century Dutch painters. And the matter of the erased coin has happened before. When a painting of Ter Borch entitled *The Parental Admonition* was recently cleaned, a partially erased coin could be made out between the thumb and forefinger of the supposed father. The painting was retitled *Brothel Scene*. In Metsu's painting, it might even be supposed that the young man has paid an early morning visit to, not the young woman, but the procuress, with the object of having his money returned. He reaches out to, not the young woman, but to the procuress. She laughingly holds up the coin to taunt him, while the unwilling object of his affections of the night before rises hastily from her bed and begins to dress.

Regardless, it is well to heed the admonition of art historians Rosenberg and Slive that "as in most matters concerning Dutch painting, in the beginning was the picture, not the word." The genius of these small Dutch genre paintings lies not in how cleverly the painter may have disguised the story, but in the very fact that an otherwise com-

monplace scene has been lifted into a singular harmony of color, line, and composition. The four figures are, for example, arranged, forefront to rear, along a diagonal that reaches from the window light source at the left edge to the door light source at the right. Two large, bulky masses of color, green at the left, red at the right, effectively balance each other, with a muted salmon midway. But it is in the contrast of textures that Metsu is the master: velvet robes, satin skirt, linen bedclothes, heavily embroidered Oriental table scarf, gleaming, carved wood chair set on a scrubbed pine floor, spaniel fur against ermine, pewter pitcher against brass candle-holder, mirror surface against silver jewel box. *The Intruder* is a tactile feast.

Of Metsu himself we know little. He was born in Leiden, The Netherlands, a university town, and was the son of a painter and perhaps a pupil of Dou. He was precocious and in his early years painted mostly religious subjects, influenced by Jan Steen and Rembrandt. At about the age of 21, he moved to the bustling commercial city of Amsterdam and turned to the elegant genre paintings for which he is so famous. He died at the age of 38 and was buried on October 24, 1667.

Gabriel Metsu (1629-1667), *The Intruder*, c 1660, Dutch. Oil on panel. 66.7 × 59.7 cm. Courtesy of the National Gallery of Art, Washington, DC; Andrew W. Mellon Collection, 1937. © 1995 The Board of Trustees of the National Gallery of Art.

continued from p. 142

GUSTAVE COURBET

Grégoire holds out a flower plucked from the bouquet, perhaps proffering it to the unseen diner whose coins lie on the counter. Her right hand rests, open, on the ledger, which contains the accounts of the customers.

Many interpretations have been offered for the action of Mère Grégoire, but none is conclusive. What is interesting to note, however, is the dialectic in the painting and Courbet's use of shapes. For example, Mme Andler's hands and arms are outstretched and could easily come together to complete the circle of an embrace. But her body presses away from an embrace, against the back of the bench. Likewise, her ample body with her large bosom gives the impression of roundness and softness. The roundness is carried

further by the large head with its hair gathered softly at the neck; by the circles of the collar and cuffs, scalloped though they be; by the flowers, both as a bouquet and individually; by the brooch at her throat; by the earrings; by the belly of the vase; and by the coins. All of this is contrasted with the strong horizontals, verticals, and obliques of the support structure: the bench, the wall panel at the left, and the countertop. Moreover, although Courbet was never praised for his composition, even here we find he has circumscribed the major, lighted elements—the face, the two hands, and the bouquet—within a circle. For example, if one takes as the center of the painting a point just above and to the right of Mme Andler's right breast and extends the radius out far enough and imagines a circle drawn with this radius, it will be found that of these four lighted elements, each falls into one quadrant of the circle.

In 1870, a decisive event, one that he had nothing to do with, occurred in Courbet's life. The Franco-Prussian War was declared. Napoleon III was defeated almost immediately at Sedan, and the Commune took over Paris. As a Socialist, Courbet was made an official, in charge of art. When the Communards pulled down the monument to Napoleon Bonaparte, the Vendôme Column, the Versailles government, next in office, laid the charge at Courbet's door. He was fined, imprisoned, and released after six months. Later, the new government ordered the rebuilding of the Column, with the cost of more than 300,000 francs to be charged to Courbet as the official in charge of the monument at the time of its destruction. Because he could not pay, Courbet fled from Ornans across the Jura Mountains to Switzerland, where he settled at La Tour de Peilz near Vevey on Lac Léman. Later, through negotiation, it was agreed he should pay the 300,000-plus francs at the rate of 10,000 francs yearly in two installments of 5000 francs each, commencing on January 1, 1878. He could also return to France. But the years of eating and drinking had made an invalid of Courbet. He had severe alcoholic cirrhosis, his girth had increased to 58 inches, and he needed frequent abdominal taps, which yielded up to 20 liters of ascitic fluid at a time. He died at La Tour at 6 in the morning on December 31, 1877, one day before the first payment to the government was due. He was 58. His 82-year-old father, Régis, having crossed the Jura Mountains only the night before, was at his side.

continued from p. 211

---

continued from p. 144

THOMAS EAKINS

every tendon expressing the horror and fear on the face we do not see; his, bloodied, holding the scalpel relaxed but firmly, totally in control of the entire amphitheater as he turns to address the students. There is no fear in these hands, only confidence and control.

Eakins was unappreciated, misunderstood, neglected, even persecuted during his lifetime, but now, almost 70 years after his death, praise swells with each new exhibition of his work. *The Gross Clinic*, for example, was rejected by the artists' committee for the Centennial. Instead, it was hung in the medical section. Only after Eakins had died did the art critic for the *New York Sun* call the painting "not only one of the greatest pictures to have been produced in America, but one of the greatest pictures of modern times anywhere." Today Soyer considers it "the most powerful painting ever painted in America." In his own large canvas, *Homage to Eakins*, Soyer shows Eakins' biographer standing, much like Gross, amid a group of contemporary American realist painters seated around a long table. On the wall behind them he has painted *The Gross Clinic*.

Thomas Eakins (1844-1916), *The Gross Clinic*, 1875, American. Oil on canvas. 243.8 × 198.2 cm. Courtesy of Jefferson Medical College, Thomas Jefferson University, Philadelphia, Pennsylvania.

---

continued from p. 146

HENRI ROUSSEAU

able for his daughter. Some say this rejection is what led finally to Rousseau's death, on September 2, 1910, of general bodily neglect and gangrene. In his will, he left Léonie all of his paintings.

Tropical Forest With Monkeys was painted in these last months of Rousseau's life. It shows one of his many exotic landscapes, lush, tropical, virgin, like a garden where no one has walked. Yet there is about to be an interruption of some sort, for the monkeys are on the alert. Two sit in the foreground fishing in the stream, gazing directly at the source of the disturbance. As yet they show no fear; they are merely puzzled, with the curiosity of the innocent. A third, more wary, remains in his tree, also curious, but hesitant and braced for action. Two others rush to investigate, arcing across the jungle on the graceful branches. Brilliant leaves, exotic flowers, and a stream in the foreground seem to form a protective barrier against any intrusion. On the other hand, the garden has already been penetrated; in the lower left, entwined about the tree, just beyond the flaming leaves, is the serpent, poised to strike. This is the garden, in its last delicious moment of indecision before yielding up its innocence.

Rousseau's paintings evoke feelings that have become deeply buried by layers of years. They are like the small and speechless child who one day suddenly utters—in direct, childish terms—some obvious but extraordinarily profound observation. Is this child a special genius who has discovered some new and astonishing truth? Or has it merely uttered something that everyone has always known but which has become disguised in memory and finally forgotten? Perhaps this was the fascination of the sophisticated Paris art world for Rousseau at the beginning of the century; perhaps it is the source of the continuing fascination at the end of the century.

Henri Rousseau (1844-1910), *Tropical Forest With Monkeys*, 1910, French. Oil on canvas. 129.5 × 162.6 cm. Courtesy of the National Gallery of Art, Washington, DC; John Hay Whitney Collection, 1982. © 1995 The Board of Trustees of the National Gallery of Art.

---

continued from p. 150

GEORGE WESLEY BELLOWS

quality to it, a sense of the unreality that accident victims often describe: "Everything was happening in slow motion," "It took a very long time," "I could watch myself falling." The powerful vertical of Firpo in purple trunks dominates the painting, his upright body and taut muscles as solidly based as an Egyptian pyramid, his face as inscrutable as that of a sphinx. Below him, almost falling out of the picture plane, Dempsey's body crumples ignominiously through the ropes, the well-developed muscles as powerless as the sagging rope, his arms and legs flailing in diagonals, his now useless left hook catching attention at the center of the painting. At the right, the referee serves as a foil to the action, as he points the count with the precision and interest of an automatic measuring device. His diagonal torso and limbs emphasize his role of supporting actor, and not protagonist, in the drama. In midground the spectators are accessory to the scene as they clamor for the blood they paid for. In the foreground the press is momentarily stunned as the "big story" is thrust upon them. And in the background, the spectral lights witness silently, like so many shrouded ghosts. The violence of the fight is emphasized by the color scheme, the fuchsia of Firpo's trunks reflected in the referee's shirt, deepened in the jacket of the reporter third from the left, and carried into the skin tones of all, fighters, referee, spectators, and press. These tones are set against an almost patina-like background of blurred green-black, an appropriate contrast for the action.

Bellows was interested in presenting the dramatic truth in his boxing paintings, but not in depicting the technical niceties of the ring. Thus, when questioned on an inaccuracy in another fight painting, he replied, "I don't know anything about boxing. I am just painting two men trying to kill each other." In *Dempsey and Firpo*, Firpo is shown swinging his left, whereas it was his right that put Dempsey through the ropes. His left elbow was, in fact, ailing. Likewise, when questioned about the morality of prizefighting, Bellows professed to be disinterested. "But let me say," he added, "the atmosphere around the fighters is a lot more immoral than the fighters themselves."

Dempsey and Firpo, completed in June 1924, was one of Bellows' last paintings. Shortly after New Year's Day, 1925, he was stricken with appendicitis. He died at Postgraduate Hospital, New York City, on January 8, aged 42 years.

George Wesley Bellows (1882-1925), *Dempsey and Firpo*, 1924, American. Oil on canvas. 129.5 × 160.7 cm. Courtesy of the Whitney Museum of American Art, New York, New York; purchased with funds from Gertrude Vanderbilt Whitney.

continued from p. 152

AMEDEO MODIGLIANI

These lines—along the shoulders and along the neckline of the dress—form a square, which frames the neck with its chins. Most interesting, however, is the cigarette, almost unnoticed, that Madame Amédée holds in her right hand. A line drawn upward along its length forms a direct diagonal with her mouth. The cigarette is also placed curiously, in her lap, perhaps suggesting another symbolism, perhaps Modigliani's private commentary on Madame Amédée. Finally, the masculine tone of the painting is suggested by the background with its tones of brown, and by its strong angularity, noted especially in the right angles of the chair and the picture frame.

Modigliani's life was tragic. Yet, like others afflicted—van Gogh, Utrillo, and Munch in his own time, and Botticelli, Parmigianino, and Michelangelo before him—he could get it all together in his art.

Amedeo Modigliani (1884-1920), *Madame Amédée (Woman With Cigarette)*, 1918, Italian. Canvas. 100.3 × 64.8 cm. Courtesy of the National Gallery of Art, Washington, DC; Chester Dale Collection, 1963 © 1995 The Board of Trustees of the National Gallery of Art.

continued from p. 158

SIR JOHN LAVERY

passion, and involvement. In terms of color, the red and white flowers in midground and background set off the blue and green medicine bottles in the foreground. The starkness of the scene is relieved by the red shades on the hanging ceiling lamps, the heavy green drapes at the windows, and the gaily striped blankets covering the beds. Each of these objects also takes a pyramidal shape, contrasting with the largely white horizontal, vertical, and oblique lines. *Sister Juliet* is indeed a charming version of color and design.

After the war Sir John became a society portraitist, working until World War II. At the age of 84, he published his autobiography, a gossipy account of his life and those he had known, and notable for its merciless self-honesty and sardonic humor. He died the following year at the home of his sister in County Kilkenny, Ireland.

Sir John Lavery (1856-1941), *Sister Juliet*, 1918, Irish. Oil on canvas. 64 × 76 cm. Courtesy of Christopher Gibbs Ltd, London, England.

continued from p. 166

GRANT WOOD

leaves, which suggest the river with its tributaries. The golden corn shocks suggest the fecundity of the earth as mother, while the preponderance of greens and the overall greenish cast hint at eternity through perpetual renewal of the feminine. Wood was to repeat some of these same decorative motifs a year later in *American Gothic*—the sansevieria, the begonia, the brooch, the collar on the dress, the rickrack on the apron.

In later years Wood taught his students at the University of Iowa to divide their sketches into thirds, both horizontally and vertically, and then to place the most important parts of the sketch along a line that connected any two points on the grid. At the time he painted *Woman With Plant(s)*, however, Wood was marking his canvases into fourths horizontally and vertically. Thus, in this case, Wood has, like Renaissance painters, given special emphasis to the nares, the chin, and to the wedding band on the left hand. He has, in fact, painted a history in a face and hands.

Wood's best known painting, *American Gothic*, followed a year later, and he was at the height of his popularity between 1930 and 1934. After that he was involved in local disputes at the University over Regionalism in art versus Internationalism and Modernism. In 1935, at the age of 44, he married and moved from Cedar Rapids to Iowa City with his wife and his mother. Six months later his mother died. The marriage ended in divorce in 1939. Thomas Hart Benton, in a 1951 essay on Regionalism in painting, recounts Wood's last days: "When I went to see him in 1942 as he lay dying of liver cancer in an Iowa hospital, he told me that when he got well he was going to change his name, go where nobody knew him and start all over again with a new style of painting." Wood died at the University of Iowa Hospital a few days later, just hours short of reaching his 51st birthday.

Grant Wood (1891-1942), *Woman With Plant(s)*, 1929, American. Oil on upsom board. 52.1 × 45.4 cm. Courtesy of the Cedar Rapids Museum of Art, Cedar Rapids, Iowa; Art Association purchase.

continued from p. 168

VINCENT VAN GOGH

Irises is the former. Flowers fill the entire canvas, which is without a horizon, as though van Gogh were looking down on them from a window. Indeed, he probably was, for in the early days of his stay he did not go outside but stayed in his room with its barred window. A line of purple irises enters at the left, then divides into broad patches of purple that fill the upper- and lower-right quadrants. In the corresponding quadrants on the left are the hot complementary oranges, yellows, and reds of marigolds and earth, while cutting across the entire canvas is a swatch of ice-green leaves, each carefully outlined in blue or purple. At the left, upright and lonely as a vestal virgin, is a single pure white iris, an anomalous saint in a world of common purple. Perhaps that is how van Gogh saw himself: singular and superior in a world of common people. In a letter to Theo a few months later, he reproached himself for his cowardice in so quietly allowing the police to close the yellow house in Arles and commit him to the hospital. "I ought rather to have defended my studio," he wrote, "even if it meant fighting with the police and the neighbors. Others in my place would have used a revolver, and certainly if as an artist one had killed some rotters like that, one would have been acquitted."

To van Gogh color was everything. He sought to express his moods by its symbolism. Whereas in Arles he had been seeking the highest yellow he could master, in the Saint-Rémy *Irises* he seems to be seeking the potentialities of its complement, bluish-purple. He tries all the gradations possible, from a deep midnight shade to the faint, almost white, pale shade of a washed-out daytime sky. In going from his high yellows of Arles to the deep blues of Saint-Rémy, it is as though he sees himself going from the heights of ecstasy to the depths of night, or from the unlimited possibilities at the day's rebirth to the unknown infinity that lies behind the night. It is the same blue that he used in his portrait of Dr Gachet, painted a year later, shortly before he died.

Van Gogh greatly admired and was influenced by Japanese prints. But whereas the irises of Hiroshige are serene and tranquil, calming to the spirit, van Gogh's are agitated,

continued from p. 213

powerful, and striving. Again, they perhaps suggest van Gogh himself. The delicate blossoms are easily bruised, but their stalks are anchored firmly in the soil and from them new and equally beautiful blossoms will arise after each storm. So, too, did van Gogh's genius reassert itself after each bout of illness, its freshness unimpaired by any violence of the past.

Van Gogh's failing, if it can be called that, was that he aspired to sainthood, which is to say he aspired to perfection and to total expression of the ultimate—not to sainthood in the Church, of which his father had been a minister, but to sainthood in the temple of art. He drove himself to agonies of body and soul seeking the ecstasies he knew existed; in the end it was he who became the sacrifice. But he left on the altar a body of color and harmonies that falls just short of the divine.

Vincent van Gogh (1853-1890), *Irises*, 1889, Dutch. Oil on canvas. 71 × 93 cm. Courtesy of The J. Paul Getty Museum, Malibu, California.

continued from p. 174

VINCENT VAN GOGH

("green earth") before applying flesh tones and drapery colors. Always, advised a major treatise on painting of that time, when the surface colors are applied, this *terra verde* must be allowed to show through the flesh tones, an effect that van Gogh has exaggerated in the mother's face. Is it possible then, that, recalling his minister father, and his own evangelist days among the poor, he was covertly painting a religious subject, a secular Madonna and Child borrowed from the Renaissance tradition? Was the child van Gogh himself?

It was not the choice of subject alone, however, that determined van Gogh's expression. Van Gogh spoke primarily by means of color. It was a symbolic language whose grammar he labored to develop. But, as he himself said, he had no interest in trying to reproduce the colors that were before his eyes. Rather, he used color arbitrarily "in order to express myself forcibly." Earlier that summer he had begun using

pairs of complementaries; red against green, blue against orange, yellow against violet. And he had reached what he later recalled as his "high yellow note." In *Madame Roulin and Her Baby* we see this language: Madame Roulin's green dress boldly outlined in red, the blue-green of the infant's dress against the intense yellow-orange of the background, and the complexion of the baby a subtle opposition of pale yellow and delicate lilac. The large expanse of white in the dress absorbs and reconciles the opposites, allowing the viewer's eye to rest and be still.

It is also interesting to note that the predominant yellow, white, green, and red of *Madame Roulin and Her Baby* are the same colors Vincent had named twice during the summer in letters to Theo to describe his much-loved Yellow House: "My house here is painted the yellow color of fresh butter on the outside with glaringly green shutters… completely whitewashed inside…floor…of red bricks." When one recalls that a home is commonly a symbol of the self and of a desire for security, and that van Gogh used these same colors in a painting of a mother and infant less than three weeks before his mental and emotional collapse, one begins to hear what he is saying. Traditionally, such a painting would arouse feelings of warmth and security, but this painting shows a distant mother and a precariously perched baby. It was also a precariously perched Vincent who made the painting. Nevertheless, van Gogh was still hoping for yet another fresh start, for "a rebirth." The large expanse of yellow, like the suns he painted over his fields, is an attempt to bring light to darkness, to recreate himself yet again from the chaos he felt building within.

At the time of the portrait Gauguin had been living with van Gogh in the Yellow House for six weeks. But the relationship had already soured and by mid-December Gauguin was threatening to leave. Joseph Roulin, on whom van Gogh had come to rely heavily, was being transferred to Marseilles. Not only was Christmas approaching, but the skies in Arles turned dark; in the six days immediately preceding Christmas it rained day and night. Ten times the normal rainfall for December was registered. Two days before Christmas Gauguin moved out. Van Gogh collapsed and severed his left ear.

During the 444 days of 1888-1889 van Gogh spent in Arles he reached the zenith of

his career, as recorded in the 200 paintings, 100 drawings, and 200 letters—noted for their self-revelation and perspicacity—he produced while there. But as slowly as his sun had risen, so suddenly did it set. In April 1889, van Gogh committed himself to the nearby insane asylum at Saint-Rémy, and in July 1890, back in the north again, at Auvers-sur-Oise, he shot and killed himself. He had been a painter for only a decade. He had sold one painting.

Vincent van Gogh (1853-1890), *Madame Roulin and Her Baby*, 1888, Dutch. Oil on canvas. 63.5 × 51 cm. Courtesy of The Metropolitan Museum of Art, New York, New York; Robert Lehman Collection, 1975. © 1980 by The Metropolitan Museum of Art.

continued from p. 176

PABLO PICASSO

paintings (as also do the shapes of color on the female figure), is also the liturgical color of Lent. More interesting, however, are the large light and dark shapes on either side of the central blue strip. Here there is an indication that this painting may also be seen as a meeting of opposites or as a reconciliation of conflicts in the creation of something new. The light and dark shapes may be seen, for example, as dawn and evening, reconciled in the blue of day, or man and woman reconciled in the creation of a child. (As this was painted, Picasso's and Olga's son, Paulo, was celebrating his second birthday.) Or, the pleasure of food against the pain of the Lenten fast, or sexual desire against spiritual intellect; in short, a counterpoint of flesh and spirit.

Composition for a Mardi Gras Ball is an innocent painting, just as the decade following World War I was innocent. The 1920s were, in fact, one long Mardi Gras fancy dress ball after the winter of the war. But with the dawn came Ash Wednesday. Before the next decade was out, Picasso was painting *Guernica*.

Pablo Picasso (1881-1973), *Composition for a Mardi Gras Ball*, 1923, Spanish. Oil on canvas. 289.6 × 213.4 cm. Courtesy of The Chrysler Museum, Norfolk, Virginia; gift of Walter P. Chrysler, Jr.

continued from p. 180

THOMAS EAKINS

directly to the surgical instrument in White's hand and to the patient's breast, thereby tying Agnew to the action. But the key to the drama is the figure of the nurse on the right. Besides Agnew's, hers is the only other upright figure in the painting. The others are sitting, lying, stooped, or otherwise bent from their full heights. If one allows for the nurse's cap, she is almost the same height as Agnew. Placed as she is, she forms a counterforce to Agnew in the circle of the pit. She is also a counterbalance to the patient. Whereas the body of the young man asleep in the top row parallels and emphasizes that of the unconscious horizontal patient at the bottom of the painting, the figure of the nurse, the only other woman in the painting, forms a strong perpendicular contrast to it. Nor is the emotional drama lost, as the buxom country girl glowing with good health attends a woman little older than herself who has lost a breast.

Like its predecessor, *The Agnew Clinic* was met with disapproval by both peers and public. As a result, it remains today with its original owner, hanging in a foyer of the University of Pennsylvania, just as *The Gross Clinic* remains hanging at the Jefferson Medical College.

Thomas Eakins (1844-1916), *The Agnew Clinic*, 1889, American. Oil on canvas. 331.5 × 189.2 cm. Courtesy of the University of Pennsylvania School of Medicine.

continued from p. 184

CLAUDE MONET

Renoir got 18, and Pissarro, 13. Monet's total sales came to 20 francs. The rest was scattered among the 26 other participants, not a very auspicious beginning for the major art movement of the 19th century. Today, with eyes educated by a century of lightened palettes and grown used to indistinct outlines, the absence of black, brilliant colors, and short brush strokes, things are seen quite differently. Impressionism has become one of the most universally loved movements in art.

Claude Monet (1840-1926) *Wild Poppies*, 1873, French. Oil on canvas. 50 × 65 cm. Courtesy of the Musée d'Orsay, Paris, France.

continued from p. 186

ÉDOUARD MANET

20th century, look *at* a surface covered with color. The subject is the painting itself. Manet was its father. His tragedy is that he insisted on his principles and at the same time insisted on the acclaim of a public that did not accept them.

Édouard Manet (1832-1883), *Le Bon Bock*, 1873, French. Oil on canvas. 94.6 × 83.3 cm. Courtesy of the Philadelphia Museum of Art, Philadelphia, Pennsylvania; The Mr and Mrs Carroll S. Tyson, Jr, Collection.

continued from p. 188

GIOVANNI FRANCESCO BARBIERI (IL GUERCINO)

tumultuous baroque of Guercino's early years, but the calm classicism of his later years. His work has been perhaps best characterized as baroque-classical.

The legend of Luke the painter that grew up alongside the tradition of Luke the physician endures to this day, for Luke is the patron of both physicians and artists.

Giovanni Francesco Barbieri (called Guercino) (1591-1666), *St Luke Displaying a Painting of the Virgin*, 1652-1653, Emilian. Oil on canvas. 221 × 180.3 cm. Courtesy of the Nelson-Atkins Museum of Art, Kansas City, Missouri; purchase.

continued from p. 190

MARSDEN HARTLEY

wreck to the ground. The large red circle with the three bursts of flame would seem to symbolize the three explosions and the blazing dirigible. Other symbols can be read in various ways. The red, green, white, and yellow disks were probably prompted by similar disks used frequently by Delaunay, and which appeared in his homage painting to the French aviator Blériot. The red and green squares are, according to Rönnebeck, reminders of von Freyburg, who liked to play chess. Crosses, especially the Prussian Iron Cross, were also frequently used by Hartley to symbolize von Freyburg specifically or the military in general. In *The Aero* they have become the Geneva cross, symbolizing the dead and wounded, or, for Hartley's part, neutrality. The paddlelike motifs, which also appear in a number of paintings, represent the epaulets of a German officer's uniform. Other elements of the painting give an impression of the pomp and pageantry of the military, with its waving banners and gold-braided uniforms.

When war was declared in August 1914, Hartley stayed on in Germany. Shortly thereafter von Freyburg was killed in action, for Hartley an almost unbearable grief. The following year, beset by food shortages and economic difficulties, Hartley returned to the United States. He was 38, and for the next 20 years would be a wanderer again. When he died at the age of 66, his search had produced more than a thousand paintings, four books, and numerous articles and poems. And he had returned to Maine, whence he came, to paint once again its austere and powerful landscapes and its people, but this time they were filtered through a lifetime of experience. Here he at last had found the means of expressing the vision of truth that was uniquely his.

Marsden Hartley (1877-1943), *The Aero*, 1914, American. Canvas. 100.3 × 81.2 cm. Courtesy of the National Gallery of Art, Washington, DC; Andrew W. Mellon Fund, 1970. © 1995 The Board of Trustees of the National Gallery of Art.

continued from p. 196

FRA ANGELICO

Little can be said about an Angelico painting that has not already been repeated many times. In his 16th-century biography of Angelico, Vasari gives special mention to the Cosmas and Damian *predella*, saying that "figures more delicate or more judiciously arranged can hardly be conceived." In the mid-19th century, Ruskin called his pictures "simply so many pieces of jewellery" and "opals among marbles." More recently, in the early 20th century, Berenson referred to Angelico's "perfect certainty of purpose, utter devotion to his task, and a sacramental

continued from p. 215

earnestness in performing it." In our own time, Canady has called him the "last and sweetest and purest voice that medieval faith produced in Italy." Perhaps the miracle of Angelico is that at a distance of five and a half centuries from *The Healing of Palladia* we can still appreciate colors that remain as clear as a bell sounding over the Tuscan valley, a line that flows like Gregorian chant from a choir of monks, and space that is as free and uncluttered as the nave of a Roman church. Angelico is a moment of grace across the face of the world.

When Fra Angelico, still known to his companions as Fra Giovanni da Fiesole, died in Rome on February 18, 1455, the great Italian humanist Lorenzo Valla wrote the epitaph: "For some works I shall survive on earth and for others in heaven." It was perhaps prophetic. In 1983, Pope John Paul II declared Fra Angelico "Blessed," the last stage in the Roman Catholic process of canonization before sainthood, and in 1984 Beato Angelico was declared patron of artists, in particular, painters.

Fra Angelico (1387-1455), *The Healing of Palladia by Saint Cosmas and Saint Damian,* c 1438-1443, Florentine. Tempera on panel. 36.5 × 46.7 cm. Courtesy of the National Gallery of Art, Washington, DC; Samuel H. Kress Collection, 1952. © 1995 The Board of Trustees of the National Gallery of Art.

---

continued from p. 198

EDVARD MUNCH

In painting *The Sick Child,* Munch struggled so to portray his emotions and mood honestly that he painted, scraped, and repainted the canvas countless times. The figures of the woman and the girl have finally been gouged into the heavily painted surface, rather than being laid on in strokes. In fact, Munch was able to complete the painting only after a year of such struggle when, one day, he looked at it through the eyelashes of his partially lowered lids. He then took the handle of his brush and scratched over the surface the grid pattern he had seen through his lashes. He could, as it were, look at death only by dimming his vision. Nor even then could he look death full in the face, but only askance: death in profile, mourning across the top of a head. Only by averting his eyes and dimming his vision could he finally acknowledge a universal experience of human life. Yet, although he cannot look directly, neither does he walk away. He remains present to the dying girl and the grieving woman, just as they remain present to each other; in so doing, he has redeemed his own grief and has transformed it into art.

In spite of frequent illness, both emotional and physical, and a greatly troubled life, Munch lived on in Norway until shortly after his 80th birthday. He died of pneumonia at his home in Ekely on January 23, 1944.

Edvard Munch (1863-1944), *The Sick Child,* 1886, Norwegian. Oil on canvas. 120 × 119 cm. Courtesy of Nasjonalgalleriet, Oslo, Norway. © 1995 The Munch Museum/The Munch Ellingsen Group/Artists Rights Society, New York, New York.

INDEX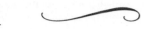